Baillière's
CLINICAL
GASTROENTEROLOGY
INTERNATIONAL PRACTICE AND RESEARCH

Baillière's

CLINICAL GASTROENTEROLOGY

INTERNATIONAL PRACTICE AND RESEARCH

Volume 9/Number 2
June 1995

Coeliac Disease

P. D. HOWDLE BSc, MD, FRCP
Guest Editor

Baillière Tindall
London Philadelphia Sydney Tokyo Toronto

This book is printed on acid-free paper.

Baillière Tindall   24–28 Oval Road
W. B. Saunders   London NW1 7DX, UK
Company Ltd
          The Curtis Center, Independence Square West
          Philadelphia, PA 19106–3399, USA

          55 Horner Avenue
          Toronto, Ontario M8Z 4X6, Canada

          Harcourt Brace & Company,
          Australia
          30–52 Smidmore Street, Marrickville, NSW 2204, Australia

          Harcourt Brace & Company,
          Japan Inc.
          Ichibancho Central Building,
          22–1 Ichibancho, Chiyoda-ku, Tokyo 102, Japan

ISSN 0950–3528

ISBN 0–7020–1953–4 (single copy)

Baillière's Clinical Gastroenterology is published four times each year by Baillière Tindall. Prices for Volume 9 (1995) are:

TERRITORY	ANNUAL SUBSCRIPTION	SINGLE ISSUE
Europe including UK	£94.00 (Institutional) post free £80.00 (Individual) post free	£30.00 post free
All other countries	Consult your local Harcourt Brace & Company Office	

The editor of this publication is Ian Bramley, Baillière Tindall, 24–28 Oval Road, London NW1 7DX, UK.

Baillière's Clinical Gastroenterology is covered in Index Medicus, Current Contents/Clinical Medicine, the Science Citation Index, SciSearch and Research Alert.

Baillière's Clinical Gastroenterology was published from 1972 to 1986 as *Clinics in Gastroenterology*

Typeset by Phoenix Photosetting, Chatham.
Printed and bound in Great Britain by the University Printing House, Cambridge, UK.

Contributors to this issue

PAUL J. CICLITIRA MD, PhD, FRCP, Professor of Gastroenterology, United Medical and Dental School of Guy's and St. Thomas', The Rayne Institute, Gastroenterology Unit, Division of Pharmacology, St. Thomas' Hospital, Lambeth Palace Road, London SE1 7EH, UK.

GINO R. CORAZZA MD, Associate Professor of Medicine, University of L'Aquila, Via S. Sisto 22E, 67100 L'Aquila, Italy.

PETER T. CROWE BA, Senior Research Technician, University Department of Medicine, Hope Hospital, Eccles Old Road, Salford, Greater Manchester M6 8HD, UK.

ANNE FERGUSON FRCP, FRCPath, FRSE, Professor of Gastroenterology, University of Edinburgh; Honorary Consultant Gastroenterology, Western General Hospital NHS Trust, Edinburgh EH4 2XU, UK.

LIONEL FRY BSc, MD, FRCP, Dermatology Department, St. Mary's Hospital, Praed Street, London W2 4AN, UK.

GIOVANNI GASBARRINI MD, Professor of Medicine, Universitá Catolica del Sacro Cuore, Largo Gemelli 8, 00168 Roma, Italy.

PETER D. HOWDLE BSc, MD, FRCP, Senior Lecturer in Medicine and Consultant Physician, Division of Medicine, St. James's University Hospital, Leeds LS9 7TF, UK.

JAMES M. LITTLEWOOD MD, FRCP, FRCPE, DCH, Consultant Paediatrician, St. James's University Hospital, Leeds LS9 7TF; Senior Clinical Lecturer, Leeds University, UK.

MARKKU MÄKI MD, Paediatric Gastroenterologist, Senior Researcher, Department of Clinical Science, University of Tampere, PO Box 607, FIN-33101 Tampere, Finland.

MICHÁEL N. MARSH DSc, DM, FRCP, Reader in Medicine, University of Manchester (School of Medicine) and Consultant Physician, University Department of Medicine, Hope Hospital, Eccles Old Road, Salford, Greater Manchester M6 8HD, UK.

M. RICHARD TIGHE MBBS, MRCP, Senior Registrar, Gastroenterology, Division of Pharmacology, United Medical and Dental Schools of Guy's and St. Thomas' Hospitals, London SE1 7EH, UK.

LUDWIK K. TREJDOSIEWICZ BSc, PhD, Senior Lecturer in Immunology, Division of Medicine, St. James's University Hospital, Leeds LS9 7TF, UK.

HERBERT WIESER MD, German Research Institute of Food chemistry, Lichtenbergstrasse 4, D-85748 Garching, Germany.

DENNIS H. WRIGHT BSc, MD, FRCPath, Professor, University Department of Pathology, Southampton General Hospital, Tremona Road, Southampton SO16 6YD, UK.

Table of contents

PREVIOUS ISSUES

FORTHCOMING ISSUE

Preface

Coeliac disease continues to hold a fascination for gastroenterologists and clinical scientists. This is perhaps because although great strides have been made in understanding the pathology, in making an adequate diagnosis and in recognizing the many clinical manifestations, the final pieces of the jigsaw have yet to fall into place. These are concerned with questions of pathogenesis and the involvement of specific prolamin peptides. The search for answers to these questions has stimulated much basic research into immune mechanisms, cereal chemistry and molecular and cell biology. Arising out of such work in coeliac disease, our understanding of mucosal architecture and function in general has been increased.

It is timely, therefore, that *Baillière's Clinical Gastroenterology* should publish a volume on coeliac disease. It is 20 years since the volume on coeliac disease in *Clinics in Gastroenterology* appeared and there have been many significant developments since then.

The chapters in this volume fall into two distinct groups. First, there are chapters mainly concerned with pathogenesis, and second, chapters describing many clinical aspects of coeliac disease. Finally, Anne Ferguson looks into the future and tries to predict where research and clinical practice might be leading us.

One interesting area of controversy which emerges from these chapters is that of 'latent' coeliac disease. Anne Ferguson very definitely regards it as an asymptomatic state in patients with no small intestinal pathology who will eventually develop an abnormal small intestinal mucosa. These patients are 'potential' coeliac patients. Michael Marsh takes a contrary view that latent coeliac patients are certainly asymptomatic but do have a mucosal lesion, which can vary from mild to severe; these are 'silent' coeliac patients. I leave it to readers to make up their own minds on this point, but it is perhaps not as straightforward as one might think. There are patients with evidence of gluten-sensitivity, as shown by raised serum reticulin antibodies, or a coeliac-like intestinal antibody pattern, or a raised intraepithelial lymphocyte count who are asymptomatic with a seemingly normal small intestinal mucosa. It could be argued that they fit either definition of 'latent' coeliac disease. Such arguments about definition highlight some of the problems in trying to define coeliac disease. I still believe we need to base clinical diagnoses for practical purposes on major architectural abnormalities of the small intestinal mucosa which are related to the presence of gluten (and the other relevant prolamins) in the diet. Evidence of gluten-sensitivity may not manifest itself as clinical coeliac disease, but will alert the astute physician of the future to a range of possible clinical outcomes.

I thank the authors for their willingness to collaborate and I hope that readers will find the ideas in this volume stimulating in both research and clinical spheres, and that the recent advances described here will lead us all to a better understanding of this disease which will ultimately be of benefit to our patients.

P. D. HOWDLE

1

The precipitating factor in coeliac disease

HERBERT WIESER

The classical features of coeliac disease were described more than a century ago (Gee, 1888), but it was not until the postwar observations of Dicke (1950) that the consumption of wheat and wheat products was shown to be harmful to coeliac patients. Investigations during the following years led to the conclusion that wheat gluten, and in particular the alcohol-soluble gliadin fraction, was responsible for the harmful effect and that digestion with pepsin and trypsin did not destroy this 'toxic' effect. Rye, barley and probably oats were also considered to contain a similar fraction responsible for this toxicity, whereas rice and maize were not.

During the 1960s and 1970s relatively little progress was made towards a fundamental understanding of gluten toxicity, the main reasons being, first, the extreme complexity of gluten proteins and the lack of effective methods for separation and structural analysis, and, second, the lack of sensitive and specific in-vivo and in-vitro systems for testing toxicity.

The situation changed when highly effective analytical and preparative separation systems were introduced into cereal protein chemistry and when molecular biological methods were used to determine amino-acid sequences. Additionally, in-vivo and in-vitro methods for the evaluation of toxicity were developed that were sensitive to comparatively small amounts of proteins and peptides. This chapter reviews the remarkable progress in recent years both in the elucidation of gluten protein structure and in the relationship between coeliac toxicity and chemical structure.

CHEMISTRY OF GLUTEN PROTEINS

Four levels of the structural organization of proteins can be distinguished:

1. primary structure (amino-acid sequence)
2. secondary structure (local arrangement of the peptide backbone)
3. tertiary structure (three-dimensional structure of the whole protein)
4. quaternary structure (intermolecular aggregation of proteins).

With respect to coeliac disease, the discussion may be reduced to the first level because the native proteins can be heated or digested into peptides without loss of toxicity. Thus, the quaternary and tertiary structures of the proteins are not relevant and the local secondary structure may be changed

Baillière's Clinical Gastroenterology—
Vol. 9, No. 2, June 1995
ISBN 0–7020–1953–4

after the cleavage of peptide bonds, still leaving the primary structure intact. The following discussion therefore focuses on the primary structure.

Definition and characteristics of gluten

Gluten can be defined as the rubbery mass that remains when wheat dough is washed to remove starch granules and other soluble constituents. The physical properties of gluten (cohesivity, viscoelasticity) are of particular interest as they are responsible for the uniqueness of wheat with respect to its baking quality. Depending on the thoroughness of washing, the dry solids contain 75–85% protein and 5–10% lipids; most of the remainder is starch and non-starch carbohydrates (Wrigley and Bietz, 1988). Gluten protein is unique in terms of its amino-acid composition, which is characterized by a high content of glutamine (approximately 35 mol%), proline (15 mol%) and hydrophobic amino acids (19 mol%) and by a low content of amino acids with charged side groups. The major protein fractions of gluten are gliadin and glutenin, which can be distinguished by their different solubility in aqueous alcohol (e.g. 70% ethanol). The soluble gliadin contains mainly monomeric proteins, whereas the insoluble glutenin comprises aggregated proteins linked by disulphide bonds and non-covalent forces. Both fractions consist of numerous partially closely related protein components. Their only known function is to act as storage proteins, providing the germinating cereal seed embryo with nitrogen.

Nomenclature and classification of gluten protein components

In the classical definition of Osborne (1924), cereal storage proteins soluble in aqueous alcohols without reduction of disulphide bonds are designated as prolamins and the insoluble proteins as glutelins. Shewry et al (1984) also used the term 'prolamins' for glutelins, because they are as alcohol soluble as prolamins once the disulphide bonds have been reduced. To prevent confusion, however, the classical definitions of the terms 'prolamin' and 'glutelin' are used in this chapter.

The nomenclature of cereal protein components has been developed according to the progress of separation and is, therefore, rather confusing and inconsistent. The components of gliadin were initially classified into four groups on the basis of mobility at low pH in gel electrophoresis (α-, β-, γ- and ω-gliadins in order of decreasing mobility) (Woychik et al, 1961). Studies on N-terminal sequences, however, have shown that the electrophoretic mobility does not always reflect the protein relationships and that α- and β-gliadins fall into one group (α-type) (Bietz et al, 1977). The components of glutenin can be obtained after the reduction of disulphide bonds and grouped into low- (LMW) and high-molecular-weight (HMW) subunits based on differences in molecular mass (Bietz and Wall, 1972; Payne and Corfield, 1979). More recent studies have shown that the extraction of flour or gluten with aqueous alcohol does not lead to clear-cut fractions. Thus, glutenin subunits are found in the soluble gliadin fraction and gliadins are also present in the insoluble glutenin fraction (Shewry et al,

1983; Tao and Kasarda, 1989; Wieser et al, 1990; Köhler et al, 1993). Altogether, the classification of gluten proteins based on secondary properties (e.g. solubility, electrophoretic or chromatographic mobility) frequently fails to reveal the protein relationships.

The most important criterion for classifying proteins is the primary structure. In recent years gluten proteins have been extensively investigated by highly efficient separation techniques (e.g. two-dimensional electrophoresis, reversed-phase high-performance liquid chromatography) and by analysis of amino-acid compositions, molecular mass, and partial or complete amino-acid sequences. Based on these data, gluten protein components have been classified into three groups (Table 1) (Shewry et al, 1986; Wieser et al, 1991). The HMW group comprises the HMW subunits of glutenin and is characterized by relatively high proportions of glycine and tyrosine. Glutamine, glycine and proline account for 65–70% of total residues. The medium-molecular-weight (MMW) group consists of ω-gliadins, which contain high amounts of glutamine, proline and phenylalanine. These amino acids account for about 80% of the total composition. The sulphur-containing amino acids cysteine and methionine are absent or present in only trace amounts. The ω-gliadins were, therefore, classified by Shewry et al (1986) as the S-poor protein group. In contrast, the proteins of the LMW group have a higher content of cysteine and methionine and have consequently been designated as S-rich proteins. In most cases, their composition is in a medium range between the HMW and MMW group. The range of molecular masses (Table 1), as well as the primary structures analysed until now (see below), supports the classification of gluten proteins into three groups.

Each of these groups contains two or three different protein types with partly homologous, partly unique, structural elements (Table 1). The HMW group contains the x- and the y- type HMW subunits. Both types can be differentiated by the content of proline, cysteine and histidine, and by the molecular mass. The MMW group consists of the ω_5- and $\omega_{1,2}$-type gliadins. Pronounced differences are present in the content of glutamine, proline, phenylalanine and serine, and also in the range of molecular masses. The LMW group comprises three different protein types, the α- and γ-type gliadins and the LMW subunits of glutenin. The most significant differences between α- and γ-type gliadins can be observed in the proportions of tyrosine and phenylalanine. The LMW subunits are characterized by the highest amount of serine. The range of molecular masses of these types overlaps. As shown in Table 1, the N-terminal sequences are typical for each type, and, for this reason, the determination of N-terminal sequences is a very useful aid in the identification of gluten proteins.

Each type consists of numerous components with a high, mostly more than 90%, degree of homology. With respect to varietal variations, more than 100 different proteins from the same type exist. This heterogeneity is due to substitutions, insertions and/or deletions of single residues or oligopeptides in the peptide chain.

The distribution of total gluten protein among the different types is strongly dependent on wheat variety (genotype) and growing conditions (soil, climate, fertilization). An example is given in Table 1 for the German

Table 1. Classification and characteristics of gluten proteins (Shewry et al, 1986; Wieser et al, 1991).

| | HMW | | MMW (S-poor) | | LMW (S-rich) | | |
| | HMW subunits of glutenin | | ω-gliadins | | α-gliadins | γ-gliadins | LMW subunits of glutenin |
	x	y	ω_5	$\omega_{1,2}$	α	γ	
Partial amino-acid composition (mol%)							
Glx	35.8–38.0	35.6–36.3	55.4–56.0	42.5–44.9	35.5–41.3	32.5–37.8	35.2–41.7
Pro	12.0–13.2	9.9–11.0	19.7–19.8	24.8–27.4	14.5–18.5	16.2–17.7	11.7–13.8
Gly	17.6–20.1	17.1–18.9	0.6–0.8	0.9–2.1	1.3–2.6	2.8–2.9	2.1–3.6
Ser	5.7–8.8	6.4–7.0	2.6–3.3	5.8–6.3	4.8–6.5	4.6–6.6	7.4–10.0
Tyr	5.6–7.0	5.2–5.6	0.6–0.7	0.8–1.5	2.7–3.8	0.3–1.3	1.4–1.8
Phe	0.1–0.4	0.3–0.5	9.0–9.5	7.6–8.1	3.3–3.4	4.6–5.7	3.9–4.8
Cys	0.5–0.6	1.0–1.1	0.0	0.0	1.7–2.5	2.3–3.2	2.4–2.8
His	0.5–0.6	1.6–2.4	1.3–1.4	0.6–1.1	1.8–3.3	1.0–2.5	1.1–1.2
$M_r \times 10^{-3}$ SDS-PAGE	104–124	90–102	66–79	55–65	32	38–42	36–44
Sequencing	83–88	67–74	—	—	28–35	31–35	32–39
Most frequent N-terminal sequences	EGEASG*	EGEASR	SRLLSP	ARQLNP KELQSP	VRVPVP	NMQVDP NIQADP	RCIPGL SCISGL
Percentage of gluten protein cv. Kanzler	6.4	2.9	4.1	3.8	33.1	25.8	23.9

SDS–PAGE, sodium dodecyl sulphate–polyacrylamide gel electrophoresis.
* One-letter codes for amino acids are given in Table 2.

cultivar Kanzler. Generally, types from the LMW group are present in the greatest amount, whereas the different types of the HMW and MMW groups occur in much lower proportions.

Primary structure of gluten proteins

A milestone in the chemistry of cereal proteins was the determination of the complete amino-acid sequence of an α-type gliadin by Kasarda and co-workers (1984). Since then, a number of partial and complete sequences of gluten proteins have been determined, mostly by analysis of corresponding complementary DNA sequences. Although no complete sequences of ω-type gliadins have been reported, an indication of their primary structure can be obtained from the N-terminal sequence, molecular mass and amino-acid composition.

HMW group

In general HMW subunits consist of three domains: a non-repetitive N-terminal domain (domain A) of 82–105 residues, a repetitive central domain (domain B) 480–685 residues long and a non-repetitive C-terminal domain (domain C) with constant 42 residues (Shewry et al, 1992). Domains A and C are characterized by the presence of most or all of the cysteine residues and by the frequent occurrence of charged residues. Domain B contains repetitive hexapeptides (consensus QQPGQG; see Table 2 for one-letter-code for amino acids) as a backbone with inserted hexapeptides (e.g. YYPTSP) and tripeptides (e.g. QQP or QPG). The most important differences between the x- and y-type lie within the A and B domains. For example, the y-type has an insertion of 18 residues including two neighbouring cysteine residues in domain A. Typical repetitive units are less frequently repeated and more frequently modified in domain B of the y-type. The differences within a type are limited and are due mainly to modification of single residues and to the number and arrangement of repeats.

MMW group

Complete amino-acid sequences of ω-type gliadins have not been determined up to now. It can be concluded from amino-acid composition and N-terminal sequence studies that these proteins consist almost entirely of repetitive sequences with only short non-repetitive N-terminal sequences. The repetitive sequences of the ω_5-type start from position 14 with the units PQQQF (Kasarda et al, 1983). The N-terminal sequences of $\omega_{1,2}$-type gliadins reveal partially homologous, non-repetitive variants that are continued by repeats of the unit PQQPY and then by the most dominant units PQQPFPQQ (Shewry and Miflin, 1985).

LMW group

The structural principles of the three different types (α- and γ-type gliadins,

Table 2. Amino-acid sequences* of α- and γ-type gliadins and LMW subunits of glutenin (Kasarda et al, 1984; Okita et al, 1985; Rafalski, 1986).

Domain Ia

α	1	VRVPVPQLQPQNPSQQQPQEQVPLVQQQQFLG
γ	1	NMQVDPSGQVQWPQ
LMW	1	SCISGLERPW

Domain Ib†

α		γ		LMW	
33	QQQP–FP–PQQPYP	15	QQPVL	11	QQQPLPP
45	QPQP–FP–SQQPYL	20	LPQQPFS	18	QQ–SFS
57	QLQP–FPQPQLPYS	27	QQPQQTFP	23	QQPPFS
70	QPQP–FR–PQQPYP	35	QPQQTFP	29	QQQQQPLP–
82	QPQPQYSQPQQPIS	42	HQPQQQFP	37	QQPSFS
		50	QPQQPQQQFL	43	QQQPPFS
		60	QPQQPFP	50	QQQPILS
		67	QQPQQPYP	57	QQPPFS
		75	QQPQQPFP	63	QQQQPVLP
		83	QTQQPQQLFP	71	QQSPFS
		93	QSQQPQQPYP	77	QQQQLVLP
		103	QQPQQPFP	85	PQQQQQQLV––
		111	QTQQPQQQFP	94	QQQIP
		121	QSQQPQ–PFP		
		130	QPQQPQQSFP		
		140	QQQPS		

Domain II

α   96   QQQQQQQQQQQQQQQQQQQQ

Domain III†

α	114	ILQQILQQQLIFCMDVVLQQHNIAHGRSQV––––––LQQSTYQLLQELCCQHLWQI
γ	145	FIQPSLQQQLNPCKNLLLQQCRPVSLVSSLW–S–MIWPQSACQVMRQQCCQQLAQI
LMW	99	IVQPSVLQQLNPCKVFLQQQCSPVAMPQRLARSQM–WQQSSCHVMQQQCCQQLQQI
α	150	PEQSQCQAIHNVVHAIIL
γ	181	PQQLQCAAIHSVVHSISM
LMW	135	PEQSRYEAIRAIIYSIIL

Domain IV

α	182	HQQQKQQQQPSSQVSFQQPLQQYPLGQGSFRPSQQN
γ	217	QEQQQQQQQQQQQQQQQQGMRILLPLYQQQQVGQGTL
LMW	172	QEQQQGFVQPQQQQPQQSGQGVSQSQQQSQQQLEQCSFQQPQQQLGQQPQQQQQQQ

Domain Va†

α	218	PQAQGSVQPQQLPQFEEIRNLALQTLPAMCNVYIAPYC–TI–APFG
γ	253	VQGQGIIQPQQPAQLEAIRSLVLQTLPTMCNVYVPPECSIIKAPFA
LMW	228	VLQGTFLQPHQIAHLEAVTSIALRTLPTMCSVNVPLYSATTSVPFG

Domain Vb

α	262	IFGTN
γ	299	SIVTGIGGQ
LMW	274	VGTGVGAY

* One-letter code for amino acids: A, Ala; C, Cys; D, Asp; E, Glu; F, Phe; G, Gly; H, His; I, Ile; M, Met; N, Asn; P, Pro; Q, Gln; R, Arg; S, Ser; T, Thr; V, Val; W, Trp; Y, Tyr. Numbers indicate the position of the first amino acid per line within the complete sequence.
† Ordered to the best possible homology; – signifies a deletion.

LMW subunits of glutenin) are presented by means of three examples in Table 2. The sequences have been divided into five domains (I–V) according to Kasarda et al (1984).

The non-repetitive N-terminal sequences (*domain Ia*) are unique for each type. *Domain Ib* consists of repetitive sequences rich in glutamine, proline and aromatic amino acids. The repetitive units of the α-type consist of dodecapeptides such as QPQPFPPQQPYP, which are usually repeated five times. The typical repeat unit of the γ-type is PQQPFPQ, which is repeated up to 16 times and interspersed by Q, QQ, TQQ, LQQ or PQQ. The repetitive sequences of the LMW-type contain a series of glutamine, followed by units such as PPFS, which are frequently modified. *Domain II* is present only in the α-type and contains a polyglutamine sequence (a maximum of 18 residues of Q). *Domain III* represents long homologous sequences, which are non-repetitive, have less glutamine and proline than domain I and possess a more usual composition containing most of the cysteine residues and numerous charged or hydrophobic residues. The degree of homology in the examples of Table 2 is 43% (α/γ-type), 37% (α/LMW-type) and 55% (γ/LMW-type). *Domain IV* is less homologous than domain III, poor in proline and rich in glutamine with a maximal 15 residues of Q in series (γ-type). The sequence of LMW subunits is elongated by about 20 residues and contains one cysteine residue. *Domain V* can be divided into a homologous section Va and a short unique section Vb (C-terminal sequences). Similar to domain III, charged and hydrophobic amino-acid residues are more dominant than in the other domains; the degree of homology is 61% (α/γ), 37% (α/LMW) and 46% (γ/LMW).

Altogether, the different types of the LMW group are homologous in two of five domains, and most typically different in the N-terminal and repetitive sequences (domain I). The α- and LMW-types appear to be less related than the α/γ-types and γ/LMW-types.

Relation of gluten proteins to other cereal storage proteins

The structural features (amino-acid composition, molecular mass, N-terminal and, as far as known, complete amino-acid sequences) of the storage proteins reflect very well the taxonomic relationships of the cereals. Within the tribe of Triticeae, each of the different protein groups is present (Shewry et al, 1987) (Table 3). The aggregative HMW group comprises the

Table 3. Classification of the Triticeae storage proteins (modified from Shewry et al, 1987).

Group	Wheat	Rye	Barley
HMW	HMW subunits of glutenin (a)	HMW secalins (a)	D-hordeins (a)
MMW (S-poor)	ω-type gliadins (m)	ω-secalins (m)	C-hordeins (m)
LMW (S-rich)	LMW subunits of glutenin (a)	γ-75 kDa-secalins (a)	B-hordeins (a)
	α-type gliadins (m)	γ-40 kDa-secalins (m)	γ-hordeins (m)
	γ-type gliadins (m)		

(a), Mainly aggregative (glutelin); (m), mainly monomeric (prolamin).

HMW subunits of glutenin (wheat), the HMW secalins (rye) and the D-hordeins (barley). As well as ω-gliadins (wheat), ω-secalins (rye) and C-hordeins (barley) have been grouped into the mainly monomeric MMW group. The corresponding types of the LMW group are partly aggregative (LMW subunits of wheat, γ-75 kDa-secalins of rye, B-hordeins of barley) and partly monomeric (α- and γ-type gliadins of wheat, γ-40 kDa-secalins of rye, γ-hordeins of barley).

Studies on amino-acid sequences (Egorov, 1988) revealed that the prolamin fraction of oats (avenin) can also be classified into the LMW group because of remarkable homology within domains III and Va. These non-repetitive domains are partly homologous in a large group of seed proteins (Kreis et al, 1985). The storage proteins of maize, rice, millet and sorghum, however, do not show any significant relationship to those of the Triticeae.

RELATIONSHIP BETWEEN CHEMICAL STRUCTURE AND COELIAC TOXICITY

Early investigations

Early workers established coeliac toxicity in a series of feeding tests based on the production of symptoms such as steatorrhoea or on tests such as malabsorption of fat or xylose (for details and references see Kasarda, 1975). Soon after Dicke (1950) found that the ingestion of wheat was responsible for the symptoms of coeliac disease, it was demonstrated that rye and barley were also harmful, whereas maize, rice and buckwheat were not. There is still disagreement, however, about the coeliac toxicity of oats. Fractionation of wheat flour and testing led to the conclusion that gluten was toxic, whereas starch and albumin were not. Gliadin, the protein fraction of gluten soluble in aqueous alcohols, was found to be the most toxic factor, whereas the effect of the insoluble glutenin fraction was described, somewhat controversially, as either non-toxic or possibly toxic, but on very inadequate evidence.

The complete degradation of gliadin into free amino acids by acid hydrolysis rendered it harmless as did deamidation of glutamine side chains combined with a limited cleavage of peptide bonds. Both glutamine and proline residues were considered to be important for coeliac toxicity. Glutamine itself, however, was not toxic.

The digestion of gluten or gliadin with pepsin and trypsin alone or followed by pancreatin resulted in the retention of toxicity. Further digestion with fresh hog intestinal mucosa rendered the preparation non-toxic. Detoxification of gliadin was also achieved by exhaustive digestion with crude papain. The breakdown of the disulphide bonds in peptic–tryptic peptides by oxidation did not destroy toxicity.

Equivalent to the gliadin fraction of wheat, the prolamin fractions of rye (secalin), barley (hordeins) and probably oats (avenins) were associated with coeliac toxicity. Although the prolamin fractions of the cereals are crude mixtures of different proteins, their amino-acid compositions show a close relation to both coeliac toxicity and taxonomy of the cereals (Wieser et al, 1980).

In summary, therefore, although the early investigations were somewhat unsatisfactory with regard to both test systems and the characterization of proteins or protein digests, the following facts were established: (1) wheat, rye and barley are coeliac-toxic cereals; (2) gliadin, the prolamin fraction of wheat, is highly toxic; and (3) toxicity is not destroyed by gastropancreatic enzymes.

In-vitro models of coeliac toxicity

Most investigators would agree with Stern et al (1990) that in-vivo testing is the 'gold standard' for assessing the coeliac toxicity of proteins or peptides. But ethical considerations apart, the need for comparatively large amounts is one of the most crucial limiting factors. Even the relatively sensitive instillation test introduced by Hekkens et al (1970) requires the equivalent of several grams of gliadin per patient. For these reasons, in-vitro models were developed in order to identify toxic compounds in microgram or milligram amounts (for details and references see recent reviews by Cornell, 1988a; Troncone and Auricchio, 1991).

The organ culture of human small intestine has been proposed as providing the most reliable in-vitro approach. Intestinal mucosal tissue obtained by biopsy from patients with active enteropathy shows improvement of enzyme activity and morphology in the medium alone, but not in the presence of coeliac-toxic substances (Howdle et al, 1981). Apart from human material, cultures of the immature intestine of rat or chick fetus have been used to demonstrate the cytotoxic activity of gliadin fractions (Wood et al, 1987).

Assays based on the stimulation of peripheral blood lymphocytes from coeliac patients or the production of the leukocyte-migration inhibition factor (LMIF) were also shown to reflect coeliac toxicity and were used as screening tests. Alternatively, the production of macrophage proagulant activity (MPCA) was proposed. Another approach used the ability of coeliac-toxic compounds to disrupt rat liver lysosomes, but this test supposedly lacked specificity.

In summary, in-vitro tests cannot substitute for in-vivo testing, but are a valuable aid in the search for potentially toxic candidates that ultimately have to be tested in vivo.

Testing of gliadin fractions

Amongst the prolamin fractions, only gliadin has been investigated in detail. Hekkens et al (1970, 1978) were the first to demonstrate the toxicity of a well-defined gliadin subfraction. By means of direct instillation into the small intestine, followed by biopsy, the coeliac toxicity of A-gliadin, a group of aggregable α-type gliadins, was established. The activity of A-gliadin was supported by in-vitro test systems, e.g. an organ culture test (Falchuk et al, 1980). The analysis of A-gliadin demonstrated that covalently bound carbohydrates were absent and therefore not involved in activating coeliac disease

(Bernardin et al, 1976). Later, in-vivo and in-vitro studies indicated that all major gliadin subgroups (α-, β-, γ- and ω-gliadins in terms of electrophoretic mobility) produced toxic effects (Jos et al, 1982; Wieser et al, 1982; Ciclitira et al, 1984; Howdle et al, 1984). Studies of N-terminal amino-acid sequences, however, indicated that the fractions investigated were not necessarily pure with respect to protein type (Bietz et al, 1977; Egorov and Odintsova, 1987; Kasarda et al, 1987). Thus, the toxicity of the different gliadin types remains an open question.

Testing of gliadin peptides

The introduction of in-vitro systems for testing toxicity opened a new era in the study of gliadin peptides, as small amounts could be tested. Nevertheless, only a few attempts have been made to isolate and characterize pure peptides from gliadin and to test them for coeliac toxicity. The amino-acid sequence and origin of those peptides containing 31 residues or fewer which have been tested in one system or another, are shown in Table 4.

Jos et al (1983) obtained a pure peptide from a peptic–tryptic digest of a β-gliadin that was, in fact, an α-type gliadin. Coeliac toxicity was established by organ culture testing. Amino-acid composition and N-terminal amino-acid residues indicated that this peptide corresponds to residues 3–24 of α-type gliadins.

Wieser et al (1983) isolated pure peptides from a peptic–tryptic digest of total gliadin by means of different separation techniques. After each step, the peptide fractions were tested using LMIF and organ culture test systems. One of the toxic peptides, designated B3142, was analysed for amino-acid sequences. The results revealed a high proportion of glutamine and proline, and indicated that this peptide corresponds to residues 3–55 of α-type gliadins and was identical to residues 3–55 of A-gliadin, except that residue 31 was proline instead of leucine (Wieser et al, 1984). Conformational studies of peptide B3142 showed that β-turns were the predominant structural feature, and it was suggested that β-turn conformation may be involved in the activation of coeliac disease (Tatham et al, 1990). In subsequent work, B3142 was cleaved with chymotrypsin into two fragments (CT-1 and CT-2), which correspond to residues 3–24 and 25–55, respectively, of α-type gliadins (Wieser et al, 1986). Both peptides were shown to be as active as B3142 by organ culture testing (Table 4). The longest sequences common for both peptides were -Pro-Ser-Gln-Gln- and -Gln-Gln-Gln-Pro-. A large-scale procedure was developed to produce B3142 and peptides with related sequences in milligram amounts (Wieser and Belitz, 1992a).

De Ritis et al (1988) cleaved A-gliadin with cyanogen bromide to yield three fragments designated CN-I (residues 1–127), CN-II (128–246) and CN-III (247–266). Both large peptides were toxic in an organ culture system; CN-III was non-toxic. Peptide CN-I was further cleaved by limited chymotryptic digestion into fragments XT (1–55), XT (56–68) and XT (69–127). The first two peptides were subjected to organ culture testing and only XT (1–55) was found to be toxic. Further digestion of XT (1–55) with chymotrypsin yielded peptides XT (1–30) and XT (31–55) (Table 4). Both

Sequence*	Designation	Source	Position	Toxicity (test)†	Reference
VPVPQLQPNPSQQPQEQVPL	CT-1	Gliadin	α: 3–24	+ (OC)	Wieser et al (1986)
VQQQFPGQQQPFPPQQPYPQPQPFPSQQPY	CT-2		α: 25–55	+	
VRVPVPQLQPNPSQQPQEQVPLVQQQF	XT (1–30)	A-gliadin	α: 1–30	+	De Ritis et al (1988)
LGQQPFPPQQPYPQPQPFPSQQPY	XT (31–55)		α: 31–55	+ (OC)	
LQLQPFPQPQLPY	XT (56–68)		α: 56–68	–	
CNVYIAPYCTIAPFGIFGTN	CN-III		α: 247–266	–	
LGQGSFRPSQQN	—	Synthetic	α: 206–217	+ (LMIF, IV)	Mantzaris et al (1990, 1991)
CPQLQPQNPSQQQPQEQG	A		α: 5–22‡	+	Devery et al (1991)
CPQPFPSQQPYLQLQG	B		α: 45–60‡	+ (LMIF, MPCA)	
GSFRPSQQNPQAQG	C		α: 209–222‡	–	
CMDVVLQQHNIAHGRSQ	D	Synthetic	α: 126–142	–	
GQAIHNVHAIIMQG	E		α: 169–183‡	–	
GQQLPQFAEIRNLG	F		α: 226–239	– (MPCA)	
GFPQPQQPYQQQPG	G		γ	–	
GQQLAQIPQQLQQG	H		γ	–	
LQPQNPSQQQPQ	I		α: 8–19	+	Kocna et al (1991)
QPQPFPSQQPYL	II		α: 45–56	+	
QGSFRPSQQNPQ	III		α: 208–219	+	
LQPQNTGQQQPQ	IV	Synthetic	α: 8–19‡	+ (FCI)	
LQPQNPSAAAPQ	V		α: 8–19‡	–	
LQPQNPSNNNPQ	VI		α: 8–19‡	–	
LQPQNPSPPPPQ	VII		α: 8–19‡	–	
PSQQQP	I		α: 13–18	–	Cornell and Mothes (1993)
QQPYPQ	II		α: 40–45/77–82	–	
PQQPYPQPQP	III	Synthetic	α: 39–48/76–85	– (FCI, RLL)	
PQPFPSQQPYLQ	IV		α: 46–57	–	
RPQQPYPQPQPQ	V		α: 75–86	+	
LGQQQPFPPQQPYPQPQPF	A		α: 31–49	+	Sturgess et al (1994)
QQYPLGQGSFRPSQQNPQA	B	Synthetic	α: 202–220	– (IV)	
VPVPQLQPNPSQQPQEQ	C		α: 3–21	–	

* See Table 2 for one-letter code for amino acids.
† OC, organ culture; LMIF, leukocyte migration inhibition factor; IV, in vivo; FCI, fetal chick intestine; MPCA, macrophage proagulant activity; RLL, rat liver lysosome.
‡ Modified.

peptides were toxic, in agreement with the findings for CT-1 and CT-2 (Wieser et al, 1986).

Cornell and co-workers separated a peptic–tryptic–pancreatinic digest of gliadin with ultrafiltration and cation exchange chromatography and identi-fied a fraction, designated fraction 9, that showed coeliac toxicity as assessed by means of xylose absorption, organ culture and rat liver lysosome tests (reviewed by Cornell, 1988a). Further separation of fraction 9 by anion exchange chromatography yielded the toxic subfractions 9–1 and 9–2, whereas subfractions 9–3, 9–4 and 9–5 were non-toxic (Cornell and Max-well, 1982). The intestinal mucosa from coeliac patients in remission was unable to abolish the toxicity of subfraction 9–2, whereas control intestinal mucosa was able to do so (Cornell et al, 1988). The authors suggested that an enzyme deficiency is the most likely explanation for these effects. Two of the peptides resistant to mucosal digestion were isolated and shown to be toxic to rat liver lysosomes; their molecular mass and amino-acid composition suggested that they are hexapeptides with the sequences Pro-Ser-Glx-Glx-Glx-Pro and Glx-Glx-Pro-Tyr-Pro-Glx, respectively (Cornell, 1988b).

As indicated by the toxic peptides isolated from gliadin digests, the sequences -Pro-Ser-Gln-Gln- and -Gln-Gln-Gln-Pro- were not cleaved by pepsin, trypsin or chymotrypsin. Recent studies on the enzymatic fragmen-tation of the toxic peptide CT-1 demonstrated that these sequences were also not cleaved by pancreatin, thermolysin or endoproteinase Glu-C (Wieser and Belitz, 1992b). In contrast, papain was active against these sequences from both CT-1 and B3142 (Wieser et al, 1984), mainly splitting the peptide bonds between Gln residues. This special activity may partially explain the detoxifying effect of papain (Messer et al, 1964).

In summary, the results obtained by groups using different approaches indicate that domain I of α-type gliadins is involved in the pathogenesis of coeliac disease. The tetrapeptide sequences -Pro-Ser-Gln-Gln- and -Gln-Gln-Gln-Pro-, common for toxic peptides, are considered as key sequences for further investigation. The importance of these sequences may be sup-ported by the fact that they occur in the storage proteins of all coeliac-toxic cereals: -Pro-Ser-Gln-Gln- appears in α-type gliadins, HMW subunits of glutenin and hordeins; -Gln-Gln-Gln-Pro- appears in α-, γ- and ω-type gliadins, LMW and HMW subunits of glutenin, secalins, hordeins and avenins. As far as is known, they do not occur in storage proteins from non-toxic cereals, e.g. maize zein or rice prolamin, or in other important food proteins, e.g. milk proteins (Wieser et al, 1986).

Testing of synthetic peptides

Since 1987 synthetic peptides containing the proposed key sequences of α-type gliadins have been investigated (Table 4). Partial sequence homology between an adenovirus E1B protein and α-type gliadins including the residues -Pro-Ser-Gln- led to the proposal that human adenovirus type 12 may play a role in activating coeliac disease (Kagnoff et al, 1984). A dodecapeptide corresponding to residues 206–217 (including -Pro-Ser-Gln-Gln-) of A-gliadin and homologous to a partial sequence (residues 384–395) of the E1B protein was synthesized and tested by an indirect LMIF test and by direct instillition into the small intestine of two coeliac patients in remission (Karagiannis et al, 1987; Mantzaris et al, 1990; Mantzaris and Jewell, 1991). The results indicated toxicity in both systems. These studies were the first comparing in-vivo and in-vitro tests with a pure peptide corresponding to a gliadin sequence.

A panel of synthetic peptides homologous to specific α- and γ-type gliadin sequences was tested using an indirect LMIF test or a macrophage proagulant activity assay (Devery et al, 1991; Skerritt et al, 1991) (Table 4). The tetrapeptide Pro-Ser-Gln-Gln itself was found to be inactive, probably because of its small size, whereas an octadecapeptide and a hexadecapeptide comprising this sequence and corresponding to residues 5–22 and 45–60, respectively, of A-gliadin were active in at least one of the test systems. In contrast to the results of Karagiannis and co-workers, neither assay showed activity to a tetradecapeptide (residues 209–222 of A-gliadin) homologous to the adenovirus protein. Five other peptides, not containing -Pro-Ser-Gln-Gln-, and corresponding to sequences from domains III and V of α-type gliadins and to sequences from domain I and III of γ-type gliadins, were also inactive.

Two series of different synthetic peptides were tested for their effects in the fetal chick intestine model. The first included three dodecapeptides with sequences identical to residues 8–19, 45–56 and 208–219 of A-gliadin and four dodecapeptides with modified sequences (Kocna et al, 1991) (Table 4). The effect of peptide I (residues 8–19 including -Pro-Ser-Gln-Gln-) was most pronounced and was not lost when -Pro-Ser- was replaced by -Thr-Gly- (peptide IV). This sequence was expected to contribute to a β-turn conformation equivalent to -Pro-Ser-. The substitution of -Gln-Gln-Gln-, however, by -Ala-Ala-Ala-, -Asn-Asn-Asn- or -Pro-Pro-Pro- resulted in the loss of activity (peptides V, VI, VII). Peptides II (residues 45–56) and III (208–219), also containing -Pro-Ser-Gln-Gln-, were active, but to a lesser degree than peptide I.

For the second series of peptides, the effect on rat liver lysosomes was also used for testing toxicity (Cornell and Mothes, 1993) (Table 4). A hexapeptide (residues 13–18) and a dodecapeptide (46–57), both containing -Pro-Ser-Gln-Gln-, were non-toxic as well as two other hexa- and decapeptides not containing this sequence. A dodecapeptide corresponding to residues 75–86 was the only peptide to display appreciable activity in both assays (peptide V). This peptide was shown to be the major component of the toxic fraction 9 (Cornell et al, 1992). It was suggested that the sequences -Gln-Gln-Gln-Pro- and -Pro-Ser-Gln-Gln- are not sufficient by themselves to cause activity and that certain amino-acid residues flanking the key sequences are also required.

A recent report (Sturgess et al, 1994) describes in-vivo challenge experiments in four treated coeliac patients using synthetic gliadin peptides (Table 4). The peptide corresponding to amino acids 31–49 of A-gliadin containing the -Gln-Gln-Gln-Pro- (QQQP) motif but not the -Pro-Ser-Gln-Gln- (PSQQ) motif was shown to be toxic, but the peptides corresponding to amino acids 3–21 and 202–220 were not toxic, even though the former

contained both PSQQ and QQQP, the latter PSQQ. These results raise
doubts about the importance of the PSQQ sequence but support the possible
toxicity of QQQP. They also do not support the results of Mantzaris et al
(1991) concerning the toxicity of the adenovirus 12 homologous sequence in
the peptide containing the 202–220 residues. Clearly these important but
somewhat contradictory results need confirmation by other workers.

SUMMARY

In recent years, remarkable progress has been made in the elucidation of
cereal protein structure and its relation to coeliac toxicity.

Gluten proteins of wheat can be classified according to their primary
structure into high-, medium- and low-molecular-weight (HMW, MMW,
LMW) groups. Each of these groups contains two or three different protein
types having partly homologous, partly unique, structural elements: x- and
y-type HMW subunits of glutenin (HMW group), ω_5 and $\omega_{1,2}$-type gliadins
(MMW group) and α-type gliadins, γ-type gliadins and LMW subunits of
glutenin (LMW group). Numerous proteins from the same type do exist with
only a few modifications of the amino-acid sequence. The structure of the
HMW and LMW group proteins can be divided into three and five domains,
respectively. Most typical for each type and unique for cereals are the
glutamine- and proline-rich domains containing repetitive sequences
(HMW group: domain B; LMW group: domain I). ω-type gliadins consist
almost entirely of repetitive sequences. Rye and barley, closely related to
wheat, have protein types homologous to those of wheat.

Early investigations showed that wheat gluten and, in particular, the
alcohol-soluble gliadin fraction contained the factor toxic for coeliac
patients. Equivalent protein fractions of rye, barley and probably oats were
also considered to be toxic. The effects of toxic proteins were not destroyed
by digestion with pepsin, trypsin and pancreatin. In-vivo (instillation)
testing established the toxicity of α-type gliadins, and in-vitro (organ culture) testing of gliadin peptides demonstrated that the N-terminal region
(domain I) of α-type gliadins is involved in activating coeliac disease. The
longest sequences common for toxic peptides were found to be -Pro-Ser-
Gln-Gln- and -Gln-Gln-Gln-Pro-. Various in-vitro tests and two in-vivo
studies on synthetic peptides support the importance of one or both of these
sequences. They do not occur in non-toxic food proteins and are characterized by their ability to form a β-turn conformation. Although these
sequences are probably not sufficient for toxicity in themselves, and other
amino-acid residues are additionally required, they could serve as the starting point for further investigation.

REFERENCES

Bernardin JE, Saunders RM & Kasarda DD (1976) Absence of carbohydrate in celiac-toxic
    A-gliadin. *Cereal Chemistry* **53**: 612–614.
Bietz JA & Wall JS (1972) Wheat gluten subunits: molecular weights determined by sodium
    dodecyl sulfate–polyacrylamide gel electrophoresis. *Cereal Chemistry* **49**: 416–430.

Bietz JA, Huebner FR, Sanderson JE & Wall JS (1977) Wheat gliadin homology revealed through N-terminal amino acid sequence analysis. *Cereal Chemistry* **54**: 1070–1083.

Ciclitira PJ, Evans DJ, Fagg NLK et al (1984) Clinical testing of gliadin fractions in coeliac patients. *Clinical Science* **66**: 357–364.

Cornell HJ (1988a) Wheat proteins and celiac disease. *Comments in Agriculture and Food Chemistry* **1**: 289–313.

Cornell HJ (1988b) Amino acid composition of peptides remaining after in vitro digestion of a gliadin sub-fraction with duodenal mucosa from patients with coeliac disease. *Clinica et Chimica Acta* **176**: 279–290.

Cornell HJ & Maxwell RJ (1982) Amino acid composition of gliadin fractions which may be toxic to individuals with coeliac disease. *Clinica et Chimica Acta* **123**: 311–319.

Cornell HJ & Mothes T (1993) The activity of wheat gliadin peptides in in vitro assays for coeliac disease. *Biochimica et Biophysica Acta* **1181**: 169–173.

Cornell HJ, Auricchio RS, de Ritis G et al (1988) Intestinal mucosa of celiacs in remission is unable to abolish toxicity of gliadin peptides on in vitro developing fetal rat intestine and cultured atrophic celiac mucosa. *Pediatric Research* **24**: 233–237.

Cornell H, Wieser H & Belitz H-D (1992) Characterization of the gliadin-derived peptides which are biologically active in coeliac disease. *Clinica et Chimica Acta* **213**: 37–50.

Devery JM, Bender V, Penttila I & Skerritt JH (1991) Identification of reactive synthetic gliadin peptides specific for coeliac disease. *International Archives of Allergy and Applied Immunology* **95**: 356–362.

Dicke WK (1950) *Coeliac disease. Investigation of the harmful effects of certain types of cereals on patients with coeliac disease.* PhD thesis, University of Utrecht (in Dutch).

Egorov TA (1988) The amino acid sequence of the 'fast' avenin component (*Avena sativa* L.) *Journal of Cereal Science* **8**: 289–292.

Egorov TA & Odintsova TI (1987) Microsequence analysis of prolamins with gas phase protein sequencer. In Lasztity R & Bekes F (eds) *Proceedings of the 3rd International Workshop on Gluten Proteins*, pp 434–439, Singapore: World Scientific.

Falchuk ZM, Nelson DL, Katz AJ et al (1980) Gluten sensitive enteropathy: influence of histocompatibility type on gluten sensitivity in vitro. *Journal of Clinical Investigation* **66**: 227–233.

Gee S (1888) On the coeliac affection. *St Bartholomew's Hospital Reports* **24**: 17–20.

Hekkens WTJM (1978) The toxicity of gliadin, a review. In MacNicholl B, McCarthy CF & Fottrell PE (eds) *Perspectives in Coeliac Disease*, pp 3–14. Lancaster: MTP Press.

Hekkens WTJM, Haex AJC & Willighagen RGJ (1970) Some aspects of gliadin fractionation and testing by a histochemical method. In Booth CC & Dowling RH (eds) *Coeliac Disease. Proceedings of the International Coeliac Symposium*, pp 11–19. Edinburgh: Churchill Livingstone.

Howdle PD, Corazza GR, Bullen AW & Losowsky MS (1981) Gluten sensitivity of small intestinal mucosa in vitro: quantitative assessement of histologic charge. *Gastroenterology* **80**: 442–450.

Howdle PD, Ciclitira PJ, Simpson FG & Losowsky MS (1984) Are all gliadins toxic in coeliac disease? An in vitro study of α-, β-, γ- and ω-gliadins. *Scandinavian Journal of Gastroenterology* **19**: 41–47.

Jos J, Charbonnier L, Mosse J et al (1982) The toxic fraction of gliadin digests in coeliac disease. Isolation by chromatography on Biogel P-10. *Clinica et Chimica Acta* **119**: 263–274.

Jos J, de Tand MF, Arnaud-Battandier F et al (1983) Separation of pure toxic peptides from a β-gliadin subfraction using high-performance liquid chromatography. *Clinica et Chimica Acta* **134**: 189–198.

Kagnoff MF, Austin RK, Hubert JJ et al (1984) Possible role for a human adenovirus in the pathogenesis of celiac disease. *Journal of Experimental Medicine* **160**: 1544–1557.

Karagiannis JA, Priddle JD & Jewell DP (1987) Cell-mediated immunity to a synthetic gliadin peptide resembling a sequence from adenovirus 12. *Lancet* **i**: 884–886.

Kasarda DD (1975) Celiac disease: malabsorbtion of nutrients induced by a toxic factor in gluten. In Friedman M (ed.) *Protein Nutritional Quality of Foods and Feeds*, part 2, pp 565–593. New York: Marcell Dekker.

Kasarda DD, Autran J-C, Lew EJ-L et al (1983) N-terminal amino acid sequences of ω-gliadins and ω-secalins. Implications for the evolution of prolamin genes. *Biochimica et Biophysica Acta* **747**: 138–150.

Kasarda DD, Okita TW, Bernardin JE et al (1984) Nucleic acid (cDNa) and amino acid sequences of α-type gliadins from wheat (*Triticum aestivum*). *Proceedings of the National Academy of Sciences of the USA* **81:** 4712–4716.

Kasarda DD, Adalsteins AE & Laird NF (1987) γ-Gliadins with α-type structure coded on chromosome 6B of the wheat (*Triticum aestivum* L.) cultivar 'Chinese Spring'. In Lasztity R & Bekes F (eds) *Proceedings of the 3rd International Workshop on Gluten Proteins*, pp 20–29. Singapore: World Scientific.

Kocna P, Mothes T, Krchnak V & Fric P (1991) Relationship between gliadin peptide structure and their effect on the fetal chick duodenum. *Zeitschrift für Lebensmittel-Untersuchung und -Forschung* **192:** 116–119.

Köhler P, Belitz H-D & Wieser H (1993) Disulphide bonds in wheat gluten: further cystine peptides from high molecular weight (HMW) and low molecular weight (LMW) subunits of glutenin and from γ-gliadins. *Zeitschrift für Lebensmittel-Untersuchung und -Forschung* **196:** 239–247.

Kreis M, Forde BG, Rahman S et al (1985) Molecular evolution of the seed storage proteins of barley, rye and wheat. *Journal of Molecular Biology* **183:** 499–502.

Mantzaris GJ & Jewell DP (1991) In vivo toxicity of a synthetic dodecapeptide from A-gliadin in patients with coeliac disease. *Scandinavian Journal of Gastroenterology* **26:** 392–398.

Mantzaris GJ, Karagiannis JA, Priddle JD & Jewell DP (1990) Cellular hypersensitivity to a synthetic dodecapeptide derived from human adenovirus 12 which resembles a sequence of A-gliadin in patients with coeliac disease. *Gut* **31:** 668–673.

Messer M, Anderson CM & Hubbard L (1964) Studies on the mechanism of destruction of the toxic action of wheat gluten in coeliac disease by crude papain. *Gut* **5:** 295–303.

Okita TW, Cheesbrough V & Reeves CD (1985) Evolution and heterogeneity of the α-/β-type and γ-type gliadin DNA sequences. *Journal of Biological Chemistry* **260:** 8203–8213.

Osborne TB (1924) *The Vegetable Proteins*, 2nd edn. London: Longmans, Green.

Payne PI & Corfield KG (1979) Subunit composition of wheat glutenin proteins isolated by gel filtration in a dissociating medium. *Planta* **145:** 83–88.

Rafalski JA (1986) Structure of wheat γ-gliadin genes. *Gene* **43:** 221–229.

De Ritis G, Auricchio S, Jones HW et al (1988) In vitro (organ culture) studies of the toxicity of specific A-gliadin peptides in celiac disease. *Gastroenterology* **94:** 41–49.

Shewry PR & Miflin BJ (1985) Seed storage proteins of economically important cereals. In Pomeranz Y (ed.) *Advances in Cereal Science and Technology*, vol. VII, pp 1–83. St Paul: American Association of Cereal Chemists.

Shewry PR, Miflin BJ, Lew EJ-L & Kasarda DD (1983) The preparation and characterization of an aggregated gliadin fraction from wheat. *Journal of Experimental Botany* **34:** 1403–1410.

Shewry PR, Miflin BJ & Kasarda DD (1984) The structural and evolutionary relationships of the prolamin storage proteins of barley, rye and wheat. *Philosophical Transactions of the Royal Society of London. Series B: Biological Sciences* **304:** 297–308.

Shewry PR, Tatham AS, Forde J et al (1986) The classification and nomenclature of wheat gluten proteins: a reassessment. *Journal of Cereal Science* **4:** 97–106.

Shewry PR, Field JM & Tatham AS (1987) The structure of cereal seed storage proteins. In Morton ID (ed.) *Cereals in a European Context*, pp 421–437. Chichester: Ellis Harwood.

Shewry PR, Halford NG & Tatham AS (1992) High-molecular-weight subunits of wheat glutenin. *Journal of Cereal Science* **15:** 105–120.

Skerritt JH, Devery JM & Hill AS (1991) Chemistry, coeliac-toxicity and detection of gluten and related prolamins in foods. *Panminerva Medicine* **33:** 65–74.

Stern M, Stallmach A, Gellermann B & Wieser H (1990) In vitro testing of gliadin peptides. In Kumar PJ and Walker-Smith JA (eds) *Coeliac Disease: 100 years*, pp 148–151. University of Leeds.

Sturgess R, Day P, Ellis HJ et al (1994) Wheat peptide challenge in coeliac disease. *Lancet* **343:** 758–761.

Tao HP & Kasarda DD (1989) Two-dimensional gel mapping and *N*-terminal sequencing of LMW glutenin subunits. *Journal of Experimental Botany* **40:** 1015–1020.

Tatham AS, Marsh MN, Wieser H & Shewry PR (1990) Conformational studies of peptides corresponding to the coeliac-activating regions of wheat-α-gliadin. *Biochemical Journal* **270:** 313–318.

Troncone R & Auricchio S (1991) Gluten-sensitive enteropathy (celiac disease). *Food Reviews International* **7:** 205–231.

Wieser H & Belitz H-D (1992a) Coeliac active peptides from gliadin: large-scale preparation and characterization. *Zeitschrift für Lebensmittel-Untersuchung und -Forschung* **193:** 428–432.

Wieser H & Belitz H-D (1992b) Isolation and enzymatic fragmentation of the coeliac-active gliadin peptide CT-1. *Zeitschrift für Lebensmittel-Untersuchung und -Forschung* **195:** 22–26.

Wieser H, Seilmeier W & Belitz H-D (1980) Vergleichende Untersuchungen über partielle Aminosäuresequenzen von Prolaminen und Glutelinen verschiedener Getreidearten. I. Proteinfraktionierung nach Osborne. *Zeitschrift für Lebensmittel-Untersuchung und -Forschung* **170:** 17–26.

Wieser H, Springer G, Belitz H-D et al (1982) Toxicity of different wheat gliadins in coeliac disease. *Zeitschrift für Lebensmittel-Untersuchung und -Forschung* **175:** 321–326.

Wieser H, Belitz H-D, Ashkenazi A & Idar D (1983) Isolation of coeliac-active peptide fractions from gliadin. *Zeitschrift für Lebensmittel-Untersuchung und -Forschung* **176:** 85–94.

Wieser H, Belitz H-D & Ashkenazi A (1984) Amino acid sequence of the coeliac active peptide B3142. *Zeitschrift für Lebensmittel-Untersuchung und -Forschung* **179:** 371–376.

Wieser H, Belitz H-D, Idar D & Ashkenazi A (1986) Coeliac activity of the gliadin peptides CT-1 and CT-2. *Zeitschrift für Lebensmittel-Untersuchung und -Forschung* **182:** 115–117.

Wieser H, Seilmeier W & Belitz H-D (1990) Characterization of ethanol-extractable reduced subunits of glutenin separated by reversed-phase high-performance liquid chromatography. *Journal of Cereal Science* **12:** 63–71.

Wieser H, Seilmeier W & Belitz H-D (1991) Klassifizierung der Proteinkomponenten des Weizenklebers. *Getreide, Mehl, Brot* **45:** 35–38.

Wood GM, Howdle PD & Losowsky MS (1987) Organ culture of foetal rat small intestine for testing gluten toxicity—a reappraisal. *British Journal of Experimental Pathology* **68:** 25–34.

Woychik JH, Boundy JA & Dimler RJ (1961) Starch gel electrophoresis of wheat gluten proteins with concentrated urea. *Archives of Biochemistry and Biophysics* **94:** 477–482.

Wrigley CW & Bietz JA (1988) Proteins and amino acids. In Pomeranz Y (ed.) *Wheat: Chemistry and Technology*, vol. I, pp 159–275. St Paul: American Association of Cereal Chemists.

Addendum

The adenovirus 12 hypothesis

PETER D. HOWDLE

As an addendum to the discussion of the precipitating factor in coeliac disease, it is important to review the theory that adenovirus 12 could be implicated in the pathogenesis. Although this theory is probably untenable, it is an interesting hypothesis which has generated a lot of discussion.

There is no doubt that gliadin and related prolamins are responsible for the small intestinal lesion being manifest in coeliac disease, but it has been suggested that other environmental factors may be involved. This is supported by genetic data (see Chapter 2) which show that, although there are specific associations with coeliac disease, there are many individuals with a similar haplotype who do not have the disease. There are also good reports of discordance for coeliac disease in identical twins. It has been proposed, therefore, that another environmental trigger may be necessary for expression of the disease.

In 1984 Kagnoff et al suggested that a possible infection with an enteric adenovirus could be an environmental factor involved in the causation of coeliac disease. They showed immunological cross-reactivity between an early protein (E1B-58 kDa) of adenovirus 12 (Ad12) and gliadin. Amino-acid sequence analysis showed a region of homology between the two proteins, with eight of 12 amino acids being identical. Kagnoff and colleagues suggested that previous infection with this enteric adenovirus could lead to the development of coeliac disease in susceptible individuals on exposure to gliadin, the immunological cross-reactivity being the basis of the pathogenesis. In support of this, neutralizing antibody titres specific to Ad12 were found to be raised in coeliac patients (Kagnoff et al, 1987), implying that coeliac patients had an increased prevalence of Ad12 infection. The antibody measured in these studies, however, was directed against viral coat proteins and not against the E1B-58 kDa protein.

Further support for the hypothesis came from Karagiannis et al (1987) and Mantzaris et al (1990), who showed that treated coeliac patients had a cell-mediated immune response in the peripheral blood to synthetic gliadin and viral peptides of the homologous sequence. There is no evidence yet available of T-cell reactivity to the E1B protein itself.

We sought evidence of persisting Ad12 infection in coeliac patients by using the polymerise chain reaction to analyse small intestinal mucosa for the gene specific for the E1B-58 kDa protein. This was present in 4 of 18 coeliac patients, but also in 2 of 24 control patients (Mahon et al, 1991).

There is thus a low prevalence of such infection in both groups of patients, but certainly no significantly increased incidence in those with coeliac disease. These results suggest that persistent Ad12 infection is not a major element in the pathogenesis of coeliac disease.

As regards previous adenoviral infection in coeliac disease, there are recent antibody studies (Lahdeaho et al, 1993) which show increased titres in coeliac patients to a synthetic E1B homologous protein of Ad12, but also raised titres to a synthetic non-homologous protein of Ad40. These data suggest that enteric infections with adenovirus may be involved in the development of coeliac disease, but not on a basis of immunological cross-reactivity with gliadin.

Important in vivo data come from Mantzaris and Jewell (1991) and Sturgess et al (1994). The former investigators prepared a synthetic peptide of gliadin sharing the homology with the E1B-58 kDa protein of Ad12, and instilled this intraduodenally into two treated coeliac patients and two control patients. The protein produced some changes in the mucosa from the coeliac but not the control patients. This was interpreted as supporting the role of the Ad12 E1B protein in the pathogenesis of coeliac disease. However, Sturgess et al (1994), in a similar experiment, found that a synthetic gliadin peptide, also homologous to the E1B-58 kDa protein, did not cause any histological change when instilled into four treated coeliac patients. Controversy remains, therefore, about the role of adenovirus 12 in the pathogenesis of coeliac disease (Howdle and Blair, 1994).

REFERENCES

Howdle PD & Blair GE (1994) Molecular pathogenesis of coeliac disease. In Quirke P (ed.) *Molecular Biology of Digestive Disease*, pp 62–72. London: BMJ Publishing Group.

Kagnoff MF, Austin RK, Hubert JJ et al (1984) Possible role for a human adenovirus in the pathogenesis of celiac disease. *Journal of Experimental Medicine* **160**: 1544–1557.

Kagnoff MF, Paterson YJ, Kumar PJ et al (1987) Evidence for the role of a human intestinal adenovirus in the pathogenesis of coeliac disease. *Gut* **28**: 995–1001.

Karagiannis JA, Priddle JD & Jewel DP (1987) Cell-mediated immunity to a synthetic gliadin peptide resembling a sequence from adenovirus 12. *Lancet* **i**: 884–886.

Lahdeaho ML, Parkkonen P, Reunala T et al (1993) Antibodies to E1B protein-derived peptides of enteric adenovirus type 40 are associated with celiac disease and dermatitis herpetiformis. *Clinical Immunology and Immunopathology* **69**: 300–305.

Mahon J, Blair GE, Wood GM et al (1991) Is persistent adenovirus 12 infection involved in coeliac disease? A search for viral DNA using the polymerase chain reaction. *Gut* **32**: 1114–1116.

Mantzaris GJ, Karagiannis JA, Priddle JD & Jewell DP (1990) Cellular hypersensitivity to a synthetic dodecapeptide derived from human adenovirus 12 which resembles a sequence of A-gliadin in patients with coeliac disease. *Gut* **31**: 668–673.

Mantzaris G & Jewell DP (1991) In vivo toxicity of a synthetic dodecapeptide from A gliadin in patients with coeliac disease. *Scandinavian Journal of Gastroenterology* **296**: 392–398.

Sturgess R, Day P, Ellis HJ et al (1994) Wheat peptide challenge in coeliac disease. *Lancet* **343**: 758–761.

2

The gluten–host interaction

M. RICHARD TIGHE
PAUL J. CICLITIRA

Coeliac disease manifests in susceptible individuals as an enteropathy following the ingestion of certain 'toxic' cereal proteins. Serial histological sections from the jejunum of patients following gluten challenge have demonstrated the activation of lamina propria lymphocytes within 2 hours of antigen exposure, and it is this cell-mediated response that is believed to be the primary pathogenic mechanism of the small bowel lesion. This chapter reviews the current understanding of T-cell recognition of toxic gliadin antigens, together with the genetically determined influences on antigen presentation associated with the disease susceptibility.

T-cells are unable to recognize antigen directly but require the help of antigen-presenting cells. For recognition by a T-cell receptor, antigen must be presented bound to a cell-surface human leukocyte antigen (HLA) molecule. With the exception of superantigens, intracellular processing of the antigen into short peptide fragments is required before binding to the HLA molecule. Superantigens are proteins capable of binding directly between an HLA molecule and the V_β domain of the T-cell receptor (TCR). The region of HLA binding of a superantigen lies outside the antigen-binding groove of the HLA molecule, whilst the TCR interaction occurs on the germline-derived V_β domain rather than the highly polymorphic region, generated by gene rearrangement, that functions as an antigen peptide recognition site. Thus, superantigens are capable of stimulating large numbers of T cells through the expression of common V_β genes. There is no evidence to suggest that gliadins act as superantigens, and it is assumed that they are presented in a conventional manner.

HLA molecules are subdivided into two classes, reflecting the general differences in tissue expression, antigen processing and presenting pathways, and in TCR recognition. Despite these differences, the tertiary structure of HLA class I and II molecules is similar, reflecting their similar functions in antigen presentation.

HLA STRUCTURE AND PROCESSING

HLA class I molecules

The HLA class I molecule is composed of two protein chains: an α-chain of

Baillière's Clinical Gastroenterology—
Vol. 9, No. 2, June 1995
ISBN 0–7020–1953–4

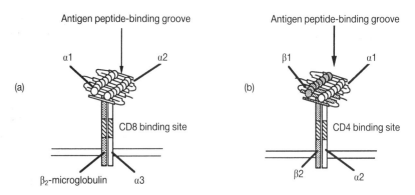

Figure 1. (a) Schematic representation of the three-dimensional structure of an HLA class I molecule, composed of β_2-microglobulin and the three-domain ($\alpha 1$, $\alpha 2$ and $\alpha 3$) HLA class I gene product. The antigen peptide-binding groove is formed by the $\alpha 1$ and $\alpha 2$ domains of the HLA gene product. (b) Schematic representation of the three-dimensional structure of an HLA class II molecule, composed of an α- and a β-chain, each derived from the HLA class II loci. The antigen peptide-binding groove is formed by the components of both α- and β- chains ($\alpha 1$ and $\beta 1$). See text for full description.

45 kDa, encoded by the class I genes, and a β-chain of 12 kDa, β_2-microglobulin (Figure 1).

The α-chain is composed of three domains, $\alpha 1$, $\alpha 2$ and $\alpha 3$. The $\alpha 3$ domain is associated with β_2-microglobulin by disulphide bonding. Both domains have hydrophobic regions indicating the membrane-spanning region of the molecule. The carboxy-termini of these two domains form the cytosolic tail of the class I molecule. The $\alpha 3$ and $\beta 2$ domains possess a binding site for the T-cell accessory molecule CD8, so that class I molecules tend to present antigen only to those T-cells bearing a CD8 molecule.

The allelic polymorphisms of the class I genes are concentrated in the $\alpha 1$ and $\alpha 2$ domains. These two domains are associated in a complex tertiary structure to form a cleft on the surface of the protein able to bind antigenic peptide (Bjorkman et al, 1987). Each domain contributes an α-helix, which forms the wall of this cleft and four β-pleated sheets which make up the cleft floor. These structures are anchored by disulphide bonding to produce a cleft approximately 37–41 Å long. The polymorphism found between HLA class I alleles is primarily centred around either residues facing into this cleft, and so interacting with the bound peptide, or residues on the top of these α-helices and directed up towards the interacting TCR. Speculation has therefore been made that polymorphisms of the HLA class I genes will alter the ability of class I molecules to bind and present certain antigens to T cells and therefore influence an individual's immune response. Detailed X-ray crystallography of class I proteins has now revealed that the class I cleft contains deep 'pockets' capable of accepting and binding certain amino-acid side chains. One characteristic of the antigen peptides, which bind to a particular HLA molecule, is the presence of certain residues able to interact with these pockets. Allelic polymorphisms of the class I loci encode for substitutions within the peptide-binding groove, so producing alterations in the size and shape of these pockets (Garrett et al, 1989; Madden et al, 1992). These changes within the cleft have been shown to affect the profile of bound peptides, as well as the binding affinities of individual peptides.

Antigen processing

Class I HLA polypeptides are synthesized and transported into the endoplasmic reticulum (ER), where they encounter β_2-microglobulin. Class I–β_2-microglobulin complexes are unstable in the absence of bound peptide. In the presence of peptide within the ER, class I molecules, β_2-microglobulin and peptide associate producing a stable trimolecular complex. This complex is transported via the Golgi apparatus to the cell surface for presentation to T-cells (Figure 2).

The peptide pool within the ER represents the range of potential peptide antigen available for binding to class I molecules. Endogenously synthesized proteins, including viral proteins, present in the cytosol are degraded into peptide components by a complex of enzymes known collectively as the proteosome complex (Glynne et al, 1991). These peptides and proteins are unable to enter the ER compartment passively, although an active peptide pump is located on the cytosolic surface of the ER. This pump, known as the transporter-associated pathway, belongs to the ATP-binding cassette family of proteins, responsible for the active transport of peptides across cellular membranes. It is composed of a heterodimer of polypeptides (TAP1 and 2), each of which has a membrane-spanning domain and an ATP-binding cassette domain (Trowsdale et al, 1990). Absence of either of these heterodimer components results in failure of peptide transport into the ER, failure to load HLA class I molecules and failure of expression of stable class I molecules on the cell surface (Spies and DeMars, 1991; Attaya et al, 1992).

HLA class II molecules

The tertiary structure of HLA class II molecules is strikingly similar to that of class I molecules (see Figure 1). Class II molecules are also heterodimeric molecules, comprising of a 33–35-kDa α-chain and a 25–29-kDa β-chain. β_2-microglobulin is not associated and the class II genes encode both α- and β-chains. In similarity to the four-domain structure of class I molecules, each α- and β-chain is organized into two domains. The *C*-terminal domains α2, and β2, correspond to the class I α3 and β_2-microglobulin respectively, and possess hydrophobic membrane-spanning sequences. In contrast to class I molecules, these *C*-terminal domains do not interact with the T-cell accessory molecule CD8, but instead will bind CD4.

The *N*-terminal domains, α1 and β1, correspond to the class I domains α1 and α2 respectively, and form an almost identical cleft-like structure for the binding of antigenic peptide, with an α-helix and four β-pleated sheets derived from each domain. Again, the majority of allele-encoded polymorphism is centred around this cleft, suggesting that this genetic variability will influence the immune response to antigens presented by the class II system. The current studies on class II structure and peptide-binding profiles are less advanced compared with class I molecules, although the recent X-ray crystallography of HLA-DR1, together with the mass spectrometry results of peptides eluted from class II molecules, support the hypothetical models developed from the class I system (Brown et al, 1993; Stern et al, 1994).

Antigen processing

Class II molecules are similarly synthesized and transported into the ER (Figure 2), where they associate into a stable trimolecular complex with a third polypeptide, known as the invariant chain (Ii) (Cresswell et al, 1987).

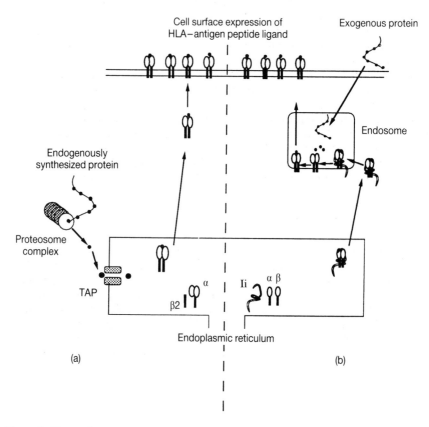

Figure 2. The antigen processing pathways for HLA class I and II molecules (see text). (a) Endogenously synthesized proteins are degraded into peptide subunits within the cytosol by the proteosome complex. Peptides are actively transported into the endoplasmic reticulum by the 'transporter associated pathway' (TAP) protein and loaded on to HLA class I molecules to form a stable trimolecular complex. HLA–peptide ligand is transported to the cell surface for expression to the T-cell receptor. (b) Exogenously synthesized protein is endocytosed into the endosome compartment and degraded into peptide subunits. HLA class II molecules are associated within the endoplasmic reticulum in the presence of the invariant chain (Ii) and are transported to the endosome. Dissociation of the invariant chain allows loading of HLA class II molecules with antigen peptide, followed by cell-surface expression to the T-cell receptor.

The invariant chain binds to the peptide binding cleft, acting as a chaperon for class II folding whilst also preventing the binding of ER peptides destined for class I molecules. The invariant chain has targeting signals that direct it and the associated class II molecule through the Golgi apparatus to the endosome compartment. The endosome contains endocytosed protein antigen and proteases in an acid environment. The low pH of the endosome facilitates dissociation of the invariant chain, leaving the class II molecule free to bind antigenic peptides derived from the proteolysis of exogenous antigen proteins. Time studies indicate that the class II molecule–invariant chain complex arrives in the endosome within 2 min of internalization, after which the class II molecule rapidly binds peptide and is transported to the cell surface for expression.

The tissue distribution of HLA class I and II expression reflects these differences in antigen processing. Class I molecules present peptides derived predominantly from endogenously synthesized proteins, which would include viral proteins. Class I molecules are therefore expressed ubiquitously on nucleated cells, allowing cytotoxic T-cells to act on virally infected cells. Class II molecules present peptides derived predominantly from exogenous endocytosed protein antigens, and their expression is therefore restricted to specialized antigen-presenting cells, although this may be upregulated by the influence of inflammatory mediators. Some cross-over may occur between the two pathways, so that, for example, endogenously synthesized antigen may also be presented by class II molecules.

MHC ORGANIZATION

The genes encoding components of the antigen-presenting system are located mainly on the short arm of chromosome 6 in the region termed the major histocompatibility complex (MHC) (Figure 3) (Trowsdale and Campbell, 1992). The class I region spans 1.5 million base-pairs (Mbp) of DNA and includes the three classical class I loci, HLA-B, -C and -A, the non-classical HLA loci, HLA-E–HLA-H, as well as genes of unknown function. It is likely that an, as yet, undetermined gene close to HLA-A is responsible for the inheritance of primary haemochromatosis. The class III

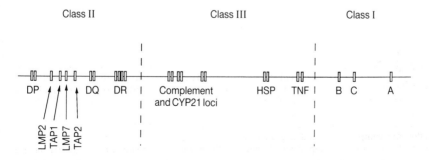

Figure 3. Schematic representation of the MHC organization on chromosome 6.

region lies centromeric to class I, spanning 1.1 Mbp of DNA. This region includes genes whose products have an immunological function, such as the tumour necrosis factor (TNF-α and TNF-β) and the heat-shock protein genes, as well as other loci whose functions appear unrelated, such as the complement genes and the steroid 21-hydroxylase gene (CYP-21), implicated in congenital adrenal hyperplasia. Many genes within this region have been described whose function remains to be characterized. The class II region lies centromeric of the class I and III regions. The three classical HLA class II loci, HLA-DR, -DQ and -DP, are encoded within this region in addition to genes involved in antigen processing for the class I presentation pathway. These genes include the TAP loci, whose products form the peptide transporter pump by which peptides gain access to the ER, and components of the proteosome complex responsible for the degradation of endogenous proteins into peptides suitable for loading into the TAP heterodimer.

One feature of the MHC, which has complicated the study of disease immunogenetics, is the tendency for the complex to be inherited *en bloc*, rather than to be divided at meiotic events. Thus, within populations, certain combinations of HLA class I, II and III alleles are often found inherited together rather than occurring by random association—a concept referred to as linkage disequilibrium. These HLA combinations are referred to as haplotypes. Speculation is made that the association of certain combinations of HLA alleles within a haplotype confers an evolutionary advantage through the complementary range of antigenic peptides that they are able to bind and present. An example of an extended HLA haplotype is the common inheritance of the alleles HLA-A1, -B8, -DR3, -DQ2 and -DP1, together with the class III region complotype alleles {SC01}.

THE PRIMARY HLA ASSOCIATION OF COELIAC DISEASE

In 1972 an association was found between the class I allele HLA-B8 and coeliac disease in both the UK and the USA (Stokes et al, 1972). Subsequent studies demonstrated that this association was with the HLA-B8, DR3 haplotype, with a stronger relative risk ascribed to the class II allele DR3 than HLA-B8 (Keuning et al, 1976). This suggested that the primary association may reside with the class II alleles and that the increase in the HLA-B8 allele is a secondary association. Studies from southern Europe, and in particular Sardinia, where the prevalence of the HLA-B8, -DR3 haplotype is low in comparison to the UK, have demonstrated an association of coeliac disease with the haplotype HLA-B18, {F1C31}, -DR3, -DQ2, indicating that the HLA predisposition resides within the common class II region rather than the differing class I or III region (Figure 4) (Rittner et al, 1984; Coniga et al, 1992).

Within the class II region, recombination events may occur at meiosis between the DP and DQ loci, but are rarely if ever seen between DQ and DR loci. An association has been described between the DP allele DPB1*0101 and coeliac disease, although this has subsequently been realized to be a secondary association due to its inheritance on a common HLA-B8, -DR3, -DQ2, -DP1 haplotype (Hall et al, 1990). A few reports have suggested associations with other DP alleles, but these have largely been refuted by other studies. The susceptibility HLA-linked locus for coeliac disease therefore appears to be located within the HLA class II region telomeric to the -DP/-DQ recombination point and centromeric to the class III region.

Within populations from southern Europe, an additional HLA class II association is seen with HLA-DR7 with a concomitantly reduced association with DR3 (Albert et al, 1978; DeMarchi et al, 1983). This is a reflection of the geographical reduction in the frequency of DR3 in control populations from north to south Europe. HLA-DR7 is associated with coeliac disease only in the presence of HLA-DR5 or -DR3, and similarly no association is found with HLA-DR5 in the absence of -DR7. A unifying hypothesis between these ethnic groups can be found among alleles at the DQ loci. DR3 haplotypes all possess the DQ alleles DQA1*0501 DQB1*0201. DR5 haplotypes also possess the DQ allele DQA1*0501, but possess a DQB1*0301 allele at the DQB locus, in place of DQB1*0201. DR7 haplotypes, in contrast, lack the DQA1*0501 allele (instead possessing a DQA1*0201 allele) but do bear the DQB1*0201 allele. A heterozygous combination of DR5/DR7 haplotypes therefore contains the same DQA1*0501 DQB1*0201

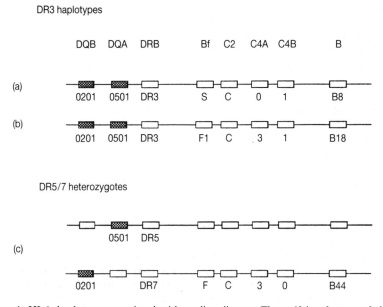

Figure 4. HLA haplotypes associated with coeliac disease. The unifying feature of these differing haplotypes is the presence of the HLA-DQA1*0501 DQB1*0201 alleles in either a *cis* or *trans* configuration. (a) HLA-B8, -DR3 haplotype found in northern European populations. (b) HLA-B18, -DR3 haplotype of southern European populations, particularly in Sardinia. (c) The heterozygous combination of HLA-DR5 and -DR7 haplotypes found in southern European populations.

alleles as DR3 haplotypes, although encoded in a *trans-* rather than a *cis*-configuration (Figure 4). This allele combination is found in 98% of patients with coeliac disease from northern Europe, and in 92% of those from southern Europe, and it is these DQA1*0501 DQB1*0201 alleles that are proposed as the primary HLA susceptibility genes (Sollid et al, 1989; Tighe et al, 1992).

ALTERNATIVE LOCI WITHIN THE MHC

Several additional genes involved in the processing of endogenous antigen for presentation to the HLA class I pathway have recently been characterized and found to be located close to the HLA-DQ loci. LMP-2 and LMP-7 are two components of the proteosome enzyme complex responsible for the degradation of cytosolic proteins before transport into the ER. The loci encoding these proteins are located between the HLA-DP and -DQ loci. Experimental evidence indicates that these genes are responsible for subtle alterations in the character of peptide subunits produced, which is reflected in the character of peptides presented by class I molecules. The *TAP1* and *2* genes encode for the heterodimeric ABC transporter molecule necessary for the active transfer of peptide antigen into the ER. A polymorphism of one of these genes in the rat encodes for substitutions in the membrane-spanning domain of the transporter protein, producing marked effects on the profile of antigens bound and presented by the class I system (Powis et al, 1992). The *TAP1* and *2* genes are also located between HLA-DP and -DQ, with the *TAP2* locus situated most telomerically adjacent to HLA-DQ. Polymorphisms of these genes are known to exist in humans, although their functional significance has yet to be determined. Speculation has been made as to the presence of these genes within the MHC, suggesting that their location allows for the inheritance of compatible class I and class I antigen-processing alleles on the same haplotype. An alternative hypothesis on their location would suggest that this offers the ability for co-ordinated upregulation of both HLA and antigen-processing genes in response to stress. It has been postulated that the observed HLA class II associations of several diseases may actually reflect a primary association with polymorphisms of either the TAP or proteosome genes.

   Several studies have examined alleles at the TAP loci for possible primary or secondary associations with coeliac disease (Colonna et al, 1992; Tighe et al, 1994). These studies conclude that a recombination hot-spot resides between TAP2 and HLA-DQ so that alleles at these loci may become separated at meiosis. Susceptibility towards coeliac disease lies telomeric to this hot-spot towards HLA-DQ, implying that any association with TAP or LMP alleles is secondary to linkage disequilibrium.

   Similarly, a recent report has examined the association of a microsatellite polymorphism located close to the TNF loci within the class III region. An initial positive association was described, suggesting an additive effect on the disease pathogenesis. In retrospect, however, the coeliac patients were collected from a geographical region where the disease is known to have a close association with the HLA-B8, -DR3, -DQ2 haplotype, and it seems probable that this TNF association is secondary to the primary DQ association within this haplotype.

ADDITIONAL HLA SUSCEPTIBILITY ALLELES

In a study of 98 Norwegian children with coeliac disease, 97 possessed the alleles DQA1*0501 DQB1*0201 (Sollid et al, 1989). The individual lacking these susceptibility genes possessed a DR4 DQ8 haplotype. Isolated cases of DR4-associated coeliac disease have been previously recognized. In 1984 an international collaborative study examined 12 DR4-positive coeliac patients (DeMarchi and Carbonara, 1984). Susceptibility appeared to be most closely associated with the HLA class II region genes, rather than the class I region. By radio-immunoassay using DQ-specific monoclonal antibodies, ten individuals were typed as DQ8 while the remaining two expressed the DQ7 antigen (Tosi et al, 1986). The study concluded that a unifying feature was the 'common DR4 antigen', although several of these individuals were subtyped to the DRB1*0401 (DR4 Dw4) specificity. The DR4 antigen is now recognized to be polymorphic, with more than 12 DRB1*04 alleles currently described. These allele polymorphisms encode for functional substitutions within the peptide-binding cleft and alter the HLA-associated predisposition towards other diseases. Rheumatoid arthritis, for example, is closely associated with the alleles DRB1*0401 and 0404, although no association is seen with DRB1*0402 and 0403 (Wordsworth et al, 1989).

Among Ashkenazi Jews in Israel, a study in 1981 noted a low association of coeliac disease with either the DR3 or DR7 antigens; in retrospect these individuals were found to lack the DQA1*0501 DQB1*0201 allele combination (Brautbar et al, 1981). Specific details of the DR3/DR7-negative individuals were not provided, although 35% of coeliac patients possessed the DR4 antigen. A second population of Ashkenazi Jews with coeliac disease has now been studied using techniques suitable for identifying allelic substitutions (the combination of amplification of the DRB1*04 gene sequence by the polymerase chain reaction, combined with sequence-specific oligonucleotide probe hybridization) (Tighe et al, 1993). Coeliac disease is associated with the susceptibility alleles DQA1*0501 DQB1*0201 in 70% of Ashkenazi Jews, while the association with a DR4 haplotype accounts for a further 20%. Subtyping demonstrates that a common DR4 haplotype is associated with coeliac disease in this ethnic group featuring the DRB1*0402 allele together with the DQA1*0301 DQB1*0302 (DQ8) alleles. This haplotype is also a prominent DR4 haplotype within the control population.

These two studies, therefore, have demonstrated that coeliac disease may be found in association with both DRB1*0401 and 0402 haplotypes and that the prominent unifying feature of these haplotypes is the presence of the DQA1*0301 DQB1*0302 (DQ8) alleles. Isolated cases from other populations confirm the association with alleles at the DQ rather than the DRB1 locus. Further evidence for a susceptibility influence of DQA1*0301

DQB1*0302 towards coeliac disease comes from the recent characterization of gliadin-specific T-cells (Lundin et al, 1993). These T-cells have been isolated and cloned from a coeliac patient heterozygous for the two haplotypes DR4 DQ7 and DR4 DQ8. This individual was therefore homozygous at the DR loci (DRB1*0401 DRB4*0101) and the DQA locus (DQA1*0301), and heterozygous at the DQB locus (DQB1*0301 and DQB1*0302). Gliadin-specific T-cells were isolated from small bowel biopsies. These T-cells were reactive to Frazer's fraction III (FF-III), a partial digest of gliadin, when the antigen was presented by antigen-presenting cells bearing the DQ8 molecule (DQB1*0302 encoded) with little or no cross-reactivity with antigen-presenting cells bearing the DQ7 molecule (DQB1*0301 encoded). This finding suggests that the DQ8 molecule is able to bind and present an antigen within gliadin for T-cell recognition. In contrast, the lack of reactivity of these T-cell clones, derived from a DQ7/DQ8 individual, to gliadin in the presence of DQ7 suggests that the binding and presentation of a gliadin antigen to this molecule is insufficient for T-cell recognition.

These studies are all supportive of the hypothesis that the DQA1*0301 DQB1*0302 alleles act as an additional genetic influence on the predisposition to coeliac disease. Cases of coeliac disease have been described within families associated with both the DQA1*0301 DQB1*0302 and DQA1*0501 DQB1*0501 DQB1*0201 genes, suggesting that any additional environmental or genetic factors influencing the disease pathogenesis are similar. Among Ashkenazi Jews, the clinical presentation of the disease does not differ between DQA1*0301 DQB1*0302 and DQA1*0501 DQB1*0201 subgroups. The low frequency of DQA1*0301 DQB1*0302 (DQ8)-associated coeliac disease in northern Europe compared with the associations of DQA1*0501 DQB1*0201 indicates a hierarchy of susceptibility, with a relatively stronger influence attached to the DQA1*0501 DQB1*0201 genes, and a weaker influence to the DQA1*0301 DQB1*0302 (DQ8) genes. In southern European countries, such as Italy, the reduction in frequency of DR3 haplotypes in the control populations is mirrored by an increase in the control frequencies of DR7. Coeliac disease remains primarily associated with the DQA1*0501 DQB1*0201 genes derived from both DR3 and DR5/7 haplotypes. In some Eastern European countries, the frequencies of both DR3 and DR7 are relatively low among the control populations, while those of DR4 DQ8 haplotypes are high. In these populations, a more prominent association with these lesser susceptibility genes may therefore be expected. Among Ashkenazi Jews, this effect is likely to be amplified by the high prevalence of coeliac disease in this population group (1:800) (Dahan et al, 1984). This high prevalence may reflect the presence of additional genetic influences outside the MHC, although environmental factors may also play a role. A similar hierarchy of susceptibility is also found in the immunogenetics of rheumatoid arthritis, with a strong influence attributable to DRB1*0401 and DRB1*0420, and a weaker influence from the alleles DR1 and DR10, the latter becoming apparent only in populations with a low prevalence of the former alleles (in the Balkans and among Ashkenazi Jews in Israel) (Wordsworth et al, 1989).

IMPLICATIONS OF THE HLA ASSOCIATIONS OF COELIAC DISEASE FOR ANTIGEN PRESENTATION

The association of coeliac disease with the alleles DQA1*0301 DQB1*0302 rather than DQB1*0301 suggests that a substitution, encoded by the DQB1*0302 allele within the antigen-binding cleft, allows the efficient binding and presentation of a gliadin antigen to pathogenic T-cells. This is further suggested by the results from gliadin-specific T-cells outlined above. DQB1*0302 encodes for four amino-acid substitutions within the β1 domain compared with DQB1*0301 to produce this alteration of antigen-binding affinity (see Figure 6a). Two substitutions at positions β13 and β26 are located on the β-pleated sheets which form the floor of the cleft in a region that is predicted in the HLA-DR1 model to form a side chain binding pocket for the antigen peptide (Figure 5). The residues β13-glycine and β26-leucine of DQB1*0302 are substituted for β13-alanine and the bulky aromatic β26-tyrosine on the DQB1*0301 allele. One substitution at position β57 is located at the 'right hand' end of the peptide-binding groove and is postulated to form a salt bridge with α76-arginine of the α₁ domain, stabilizing the tertiary structure of the groove. DQB1*0301 encodes for β57-aspartic acid, capable of forming this salt bridge. The DQB1*0302 allele, however,

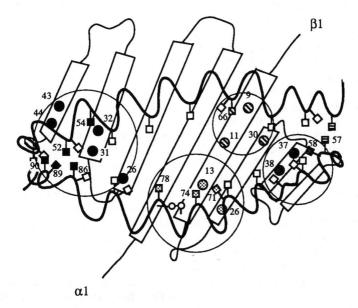

Figure 5. Structure of the HLA class II antigen-binding groove as predicted from X-ray crystallography of HLA-DR1. Pockets in the floor of the binding groove (encircled) interact with peptide side chains of the binding peptide. A prominent pocket located at the 'left' end of the groove is composed of residues α26, 31, 32, 43, 44, 52, 54 and β86, 89 and 90. Other pockets are predicted to be formed by residues α66, β9, 11 and 30; β13, 26, 71, 74 and 78; and β37, 38 and 58. Residues α76 and β57 may be involved in the formation of a salt bridge under the exiting peptide stabilizing the 'right' end of the groove.

substitutes β57-alanine, resulting in loss of this salt bridge and potentially altering the shape of the HLA molecule and hence its recognition by the TCR. The fourth substitution occurs at position β45, which is predicted to lie outside the regions of antigen peptide interaction and TCR contact. While the substitution of β57 has been postulated in the immunogenetics of insulin-dependent diabetes mellitus (IDDM), the association of coeliac disease with DR4 (DQB1*0302) haplotypes relative to DR3 (DQB1*0201) haplotypes is far less than with IDDM. It is also unclear what effect the loss of the α76–β57 salt bridge has in vivo. The first domain of the allele DQB1*0303 differs from DQB1*0302 only by the presence of an aspartic acid residue at position β57 and thus has the same β13 and β26 substitutions but is capable of forming the α76–β57 salt bridge. T-cell clones autoreactive to DQ9 (DQB1*0303) show strong cross-reactivity with DQ8 (DQB1*0302) but no cross-reactivity with DQ7 (DQB*0301). These T-cell clones are therefore able to differentiate DQ8 and DQ9 from DQ7 by means of the two substitutions within the peptide-binding groove, regardless of the presence or absence of the postulated salt-bridge.

The DQB1*0302 substitutions at positions β13, β26 and β57 are shared with the allele DQB1*0201, suggesting that a common substitution within the peptide-binding groove may unite these two HLA-DQ associations of coeliac disease. The increased effect of DQB1*0201 (with DQA1*0501) on susceptibility suggests that these substitutions alone may not be sufficient and, in particular, implying that the substitution at β57 is not solely responsible for the DQB allele association. DQB1*0201 also encodes for a unique sequence of non-polar hydrophobic residues at β37, 38, 47 and 58—a region predicted from the HLA-DR1 model to form an additional peptide side chain binding pocket (Figure 5).

This speculation has so far considered only the β_1 domain of the HLA antigen binding groove. However, for DQ molecules both α- and β-chains are polymorphic and the antigen-HLA–T-cell interaction is likely to be influenced by substitutions within both α_1 and β_1 domains. Indeed, the association of coeliac disease with the heterozygous combination of DR5 and DR7 haplotypes rather than DR7 haplotypes alone is a strong indication of the role of the DQA alleles towards the disease predisposition. The structure of HLA-DR1 reveals a deep side chain binding pocket at the 'left hand' end of the groove centred around the conserved residues α26, 32, 43 and 54 together with the DQB-conserved residues at positions β86, 88 and 89 (Figure 5). Allelic polymorphism encodes for variability at this pocket through substitutions at residues α31, 44 and 52. Position 44 is predicted to lie at the base of this pocket, with position 31 sited close to the pocket opening. A comparison of DQA sequences indicates common features between susceptible and non-susceptible DQA alleles. Unique to the DQA1*0501 allele is the encoding of a polar cysteine residue at α44, whereas most DQA alleles encode for a positively charged residue at this position. DQA1*0301 encodes for a polar glutamine residue at position α44 (Figure 6b). Additionally, DQA1*0501 also uniquely encodes for a polar glutamine residue at α31 at the opening of this pocket, in contrast to a negatively charged residue on all other alleles.

These comparisons of DQA and DQB allele sequences with the structure of HLA-DR1, whilst speculative, indicate the nature by which genetic HLA polymorphisms may influence the binding of gliadin antigen peptides and hence their T-cell recognition. Work continues at present to characterize the nature of these peptide sequences and to determine the key 'anchor' residues enabling high-affinity binding to these susceptibility molecules.

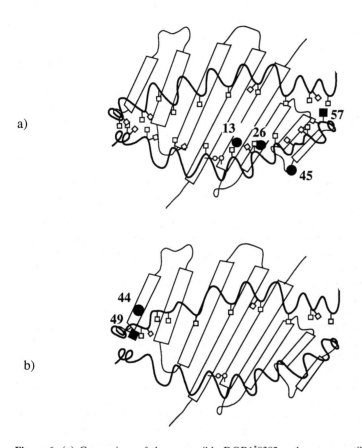

a)

b)

Figure 6. (a) Comparison of the susceptible DQB1*0302 and non-susceptible DQA1*0301 sequences. In the floor of the binding groove, DQB1*0302 encodes for the polar glycine residue at position 13 in place of a hydrophobic alanine residue and a hydrophobic leucine in place of the bulky aromatic tyrosine at position 26. The substitution of alanine (0302) at position 57 for aspartic acid (0301) results in loss of the aspartic acid–arginine salt bridge between residues α76 and β57. Residue 45 lies outside the binding groove and TCR contact region. These DQB1*0302 substitutions are also found in the susceptible DQB1*0201 sequence. (b) Unique non-conservative substitutions common to the DQA susceptibility alleles DQA1*0501 and DQA1*0301. Residue α44 lies at the base of the prominent peptide side chain-binding pocket at the 'left' end of the groove. At position α44, DQA1*0501 encodes a polar cysteine residue, DQA1*0301 encodes a polar glutamine residue whilst non-susceptible DQA alleles encode a negatively charged residue. The DQA susceptibility alleles also encode for a negatively charged arginine residue at position α49 compared with an uncharged residue on non-susceptible alleles.

T-CELL RECEPTOR

The HLA–antigen peptide ligand expressed on the cell surface of an antigen presenting cell is recognized by a T lymphocyte through interaction with the cell's T-cell receptor (TCR). The TCR is composed of two protein chains, either an α- and β-chain, or a γ- and δ-chain. The TCR gene loci exhibit a high degree of gene diversification, enabling the recombination of differing gene segments, to allow for the recognition of a large range of antigens. Each protein chain is produced by the rearrangement of variable (V), diversity (D), joining (J) and constant (C) region genes in a similar manner to the rearrangement of immunoglobulin genes. The α-gene complex lacks J-region genes, but otherwise follows the same principle. There are multiple loci at each of these V, D, J and C region genes, creating a wide possible spectrum of rearranged TCRs. For example, in humans, approximately 50 V_β, 2 D_β, 13 J_β and 2 C_β loci have been described, and allelic polymorphisms are known to occur at some of these loci. In addition to the possible recombination sequences, additional diversity is created by the random insertion or deletion of nucleotides at the sites of rearrangement—junctional diversity—so that an almost infinite number of TCR sequences can potentially be produced.

The protein structure produced by this rearranged TCR signal is thought to form a similar conformation to immunoglobulin by virtue of a similar conserved framework of residues (Davies and Bjorkman, 1988). The variable domain of immunoglobulin is also composed of a rearrangement of variable, diversity and joining sequences. The Ig variable domain has a tertiary β-barrel structure, in which a conserved framework of β-strands supports three hypervariable antigen-binding loops, termed the complementarity-determining regions (CDRs). The sequence of the rearranged TCR loci indicate that three variable sequence regions correspond in position to the immunoglobulin CDR1–3. The TCR CDR1 and 2 are derived from germline variable region genes, whilst the TCR CDR3 region is located at the V (D) J junctional sites. The CDR3 region therefore also contains the sites where junctional diversity occurs. The interaction between TCR and HLA-antigen peptide predicts that the CDR1 and 2 loops overlie the polymorphic residues of the HLA α-helices and hence their derivation from germline sequences ensures HLA recognition. The hypervariable CDR3 loop overlies the peptide antigen bound within the HLA cleft, so that the variability obtained by rearrangement and random junctional diversity will allow the recognition of a wide range of possible antigens.

During T-cell maturation in the thymus, selection occurs to ensure that the TCR sequences generated will be functional. Positive selection occurs for those TCRs that will recognize antigen when presented by an individual's HLA system, whilst negative selection allows deletion of those TCRs whose HLA affinity is high and so may lead to autoreactivity. Additional mechanisms for the suppression of potentially autoreactive TCRs also occur in the periphery, leading to T-cell anergy.

The T-cell-mediated pathogenesis of coeliac disease has led to the exploration of the small bowel T-cell repertoire and to the isolation and characterization of those T-cells reactive to gliadin antigens. Serial immuno-histochemistry studies of the coeliac jejunal mucosa following gliadin challenge has indicated that the CD4-positive T cells within the lamina propria are activated early in the immune response. The relationship between these CD-positive T cells and the HLA class II associations described above fits with the hypothesis that these cells are responsible for the recognition of gliadin, subsequently triggering the immunological response cascades.

TCR V$_\beta$ REPERTOIRE OF THE JEJUNUM IN COELIAC DISEASE

The techniques utilized in the characterization of the T-cell repertoire are outlined in view of the debates concerning quantitative polymerase chain reaction (PCR). Jejunal biopsies from untreated and treated coeliac patients and normal controls were used to examine the TCR repertoire. Biopsies were subdivided into epithelial and lamina propria compartments. Total cell messenger RNA (mRNA) was subjected to reverse transcription. In view of the differences in numbers of T cells between biopsy specimens, particularly between untreated coeliac patients and controls, complementary DNA (cDNA) concentrations were corrected for TCR-β DNA concentration before any attempts at PCR quantification. Serial dilutions of cDNA were PCR amplified with a set of C$_\beta$ primers, electrophoresed and hybridized with a C$_\beta$ probe. The TCR-β cDNA concentrations were then estimated by optical densitometry of the resultant autoradiograph. Following correction for cDNA concentration, PCR amplification was performed using 20 sets of V$_\beta$ primers in separate reactions over varying PCR cycle numbers. The results of these studies indicate that mRNA for all V$_\beta$ genes is present within both the jejunal epithelial and lamina propria compartments, and that no selection of a particular V$_\beta$ gene occurs during exposure to gliadin. These studies would tend to argue against a single gliadin-responsive pathogenic T-cell clone and would again dispel hypotheses for gliadin acting as a superantigen. They do not, however, study the VDJ region of the TCR and therefore do not answer questions concerning a common CDR3 motif responsible for the recognition of a specific gliadin peptide (Hall et al, 1992).

The examination of the VDJ region of gliadin-responsive T cells requires the isolation and cloning of these cells. A group of workers from Oslo have now succeeded in isolating these antigen-specific T cells from coeliac patients. The first clone isolated was from the peripheral blood. T-cell lines were prepared following the incubation of peripheral T lymphocytes with B cells isolated from peripheral blood in the presence of an overlapping series of peptides from the α-gliadin sequence 1–58. Reactivity of this clone to gliadin was confirmed on exposure to a peptic–tryptic digest of gliadin, FFIII, in the presence of antigen-presenting cells. This response was blocked by an anti-HLA-DQ monoclonal antibody, indicating that this clone was HLA-DQ restricted. The antigen peptide recognized by this clone was subsequently characterized as the residue sequence 31–49. Truncation of this peptide below a core residue sequence of 31–47 abrogated this recognition (Gjertsen et al, 1992).

Subsequent T-cell clones have now been identified from the jejunal mucosa of treated coeliac patients. Gliadin-sensitive T cells were isolated from jejunal biopsies by an overnight culture of the biopsy with FF-III followed by extraction of those cells displaying the interleukin 2 (IL-2) receptor (indicating T-cell activation). Cloning of these cell lines enabled the production of several gliadin-sensitive T-cell clones. These clones were all sensitive to gliadin (FF-III) and were HLA-DQ restricted. The characterization of the individual peptide epitopes has not yet been reported, although responses were not seen to the peptide 31–49. The DQ restriction was primarily to the HLA-DQA1*0501 DQB1*0201 heterodimer, although responses were seen to the DQA1*0201 DQB1*0201 heterodimer encoded on DR7 haplotypes. From the limited number of clones so far obtained, no common V_β or V_α genes, VDJ_β or VJ_α sequence motifs have been found (Lundin et al, 1993).

Additional clones mentioned above from a DR4-positive coeliac patient were restricted to the DQA1*0301 DQB1*0302 heterodimer, although again characterization of the peptide antigen epitope has not yet been fully performed.

IMPLICATIONS OF THE T-CELL CLONING STUDIES

The full implications of these studies will await the identification of the individual antigen epitopes recognized by each clone. A variety of gliadin-specific T cells appear to be present in the small bowel of coeliac patients, responding to a number of epitopes along the gliadin sequence. No particular TCR genes or rearrangements appear to be implicated consistently, although the clones do uniformly appear restricted to the HLA-DQ molecules predicted from the disease immunogenetics.

Earlier in-vitro studies have implicated a toxic epitope in domain I of A-gliadin close to residues 31–49, and this epitope is now known to be recognized by a gliadin-sensitive T-cell clone. A summation of these studies would therefore suggest that a gliadin peptide, residues 31–49, may act as a primary toxic epitope in gluten-sensitive enteropathy (Wieser et al, 1986; de Ritis et al, 1988; Ellis et al, 1993).

IN-VIVO CHALLENGES

Toxicity testing has now been performed in vivo with the peptide sequence 31–49 characterized from the initial T-cell clone. There is good circumstantial evidence from organ culture studies to suggest that this peptide may be toxic in vivo, and a monoclonal antibody directed against this sequence will cross-react only with toxic, and not non-toxic, cereals. The effect of peptide 31–49 on jejunal morphology was compared with unfractionated gliadin, and two 'control' peptides corresponding to gliadin sequences 3–21 and

202–220. Four individuals with treated coeliac disease were studied with serial jejunal biopsies taken over 6 hours following an intraduodenal instillation of 200 mg test peptide or 1 g gliadin. Each individual underwent all four challenges. The initial challenge was performed with gliadin, followed at weekly intervals by the three peptides in random order. Challenge with gliadin produced significant changes in villous height:crypt depth ratio, the enterocyte cell height and the intraepithelial lymphocyte count at 4 hours compared with $t = 0$. In contrast, peptides 3–21 and 202–220 produced no significant change in any of these parameters. Challenge with peptide 31–49 produced a significant reduction in the villous height:crypt depth ratio, a significant reduction in the enterocyte cell height and a significant rise in the intraepithelial lymphocyte count in all four individuals at 4 hours (Sturgess et al, 1994).

TOLERANCE

'Normal' healthy individuals with no histological evidence of gluten-sensitive enteropathy may have low levels of antigliadin antibodies. It is likely that, in these individuals, gliadin-specific T cells are present in the normal small bowel to help B lymphocytes to mount this antibody response. The absence of histological abnormalities would suggest these T cells are largely anergic and that the production of mucosal damage is a reflection of loss of this anergy rather than the presence of gliadin-specific T cells *per se*. Being anergic, confirmation of these T cells' presence would not be possible by current cloning techniques.

A characteristic histological finding of untreated coelic disease is an increase in the number of intraepithelial lymphocytes (IELs) within the small bowel mucosa, together with an increase in the proportion of IELs bearing a γ/δ TCR. The function of these cells remains unclear, although it has been suggested that they may play a role in immune surveillance. In-vitro studies have demonstrated that, under certain circumstances, they may recognize antigen presented by HLA molecules of either class, while other studies suggest that they recognize relatively non-polymorphic cell-surface elements, such as the heat-shock proteins. Upon in-vivo challenge with gliadin, they do not express characteristic markers of T-cell activation but do proliferate as assessed by the nuclear proliferation marker Ki-67 (Halstensen and Brandtzeag, 1993). Characterization of the γ/δ IEL T-cell repertoire has demonstrated that this expansion is heterogeneous, rather than the expansion of a disease-specific clone, and that the relative proportions of γ/δ subtypes are unaltered in coeliac disease from those in the normal small bowel (Spencer et al, 1989). Studies of other T-cell-mediated small bowel disorders, such as intestinal viral and protozoal infections, have demonstrated similar increases in the IEL γ/δ T-cell counts (Macdonald and Ferguson, 1978; Philips, 1988). An interesting hypothesis regarding the function of γ/δ IEL has been proposed following experimental work in a mouse model (Fujihashi et al, 1992). (The mouse model may not be directly comparable because a higher proportion of gut T cells bear a γ/δ TCR compared with that in humans.) In the mouse, immune tolerance develops to orally ingested dietary antigens so that little immune response results from subsequent systemic challenge with the antigen. Transfer of antigen-specific γ/δ TCR IELs from a tolerant mouse to the systemic circulation of a second tolerant mouse abrogates this oral tolerance to the antigen, allowing an immune response to be mounted towards the antigen. The authors speculate that the function of the γ/δ IEL in the normal gut may be to allow the local immune system to escape systemic immune tolerance, so allowing it to address orally encountered antigens. This would be achieved through interactions between the IELs and the lamina propria CD4-positive T cells, and allows for the production of secretory IgA. The finding that γ/δ IEL numbers are increased during T-cell-mediated immune responses to gut protozoal and viral infections may support this hypothesis. At present, however, the precise function of the IEL in humans is unknown, and their role in the disease pathogenesis uncertain.

SUMMARY

Work continues to progress in the unravelling of the molecular interactions involved in the pathogenesis of coeliac disease. The immunogenetics of the disease implicate certain HLA DQ alleles as necessary for subsequent disease development. These HLA molecules have been shown to be necessary in the binding and presentation of gliadin peptides to antigen-specific T cells. Current work is examining the precise HLA–antigen interaction that may lead to the development of antigen-blocking agents. The isolation of antigen-specific T cells has led to the confirmation of a toxic T-cell epitope of the gliadin protein (residues 31–49) and it would appear likely that additional toxic epitopes may be similarly characterized in the near future. No common TCR motifs have so far been detected, although these may become apparent as this work progresses. The gliadin peptide sequence, residues 31–49, has now been demonstrated to be toxic in vivo. Additional toxic T-cell epitopes may also be present within gliadins, but this identification of a toxic gliadin sequence for the first time raises the possibility of future manipulation of the wheat genome (and other toxic cereals) that could lead to the development of new graminae cereals with the properties of wheat, but which do not induce toxicity in patients with coeliac disease.

Acknowledgement

M.R.T. is a Wellcome Trust Clinical Research Fellow.

REFERENCES

Albert ED, Harms K, Bertele R et al (1978) B-cell alloantigens in coeliac disease. In McNicholl B, McCarthy CF & Footrell BP (eds) *Perspectives in Coeliac Disease. Proceedings of the Third International Symposium, 1977*, pp 123–129 Lancaster: MTP Press.

Attaya M, Jameson S, Martinez CK et al (1992) Ham-2 corrects the class I antigen-processing defect in RMA-S cells. *Nature* **355**: 674–649.

Bjorkman PJ, Saper MA, Samraouri B et al (1987) The foreign antigen binding site and T cell recognition regions of class I histocompatibility antigens. *Nature* **329**: 512–518.

Brautbar C, Freier S, Ashkenazi A et al (1981) Histocompatibility determinants in Israeli Jewish patients with coeliac disease: population and family study. *Tissue Antigens* **17**: 313–322.

Brown JH, Jardensky TS, Gorga JC et al (1993) Three-dimensional structure of the human class II histocompatibility antigen HLA-DR1. *Nature* **364**: 33–39.

Colonna M, Bresnahan M, Bahram et al (1992) Allelic variants of the human putative peptide transporter required for antigen processing. *Proceedings of the National Academy of Sciences USA* **89**: 3932–3936.

Coniga M, Frau F, Lampis et al (1992) A high frequency of the A30, B18, DR3, DRw52, DQw2 extended haplotype in Sardinian celiac patients: further evidence that disease susceptibility is conferred by DQA1*0501, B1*0201. *Tissue Antigens* **39**: 78–83.

Cresswell P, Blum JS, Kelner DN & Marks MS (1987) Biosynthesis and processing of class II histocompatibility antigens. *Critical Reviews in Immunology* **7**: 31–53.

Dahan S, Slater PE, Cooper M et al (1984) Coeliac disease in the Rehovot-Ashdod region of Israel: incidence and ethnic distribution. *Journal of Epidemiology and Community Health* **38**: 58–60.

Davis MM & Bjorkman PJ (1988) T-cell receptor genes and T-cell recognition. *Nature* **334**: 145–188.

DeMarchi M & Carbonara AO (1984) DR3 and DR7-negative celiac disease. In Albert E (ed.) *Histocompatibility Testing*, pp 359–362. Berlin: Springer.

DeMarchi M, Carbonara A, Ansaldi et al (1983) HLA-DR3 and DR7 in coeliac disease: immunogenetic and clinical aspects. *Gut* **24**: 706–712.

Ellis HJ, Doyle AP, Wieser H et al (1993) Specificities of monoclonal antibodies to domain 1 of α-gliadins. *Scandinavian Journal of Gastroenterology* **28**: 212–216.

Fijihashi K, Taguchi T, Aicher W et al (1992) Immunoregulatory functions for murine intra-epithelial lymphocytes: γ/δ T cell receptor-positive (TCR⁺) T cells abrogate oral tolerance, while α/β TCR⁺ T cells provide B cell help. *Journal of Experimental Medicine* **175**: 695–707.

Garrett TPJ, Saper MA, Bjorkman PJ et al (1989) Specificity pockets for the side chains of peptide antigens in HLA-Aw68. *Nature* **342**: 692–696.

Glynne R, Powis SH, Beck S et al (1991) A proteosome-related gene between the two ABC transporter loci on the class II region of the human MHC. *Nature* **353**: 357–360.

Hall M, Lanchbury J, Bolsover W et al (1990) Coeliac disease is associated with an extended HLA-DR3 haplotype which includes HLA-DPw1. *Human Immunology* **27**: 220–228.

Hall M, Lanchbury J, Sturgess R & Ciclitira P (1992) *TCR Vβ Usage in Peripheral Blood and Small Intestinal Biopsies of Treated and Untreated Coeliac Disease Patients*. London: British Society of Immunology.

Halstensen TS & Brandtzeag P (1993) Activated T lymphocytes in the celiac lesion, non-proliferative activation (CD25) of CD⁴+ α/β cells in the lamina propria but proliferation (Ki-67) of α/β and γ/δ cells in the epithelium. *European Journal of Immunology* **23**: 505–510.

Keuning J, Pena A, Van Leeuwen A et al (1976) HLA-Dw3 associated with coeliac disease. *Lancet* **i**: 506–507.

Lundin KEA, Scott H, Hansen T et al (1993) Gliadin-specific, HLA-DQ(α1*0501, β1*0201) restricted T cells isolated from the small intestinal mucosa of celiac disease patients. *Journal of Experimental Medicine* **178**: 187–196.

Lundin KEA, Gjertsen HA, Scott H et al (1994) Gliadin-specific, HLA-DQ2 restricts T cells in coeliac disease. In Feighery C & O'Farrelly C (eds) *Gastrointestinal Immunology and Gluten-Sensitive Disease*. International Symposium on Coeliac Disease. pp 281–284. Dublin: Oak Tree Press.

Macdonald TT & Ferguson A (1978) Small intestinal epithelial cell kinetics and protozoal infection in mice. *Gastroenterology* **74**: 496–500.

Madden DR, Gorga JC, Strominger JL & Wiley DC (1992) The three dimensional structure of HLA-B27 at 2.1 Å resolution suggest a general mechanism for tight peptide binding to MHC. *Cell* **70**: 1035–1048.

Phillips AD (1989) Mechanisms of mucosal injury: human studies. In Farthing MJG (ed.) *Viruses and the Gut. Proceedings of the Ninth BSG.SK&F International Workshop*, pp 30–40. Welwyn Garden City, Herts: Smith, Kline & French Laboratories Ltd.

Powis S, Deverson E, Coadwell J et al (1992) Effect of polymorphism of an MHC-linked transporter on the peptides assembled in a class I molecule. *Nature* **357**: 211–215.

de Ritis G, Auricchio S, Jones HW et al (1988) In vitro (organ culture) studies of the toxicity of specific A-gliadin peptides in celiac disease. *Gastroenterology* **94**: 41–49.

Rittner C, DeMarchi M, Mollenhauer E & Carbonara A (1984). Coeliac disease and C4A*QO: association secondary to HLA-DR3. *Tissue Antigens* **23**: 130–134.

Sollid L, Markussen G, Ek J (1989). Evidence for a primary association of coeliac disease to a particular HLA–DQ α/β heterodimer. *Journal of Experimental Medicine* **169**: 345–350.

Spencer J, MacDonald TT, Diss TC et al (1989) Changes in intraepithelial lymphocyte subpopulations in coeliac disease and enteropathy associated T cell lymphoma (malignant histiocytosis of the intestine). *Gut* **30**: 339–346.

Spies T & DeMars R (1991) Restored expression of major histocompatibility class I molecules by gene transfer of a putative peptide transporter. *Nature* **351**: 323–324.

Stern LJ, Brown JH, Jardensky TS et al (1994) Crystal structure of the human class II MHC protein HLA-DR1 complexed with an influenza virus peptide. *Nature* **368**: 215–221.

Stokes P, Asquith P, Holmes G et al (1972) Histocompatibility antigens associated with adult coeliac disease. *Lancet* **ii**: 162–164.

Sturgess RP, Day P, Ellis HJ et al (1994) Wheat peptide challenge in coeliac disease. *Lancet* **343**: 758–761.

Tighe MR, Hall MA, Barbado M et al (1992) HLA class II alleles associated with celiac disease susceptibility in a southern European population. *Tissue Antigens* **40**: 90–97.

Tighe MR, Hall M, Ashkenazi A et al (1993) Celiac disease among Ashkenazi Jews from Israel: a study of the HLA class II alleles and their associations with disease susceptibility. *Human Immunology* **38**: 270–276.

Tighe MR, Hall M, Cardi E et al (1994) The associations between alleles of the MHC encoded ABC transporter gene TAP2, HLA class II alleles and celiac disease. *Human Immunology* **39**: 9–16.

Tosi R, Tanigaki N, Polanco I et al (1986) A radioimmunoassay typing study of non-DQw2-associated celiac disease. *Clinical Immunology and Immunopathology* **39**: 168–172.

Trowsdale J & Campbell RD (1992) Complexity in the major histocompatibility complex. *European Journal of Immunogenetics* **19**: 43–55.

Trowsdale J, Hanson I, Mockeridge I et al (1990) Sequences encoded in the HLA class II region of the MHC related to the 'ABC' superfamily of transporters. *Nature* **348**: 741–743.

Wieser H, Belitz HD, Idar D & Ashkenazi A (1986) Coeliac activity of the gliadin peptides CT-1 and CT-2. *Zeitschrift für Lebensmittel-Untersuchung und-Forschung.* **182**: 115–117.

Wordsworth BP, Lanchbury JSS, Sakkas LI et al (1989) HLA-DR4 subtype frequencies in rheumatoid arthritis indicate that DRB1 is the major susceptibility locus within the HLA class II region. *Proceedings of the National Academy of Sciences USA* **86**: 10049–10053.

3

The humoral immune system in coeliac disease

MARKKU MÄKI

Mucosal surfaces are the major sites in the body where foreign antigens are encountered. There are normally about 10^{10} immunoglobulin-producing immunocytes per metre of human small bowel (Brandtzaeg et al, 1989). Furthermore, 80% of all immunoglobulin-producing cells in humans are located in the intestinal mucosa, and most of these are engaged in the production of dimers of immunoglobulin (Ig)A. Gut-associated lymphoid tissue (GALT) in humans seems to be capable of coping with all the foreign antigens it encounters.

This chapter focuses on gluten-induced humoral immunity in coeliac disease with particular respect to certain coeliac-disease-specific tissue auto-antibodies. First, a brief description is given of the prerequisites for antibody formation, the migration of mucosal lymphocytes, and the gut secretory IgA system.

ANTIBODY FORMATION, MIGRATION OF MUCOSAL LYMPHOCYTES AND THE GUT SECRETORY IgA SYSTEM

For antibody formation to occur the antigens must first be phagocytosed and broken down to small antigenic peptides (processing) by so-called antigen-presenting cells (APCs) (Figure 1(a)). A number of potential APCs may process foreign antigen. These are B cells, macrophages, dendritic cells and also intestinal epithelial cells (Mayer, 1991). All these cell types are abundantly present in the gut. The antigenic peptides must then be presented by products of the major histocompatibility complex (MHC), the human leukocyte antigen (HLA) class II molecules situated on the cell surfaces (DR, DP and DQ α/β heterodimers) (see Chapter 2). HLA class II molecules are largely restricted to cells involved in immune responses, and these cells can serve as APCs. Class II molecules contain a peptide-binding groove (Brown et al, 1988) where the processed peptide of 10–20 amino acids, the T-cell epitope, is situated for recognition. HLA class II molecules containing the processed peptide interact with immunocompetent T cells. These α/β T-cell receptor-bearing lymphocytes that recognize the peptide–class II complex have the CD4 molecule on the cell surface and function mainly as helper cells in the immune response (Janeway and Golstein, 1991). As a consequence of helper T-cell activation (mainly T helper 2 cells), B cells receive signals to become antibody-forming cells (Parker, 1993; Clark and Ledbetter, 1994). Cytokines are recognized to play a major role in antigen-driven antibody responses and in immunoglobulin heavy chain class 'switching' (Kagnoff, 1993). The B-cell epitope(s) of the antigen may be different from the antigen-derived processed T-cell epitope located in the groove of the HLA class II heterodimer.

The basis for intestinal immunity is the maturation cycle of specifically primed T and B cells from GALT via mesenteric lymph nodes and peripheral blood back to the intestinal lamina propria ('homing') (Figure 1(b)). Peyer's patches direct the switch of B cells into the IgA class during the maturation cycle. Delivery of antigen into Peyer's patches also results in

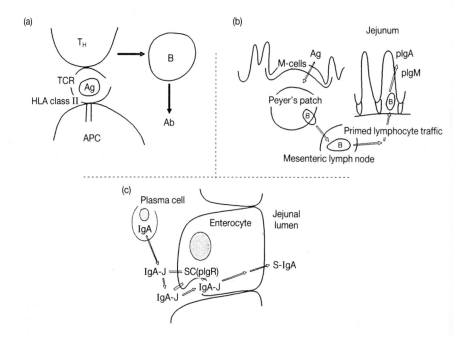

Figure 1. (a) The antigen-presenting cell (APC) presents the processed antigenic peptide (Ag) situated in the HLA class II molecule groove to T helper cells (T_H) where the T-cell receptor (TCR) recognizes the Ag–class II complex. As a consequence of the helper T-cell activation B cells receive signals to become antibody (Ab)-forming cells. (b) In the Peyer's patch the M cells transport luminal antigens (Ag) to the underlying tissue where antigen processing and presentation takes place. The primed B cells perform a maturation cycle via mesenteric lymph nodes and peripheral blood back to mucosal surfaces. In the lamina propria these primed plasma cells secrete polymeric (p) IgA and IgM. (c) The dimeric and polymeric J chains containing IgA secreted by the plasma cell bind to the epithelial cell transmembranic polyimmunoglobulin receptor (pIgR), of which the secretory component (SC) is the extracellular domain of the receptor. After endocytosis and intracellular cleavage the complex containing the IgA, J chain and SC, called secretory IgA (S-IgA), is transported into the intestinal secretions.

selective homing of antigen-specific lymphocytes to mucosal tissues (Salmi and Jalkanen, 1991). M cells, the dome of Peyer's patches, are responsible for luminal antigen sampling and transport to the underlying lymphoid tissue. M cells do not express HLA class II molecules and thus are unlikely to act as APCs (Brandtzaeg and Bjerke, 1990). Under the M cells there are abundant APCs present for active antigen handling and antigen presentation to helper T cells (Brandtzaeg et al, 1989). In diseased states, as in coeliac disease, antigen access is increased and APCs outside the Peyer's patch areas in the lamina propria may play an important role. Also, jejunal epithelial cells may function as APCs.

Primed IgA and IgM plasma cells in the lamina propria secrete dimeric and polymeric immunoglobulins (pIgs) containing the joining, J chain (Figure 1(c)). Secretory IgA contains an additional polypeptide chain, the secretory component, now known to be part of the pIg receptor. This transmembrane receptor, situated on basolateral surfaces of epithelial cells, binds both pIgA and pIgM containing the J chain and transports these immunoglobulins into intestinal secretions where they perform exclusion of luminal antigens (Brandtzaeg et al, 1989).

CIRCULATING AND INTESTINAL ANTIBODIES

Use as a screening test

Although the focus of coeliac disease screening today is on serological tests, it is the belief of the author that patients with malabsorption syndrome or an otherwise strong suspicion of coeliac disease do not require screening tests for intestinal mucosal injury but that jejunal biopsy should be the first diagnostic step. Possibly all dyspeptic patients undergoing upper gastrointestinal endoscopy should have a duodenal biopsy since a recent study showed coeliac disease to be present in 16 (2.6%) of 605 students endoscoped (Schroeder, 1990). However, the results of serum antibody tests can be helpful in coeliac patients. The effect of a gluten-free diet and the degree of mucosal healing can be monitored with the test, giving a positive result at the initial stage of the disease.

Non-invasive screening tests are also helpful in patients without malabsorption and with only a slight clinical suspicion of coeliac disease, as well as in those with coeliac disease-associated disorders. However, it should be remembered that subclinical cases of coeliac disease will not be detected by screening only selected groups of at-risk patients (Collin et al, 1990; Catassi et al, 1994; Unsworth and Brown, 1994).

Gliadin antibodies

Isotype-specific gliadin antibody tests are the most widely used today (Troncone and Ferguson, 1991). Various methods have been developed to determine these antibodies: immunofluorescence (Stern et al, 1979), enzyme-linked immunosorbent assay (ELISA) (O'Farrelly et al, 1983;

Vainio et al, 1983), diffusion-in-gel ELISA (Kilander et al, 1983), solid-phase radio-immunoassay (Ciclitira et al, 1983) and recently a strip ELISA test on a drop of whole blood (Not et al, 1993). These antibodies have frequently been found in patients with untreated coeliac disease (Burgin-Wolff et al, 1983; Savilahti et al, 1983; Levenson et al, 1985; Volta et al, 1985; Friis and Gudmand-Hoyer, 1986; Ståhlberg et al, 1986; Ascher et al, 1990; Grodzinsky et al, 1990; Scott et al, 1990; Volta et al, 1990; McMillan et al, 1991; Mäki et al, 1991c; Ferreira et al, 1992; Not et al, 1993; Bodé and Gudmand-Hoyer, 1994), but the sensitivities and specificities of the tests vary from 30% to 100% (Table 1). It would seem that both IgA- and IgG-class antibodies should be tested (Troncone and Ferguson, 1991). The different predictive values of the test in different studies are probably due to variations in patient selection and not to the tests themselves (Mäki et al, 1992).

In young children gliadin antibody tests have correlated satisfactorily with

Table 1. Sensitivity and specificity of serum gliadin antibodies in untreated coeliac disease.

Reference	Patient group	IgA class		IgG class	
		Sensitivity (%)	Specificity (%)	Sensitivity (%)	Specificity (%)
Ascher et al (1990)	Children	97	92		
Bodé & Gudmand-Hoyer (1994)	Adults	46	98	62	97
Ferreira et al (1992)	Adults	90	85	76	88
Friis & Gudmand-Hoyer (1986)	Adults	65	100	95	98
Kilander et al (1983)	Adults	67	94	78	94
	Children	100	100	100	100
McMillan et al (1991)	Adults	100	100	57	87
Mäki et al (1991c)	Adults	31	87	46	89
Not et al (1993)	Children	96	100	91	99
Ståhlberg et al (1986)	Children	90	86	94	67

Table 2. Percentage of patients positive for IgA-class gliadin antibodies with different cut-off limits for positivity. The patients are divided according to age and status of jejunal mucosa (flat mucosa, $n = 44$; normal mucosal morphology, $n = 250$).

IgA-class gliadin antibody level (ELISA units/ml)	Percentage of positive patients			
	Age < 2 years		Age 2–16 years	
	Flat mucosa	Normal mucosa	Flat mucosa	Normal mucosa
0.1	100	57	100	67
0.2	100	30	90	30
0.5	100	13	68	11
1.0	100	3	45	2
5.0	75	3	15	0

mucosal atrophy (Savilahti et al, 1983; Ascher et al, 1990; Burgin-Wolff et al, 1991), whereas in adults they often seem less predictive (Kilander et al, 1983; O'Farrelly et al, 1983; Friis and Gudmand-Hoyer, 1986; Grodzinsky et al, 1990; Scott et al, 1990; Volta et al, 1990; Mäki et al, 1991c; Uibo et al, 1993). It has also been noted that if patients have continued to consume gluten for years gliadin antibody levels gradually decrease, even to be negative in spite of pathological mucosa (Burgin-Wolff et al, 1991). When the ELISA technique is used for determining cut-off levels for serum IgG- and IgA-class gliadin antibody tests, the age of the patient should be taken into account (Table 2). For example, a high cut-off level for IgA-class antibodies can be set in young children and still attain a sensitivity of 100%, whilst at the same time false-positive results are seen in only 3% of cases. If this level is used in older children and adolescents, more than half of the cases are missed. If the cut-off level is lowered to that at which 90% of untreated coeliacs among older children are found, false-positive results must be accepted in 30%.

Gliadin antibodies are also to be found in other gastrointestinal diseases (Burgin-Wolff et al, 1983; Unsworth et al, 1983), other disorders (Kieffer and Barnetson, 1983; Finn et al, 1985; O'Farrelly et al, 1988) and in healthy individuals (Grodzinsky et al, 1990; Pettersson et al, 1993; Uibo et al, 1993). Positivity for gliadin antibodies seems to increase with age in normal individuals (Uibo et al, 1993). For example, in an adult population sample from Estonia, as many as 10% of males aged 60–69 years had high levels of IgA-class gliadin antibodies without coeliac disease, whereas no males 15–19 years old had the antibody (Uibo et al, 1993). Gliadin antibody-positive relatives of patients with coeliac disease with normal jejunal mucosa are genetically different from the probands (Mäki et al, 1991c). Recently, Pettersson et al (1993) also showed that the presence or development of gliadin antibodies is independent of the HLA genotype. Moreover, antibody activity to dietary antigens other than gluten is present in the serum of untreated patients with coeliac disease (Hvatum et al, 1992; Fälth-Magnusson et al, 1994).

Gliadin antibodies disappear during treatment with a gluten-free diet (Savilahti et al, 1983; Kilander et al, 1987) but IgG-class antibodies may persist for long periods (Weiss et al, 1983). The antibody level rises again in patients with coeliac disease when gluten is reintroduced into the diet, often several months before there is a clinical or mucosal relapse (Scott et al, 1992). Seroconversion of gliadin antibodies has been used as an indicator of mucosal relapse and timing of rebiopsy during gluten challenge (Mayer et al, 1989).

The IgG-subclass patterns to gliadin show wide individual variation, but activity occurs predominantly in the IgG_1 and IgG_4 subclasses (Ciclitira et al, 1986; Scott et al, 1992). Serum IgA antibodies to gliadin mostly comprise IgA_1, suggesting a systemic rather than a mucosal origin (Kemp et al, 1988). However, a significant relationship between the number of mucosal IgA-producing cells and the serum level of IgA-class gliadin antibodies supports a mucosal origin (Kett et al, 1990). Mascart-Lemone et al (1988) found circulating pIgA activity against gliadin in children with untreated coeliac disease. This might reflect a spillover from mucosal IgA production.

Tissue autoantibodies: reticulin, endomysium and jejunal antibodies

A new serum reticulin antibody test for detecting untreated coeliac disease was introduced in 1971 (Seah et al, 1971a, 1971b). The antigen was detected by a standard indirect immunofluorescence method using unfixed cryostat sections of rat kidney, liver and stomach as antigens. Five different immunofluorescent patterns were distinguished (Rizzetto and Doniach, 1973), and the R1-type reticulin antibodies were claimed to be specific for coeliac disease and dermatitis herpetiformis (Magalhaes et al, 1974; Eade et al, 1077). The sensitivity of the test in the detection of untreated coeliac disease has been variable and often unsatisfactory (Table 3). By measuring IgA-class R1-type reticulin antibodies, a sensitivity of 97% and a specificity of 98% were claimed (Mäki et al, 1984a). Positivity entailed a typical staining pattern in both rat kidney and liver. One-third of patients with coeliac disease were negative for IgG-class reticulin antibodies. Recent studies show the IgA-class reticulin antibody test to be reliable and valuable in assisting the early recognition of occult coeliac disease (Hällström, 1989a; Collin et al, 1990; Unsworth and Brown, 1994). It is noteworthy that the coeliac disease-specific reticulin staining pattern may be discovered in the course of routine autoantibody testing when using a compositive block of rodent tissues as substrate. Patients found in this way to be positive to the IgA class, irrespective of their clinical condition, most often have a gluten-sensitive enteropathy (Mäki et al, 1988; Collin et al, 1990, 1992a; Unsworth and Brown, 1994). The IgA-class reticulin antibody test has also been used for screening selected groups of at-risk patients, with expected results.

Table 3. Sensitivity and specificity of serum R1 type IgA-class reticulin and IgA-class endomysium antibodies in untreated coeliac disease.

Reference	Patient group	Reticulin		Endomysium	
		Sensitivity (%)	Specificity (%)	Sensitivity (%)	Specificity (%)
Ferreira et al (1992)	Adults	90	99	100	99
Hällström (1989a)	Adults	91	100	91	100
	Children	100	100	100	100
Kapuscinska et al (1987)	Children			100	100
Lazzari et al (1984)	Children	47	100		
McMillan et al (1991)	Adults			89	100
Magalhaes et al (1974)	Adults	41	100		
Mäki et al (1984a)	Children	97	98		
Mäki et al (1991c)	Adults	92*	95	92*	95
Rossi et al (1988)	Children			100	100
Sategna-Guidetti et al (1993)	Adults			93	100
Seah et al (1971b)	Children	90	100		
Volta et al (1985)	Adults	42	100		
	Children	29	100		

* Family study; one patient with selective IgA deficiency, whose IgG-class serum reticulin antibody titre was 1:8000, was missed.

Positivity clearly predicted clinically silent coeliac disease among patients with insulin-dependent diabetes mellitus (Mäki et al, 1984b; Collin et al, 1989), Sjögren's syndrome (Collin et al, 1992a) and autoimmune thyroid diseases (Collin et al, 1994). The clinician must be aware of selective IgA deficiency, where IgG-class reticulin antibodies are predictive for gluten-sensitive enteropathy (Collin et al, 1992b).

Serum from coeliac patients reacts not only with rodent tissues but also with human (Seah et al, 1971a; Kárpáti et al, 1986, 1990; Hällström 1989a) and other primate (Chorzelski et al, 1983, 1984) tissues. Hällström (1989a, 1989b) showed that all reticulin antibody-positive sera tested gave a moderate to strong immunofluorescent reticular network pattern in human jejunum, liver, lung, spleen, thymus and pancreas, but only a weak reaction in human skin, kidney and colon. Thus, reticulin antibodies in patient sera can also be tested using many human tissues as substrates. Kárpáti et al (1990) have used jejunum for the purpose and name the test the jejunal antibody test. Patient serum lacking IgA-reticulin antibodies but with IgA-class gliadin antibodies does not react with human tissue 'reticulin'. Chorzelski et al (1983, 1984) used monkey oesophagus for testing tissue antibodies in patients with coeliac disease and dermatitis herpetiformis, and named it the endomysium antibody test. Like reticulin, endoymsium antibody was found to be directed against 'reticulin-like' silver stain-positive fibres in connective tissue of the anatomical part of the monkey oesophageal smooth muscle called the endomysium (Kumar et al, 1987). This IgA-class tissue antibody test has gained popularity in recent years as it gives almost 100% sensitivity and specificity for coeliac disease (Table 3).

Reticulin (rodent-type reticulin) and endomysium (primate-type reticulin) antibody tests are highly coeliac disease-specific (Mäki, 1992; Mäki et al, 1992). Among 1312 control patients (healthy and diseased controls, children and adults) pooled from different studies, only three were reported to be positive for IgA-class reticulin antibodies (Hällström, 1989b). None of 45 patients suffering from ulcerative colitis or Crohn's disease showed IgA-class reticulin or endomysium positivity (Hällström, 1989a). One healthy blood donor of 304 tested was found to be positive; on biopsy the mucosa showed total villous atrophy with crypt hyperplasia, which also responded to a gluten-free diet (Hällström, 1989b). We have also recently learned that a positive reticulin or endomysium antibody test not only predicts undiagnosed silent coeliac disease in symptomless first-degree relatives of patients with coeliac disease, but also finds a small number of relatives with normal mucosal architecture expressing coeliac-type HLA haplotypes (A1, B8, DR3) (Mäki et al, 1991c).

Tissue antibodies in coeliac disease are gluten induced. These antibodies are found in patients with untreated coeliac disease, and they usually disappear within 1 year on a gluten-free diet (Mäki et al, 1984a; Kapuscinska et al, 1987; Hällström, 1989a). Again, a reticulin antibody test thus seems suitable for the prediction of mucosal relapse in coeliac disease (Kapuscinska et al, 1987; Mäki et al, 1989).

There seem to be some species-specific differences in the reticulin antigens (Hällström, 1989a; Valeski et al, 1990), and it is also suggested that

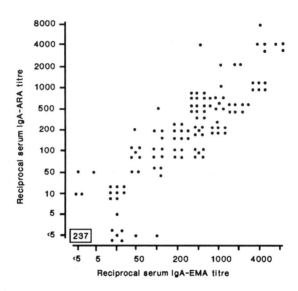

Figure 2. Correlation between R1-type IgA-class reticulin (ARA) and endomysium (EMA) antibodies. The left corner box represents 237 individuals with negative results for both tests.

within a species there might even be organ-specific differences (Valeski et al, 1990). It has recently been shown that after absorption of patient sera with rodent (rat, mouse, guinea-pig and rabbit) liver homogenates, IgA- or IgG-class reticulin antibodies can no longer be detected with rodent tissues, while human tissues and monkey oesophagus give a clear reticulin antibody staining pattern. In contrast, after absorption with human liver homo-genates, both rat and human tissues and monkey oesophagus all gave negative results (Hällström, 1989a). In clinical practice, however, patient serum gives similar results whether tested in rodent or primate tissues (Figure 2).

Reticulin and endomysium antibodies are not primarily directed against rat or monkey tissue structures but are autoantibodies directed against human 'reticulin'. Patient serum also detects molecules in human jejunum in a pattern that closely resembles the fibrillar connective tissue pattern pro-duced by silver impregnation staining (Kumar et al, 1987; Kárpáti et al, 1991). These antibodies were interpreted as being the target organ-related IgA-class autoantibodies in coeliac disease (Kárpáti et al, 1990). IgA anti-bodies in sera from patients recognize a common antigen in an amorphous component associated with collagen fibres (Kárpáti et al, 1991, 1992).

In 1973, Pras and Glynn isolated a non-collagenous reticulin component (NCRC) from kidney tissue. Rabbit antisera raised against these pig and human kidney molecules gave immunofluorescent staining patterns closely resembling those of reticulin antibodies (Pras et al, 1974). Later studies with the NCRC confirmed that histological reticulin was not a single entity (Uns-worth et al, 1982). Further studies showed that reticulin antibodies found in coeliac disease did not react with collagen type III, fibronectin or the identified NCRC (Unsworth et al, 1984).

We recently identified and purified extracellular matrix non-collagenous protein molecules from human fetal lung tissue that bound specifically to serum IgA from patients with coeliac disease (Mäki et al, 1991a). Furthermore, these coeliac disease-specific IgA-class autoantibodies were shown to be generated against a synthetic product of human fibroblasts (Marttinen and Mäki, 1993). Affinity chromatography studies showed that both the fetal lung and human fibroblast-derived molecules absorbed the IgA from patient sera responsible for the reticulin and endomysium antibody positivity but not the IgA from the same sera responsible for gliadin antibody positivity. Crude gliadin absorbed none of the IgA giving a positive tissue autoantibody test. It remains to be seen whether a fibroblast-derived coeliac disease autoantigen protein antibody ELISA test will work in coeliac disease screening.

Intestinal antibodies

Patients with untreated coeliac disease have increased numbers of IgA-, IgM- and IgG-producing plasma cells in the jejunum. The intestinal fluid also contains high levels of gliadin antibodies (Volta et al, 1988) but, in contrast to serum antibodies, levels of intestinal antibodies often remain high on a gluten-free diet (O'Mahoney et al, 1991). The fact that IgA-class reticulin antibodies have also been found in jejunal juice suggests a gastrointestinal origin for these antibodies (Mawhinney and Love, 1975). However, in serum the reticulin antibodies (primate-type reticulin, endomysium) are predominantly of the IgA_1 subclass, and the ratio of $IgA_1:IgA_2$ antibodies is similar to the proportion of total serum $IgA_1:IgA_2$, suggesting a systemic origin (Garrote et al, 1991).

Local humoral responses may be studied by determining total immunoglobulins or antibodies to dietary antigens in jejunal aspirate or gut lavage fluid (O'Mahoney et al, 1990, 1991). These studies showed that gut lavage IgA was predominantly of the secretory type. An elevated concentration of total IgA and IgM was observed in untreated coeliac disease. Intestinal fluids contained IgA and IgM gliadin antibodies as well as antibody responses to β-lactoglobulin and ovalbumin. Secretory IgM antibody activity seemed to persist during a gluten-free diet and was unrelated to enteropathy. Thus, the authors have defined this polyclonal upregulation of mucosal IgM responses seen in coeliac disease as the 'coeliac-like intestinal antibody' pattern and have used this method of assessment to identify patients with potential coeliac disease who have a normal small intestinal biopsy.

Gut immune responses to gliadin or other dietary proteins may be studied indirectly with the ELISPOT method, a solid-phase enzyme-linked immunoassay that measures the number of immunoglobulin-secreting cells in the peripheral blood or the number of specific antibody-secreting cells against dietary antigens (Forrest, 1988). The method is based on the maturation cycle of GALT-derived lymphocytes (see Figure 1(b)). After contact with intraluminal antigens, the lymphocytes travel to mesenteric lymph nodes to mature and, by way of the peripheral blood, migrate back to the gut mucosa to secrete antibodies against the priming antigen. However, it is not always the case; for example, during cow's milk challenge, in patients with cow's milk allergy, an increase in IgM-specific antibody-secreting cells against an unrelated dietary antigen, gliadin, was observed (Suomalainen et al, 1992). This may reflect increased, challenge-unrelated, antigenic permeability in the gut mucosa resulting in the formation of mucosal and circulating gliadin antibodies which are not coeliac disease specific.

Antibodies in individuals with normal jejunal mucosa

Currently we do not treat persons with positive serological tests and normal jejunal mucosal architecture. However, they may nevertheless belong to the entity 'latent coeliac disease' in which the mucosa later deteriorates to that typical of coeliac disease (Mäki et al, 1990; Ferguson et al, 1993). Clearly, the spectrum of mucosal changes due to gluten sensitivity comprises a continuum from 'normality' to the 'flat lesion' (Marsh, 1992) (see Chapter 5). Arguably, persons with latent disease should be identified and treated before there is overt coeliac disease with a manifest mucosal lesion (Arranz and Ferguson, 1993). Positive antibody tests could be markers of gluten sensitivity in such persons with normal jejunal mucosa.

In Table 4, 13 patients are listed in whom the first jejunal biopsy was thought to exclude coeliac disease but whose mucosa later deteriorated to that typical for coeliac disease. Initial serological tests may or may not be positive. Three of the four patients negative for reticulin antibodies became

Table 4. Initial morphometric small bowel biopsy findings and reticulin (ARA) and gliadin (AGA) antibodies in 13 patients excluded for coeliac disease but who later developed gluten-sensitive subtotal villous atrophy with crypt hyperplasia (proven latent coeliac disease cases). Data modified from Mäki et al (1990, 1991c), Collin et al (1993) and Holm (1993).

Patient no.	Sex	Age (years)	Villous height* (μm)	Crypt depth* (μm)	IEL	ARA (IgA)	AGA (IgA)
1	F	1	186	119	34	−	−
2	M	2	394	97	31	+	−
3	M	11	>387	NT	21	−	NT
4	F	32	506	156	14	NT	NT
5	M	35	417	112	18	+	−
6	M	8	315	166	37	+	+
7	F	24	510	190	19	+	+
8	M	49	570	90	12	+	−
9	M	52	475	70	19	−	+
10	M	62	440	90	12	+	+
11	F	45	490	70	10	−	+
12	M	66	530	70	35	+	+
13	M	22	380	125	58	+	−

* Normal values: villous height $\geqslant 300\,\mu m$; crypt depth $\leqslant 150\,\mu m$. IEL, intraepithelial lymphocytes per 100 epithelial cells (normal $\leqslant 30$); NT, not tested.

positive at the time of mucosal deterioration. However, we now conclude that a positive IgA-class reticulin antibody test in individuals with normal mucosa on biopsy should be followed up as the test seems to suggest latent coeliac disease (Mäki et al, 1990, 1991b, 1991c; Collin et al, 1993). Positivity for reticulin antibodies in patients with normal jejunal mucosal morphology predicted subsequent villous atrophy in 83% of cases (Collin et al, 1993). We have not performed aggressive gluten challenge to prove the possible existence of gluten-sensitive enteropathy in patients positive for reticulin antibodies; we rather prefer clinical follow-up while the patient continues on a normal gluten-containing diet. Gliadin antibody positivity in children with a normal jejunal mucosa predicts continuing antibody positivity without the development of overt coeliac disease (Artan R. et al, unpublished results) (Figure 3). Also, in adults, we have seen persistence of gliadin antibodies for years without development of coeliac disease. Follow-up of antibody-positive patients has shown that IgA-class gliadin antibodies predict forthcoming mucosal deterioration only in 24% and IgG-class gliadin antibodies in 0% of patients (Collin et al, 1993). It remains an open question whether or not persisting gliadin antibody positivity represents the existence of a gluten-induced disease, coeliac trait, without enteropathy. This coeliac-type gluten sensitivity in individuals with normal jejunal mucosal morphology should probably also include in its definition the susceptibility genes typical for coeliac disease (DQA1*0501 and DQB1*0201). The majority of individuals with or without abdominal symptoms but positive for gliadin antibodies most probably do not have latent coeliac disease (Uibo et al, 1993). The positive coeliac-like intestinal antibody pattern may be one further indicator of potential coeliac disease in individuals with 'normal' mucosa (O'Mahoney et al, 1990, 1991; Arranz and Ferguson, 1993; Arranz et al, 1994) (see Chapter 10).

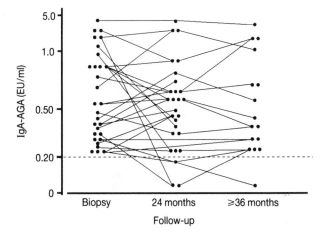

Figure 3. Follow-up of IgA-class gliadin antibodies in children suspected for coeliac disease but with normal jejunal mucosal morphology. The broken horizontal line at 0.20 ELISA units/ml represents the cut-off limit for positivity.

ANTIBODIES AND THE PATHOGENESIS OF COELIAC DISEASE

There is good evidence that the intestinal immune system is involved in the amplification and perpetuation of the morphological and functional abnormalities of the intestinal mucosa in coeliac disease. The role of antibody in the pathogenesis of coeliac disease remains unknown. As reviewed above, gliadin antibodies have frequently been found in untreated coeliac disease, but also in other gastrointestinal diseases, other systemic disorders and in healthy individuals. Neither are gliadin antibodies, in contrast to reticulin autoantibodies, distributed solely among individuals with gene markers of coeliac disease susceptibility (Mäki et al, 1991c; Pettersson et al, 1993). However, it seems that several DR specificities can present gliadin peptides to T helper cells. Gliadin antibodies in coeliac disease could still play some role therefore in the pathogenesis. Halstensen et al (1992) showed that gluten induces IgG-mediated subepithelial complement activation. The deposition was shown to be correlated with the number of mucosal IgG cells and the serum levels of gluten-specific IgG antibodies. Gluten might thus, via immunoglobulin-mediated subepithelial complement activation, damage the surface epithelium in coeliac disease. On the other hand, such deposition was found not to be specific for coeliac disease. Gliadin antibody could also cause intestinal injury through a cell-mediated cytotoxic reaction in which the antibody recognizes gliadin peptides bound to mucosal structures (Unsworth et al, 1987) and directs an antibody-dependent cell-mediated cytotoxic reaction.

Many diseases involving immunological dysfunction, notably the autoimmune diseases, are specifically associated with certain MHC polymorphic alleles. Family studies have shown the HLA class II molecule DQ to be the restriction element for reticulin and endomysium autoantibodies (Mäki et al, 1992). The antigen in human jejunum for these tissue autoantibodies is situated in the area underlying the epithelial basement membrane. In untreated coeliac disease, IgA deposits have been demonstrated by both light and electron microscopy levels in the same area (Shiner and Ballard, 1972; Lancaster-Smith et al, 1977; Rantala et al, 1985; Kárpáti et al, 1988). IgA was also found to be deposited on a subepithelial fibroblast (Rantala et al, 1985). Fibroblasts form part of the connective tissue infrastructure of the lamina propria. The sheath of fibroblasts lies in close contact with the intestinal epithelial cells and these cells replicate and migrate in parallel and in approximate synchrony with the replicating and migrating crypt epithelial cells. Fibroblasts are also known to synthesize not only extracellular matrix proteins, collagen and procollagen, but also non-collagenous proteins, many of which have paracrine functions. Therefore, our observation that coeliac disease-specific tissue antibodies are generated against a synthetic product of human fibroblasts (Marttinen and Mäki, 1993) may be of pathogenetic importance.

The *autoimmune hypothesis for coeliac disease pathogenesis* is based on the identification of self-peptides triggering the production of reticulin and endomysium autoantibodies (Mäki et al, 1991a). According to this hypothesis, all the crucial elements, that is the trigger (gliadin), the susceptibility

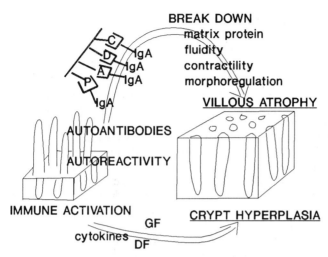

Figure 4. The pathogenetic events leading to the typical coeliac disease mucosal lesion could develop along two lines, one leading to villous atrophy, the other to crypt hyperplasia. The coeliac disease-specific tissue autoantibodies would be involved in the pathogenesis by binding to their subepithelial antigens in the lamina propria, the fibroblast-derived extracellular non-collagenous matrix proteins (coeliac disease autoantigen proteins, CDAP) and thus cause a breakdown of important physiological functions. Gluten-triggered immune activation possibly involving an autoreactive T-cell population is also hypothesized to be responsible for crypt hyperplasia. The effect of released cytokines might be involved in the process, as well as growth factor (GF) and differentiation factor (DF).

MHC class II genes (DQA/DQB) and the autoantigen, are present for auto-immunity to occur. Specific HLA class II molecules on APCs, especially DQ2, could present self-peptides, thus activating the autoreactive T-cell population. These self-peptides could be the fibroblast-derived extracellular matrix proteins (Marttinen and Mäki, 1993). Coeliac disease is indeed self-perpetuating if the specific trigger, gliadin, is not excluded. In other auto-immune diseases the triggers are so far unknown and thus cannot be excluded.

Figure 4 suggests a scheme for the pathogenesis of villous atrophy due to the production of autoantibodies. In the coeliac lesion the immunoglobulins would bind to their antigens causing a breakdown of many of the physio-logical functions of the fibroblasts and their products. On the other hand, the production of coeliac disease-specific autoantibodies may be just an epiphe-nomenon, and there are arguments against autoimmune mechanisms being operative in the pathogenesis of coeliac disease (Marsh et al, 1993). How-ever, it remains to be seen whether or not fibroblast-derived coeliac disease autoantigens are important morphoregulatory paracrine factors.

SUMMARY

IgA is transported into intestinal secretions to perform exclusion of luminal antigens. The prerequisites are antigen sampling by the Peyer's patch M cells, antigen processing by antigen-presenting cells, and presentation of antigenic peptides by HLA class II molecules to immunocompetent T cells. The basis for intestinal immunity is the maturation cycle of specifically primed T and B cells from the gut-associated lymphoid tissue via mesenteric lymph nodes and peripheral blood back to the intestinal lamina propria.

In coeliac disease, patients are sensitized against gluten and serum gliadin antibodies are often detected. Gliadin antibodies are also found in other gastrointestinal diseases, other disorders and in healthy individuals not carrying the coeliac disease-specific DQA/DQB alleles. On the other hand, serum reticulin and endomysium autoantibodies are both sensitive and highly disease-specific. Positivity in patients with normal jejunal morphology indicates latency of coeliac disease. These tissue autoantibodies are directed against fibroblast-derived extracellular matrix proteins. The immune system is involved in the amplification and perpetuation of the abnormalities of the intestinal mucosa in coeliac disease. The role of antibody in the pathogenesis remains unknown. The author hypothesizes gluten-triggered autoimmune mechanism to be operative.

Acknowledgements

The Coeliac Disease Study Project is supported by the Medical Research Council, the Academy of Finland and the Sigrid Jusélius Foundation.

REFERENCES

Arranz E & Ferguson A (1993) Intestinal antibody pattern of celiac disease: occurrence in patients with normal jejunal biopsy histology. *Gastroenterology* **104**: 1263–1272.

Arranz E, Bode J, Kingstone K & Ferguson A (1994) Intestinal antibody pattern of coeliac disease: association with gamma/delta T cell receptor expression by intraepithelial lymphocytes, and other indices of potential coeliac disease. *Gut* **35**: 476–482.

Ascher H, Lanner Å & Kristiansson B (1990) A new laboratory kit for anti-gliadin IgA at diagnosis and follow-up of childhood celiac disease. *Journal of Pediatric Gastroenterology and Nutrition* **10**: 443–450.

Bodé S & Gudmand-Hoyer E (1994) Evaluation of the gliadin antibody test for diagnosing coeliac disease. *Scandinavian Journal of Gastroenterology* **29**: 148–152.

Brandtzaeg P & Bjerke K (1990) Immunomorphological characteristics of human Peyer's patches. *Digestion* **46 (supplement 2)**: 262–273.

Brandtzaeg P, Halstensen TS, Kett K et al (1989) Immunobiology and immunopathology of human gut mucosa: humoral immunity and intraepithelial lymphocytes. *Gastroenterology* **97**: 1562–1584.

Brown JH, Jardetzky T, Saper MA et al (1988) A hypothetical model of the foreign antigen binding site of class II histocompatibility molecules. *Nature* **332**: 845–850.

Burgin-Wolff A, Bertele RM, Berger R et al (1983) A reliable screening test for childhood celiac disease: fluorescent immunosorbent test for gliadin antibodies. *Journal of Pediatrics* **102**: 655–660.

Burgin-Wolff A, Gaze H, Hadziselimovic F et al (1991) Antigliadin and antiendomysium antibody determination for coeliac disease. *Archives of Disease in Childhood* **66**: 941–947.

Catassi C, Rätsch I-M, Fabiani E et al (1994) Coeliac disease in the year 2000: exploring the iceberg. *Lancet* **343**: 200–203.

Chorzelski TP, Sulej J, Tschorzewska H et al (1983) IgA class endomysium antibodies in dermatitis herpetiformis and coeliac disease. *Annals of the New York Academy of Sciences* **420**: 325–334.

Chorzelski TP, Beutner EH, Sulej J et al (1984) IgA-antiendomysium antibody: a new immunological marker of dermatitis herpetiformis and coeliac disease. *British Journal of Dermatology* **111:** 395–402.

Ciclitira PJ, Ellis HJ & Evans DJ (1983) A solid phase radioimmunoassay for measurement of circulating antibody titres to wheat gliadin and its subfractions in patients and adult coeliac disease. *Journal of Immunological Methods* **62:** 231–235.

Ciclitira PJ, Ellis HJ, Richards D & Kemeny DM (1986) Gliadin IgG subclass antibodies in patients with coeliac disease. *International Archives of Allergy and Applied Immunology* **80:** 258–261.

Clark EA & Ledbetter JA (1994) How B and T cells talk to each other. *Nature* **367:** 425–428.

Collin P, Salmi J, Hällström O et al (1989) High frequency of coeliac disease in adult patients with type-I diabetes. *Scandinavian Journal of Gastroenterology* **24:** 81–84.

Collin P, Hällström O, Mäki M et al (1990) Atypical coeliac disease found with serologic screening. *Scandinavian Journal of Gastroenterology* **25:** 245–250.

Collin P, Korpela M, Hällström O et al (1992a) Rheumatic complaints as a presenting symptom in patients with coeliac disease. *Scandinavian Journal of Rheumatology* **21:** 20–23.

Collin P, Mäki M, Keyriläinen O et al (1992b) Selective IgA deficiency and coeliac disease. *Scandinavian Journal of Gastroenterology* **27:** 367–371.

Collin P, Helin H, Mäki M et al (1993) Follow-up of patients positive in reticulin and gliadin antibody tests with normal small-bowel biopsy findings. *Scandinavian Journal of Gastroenterology* **28:** 595–598.

Collin P, Salmi J, Hällström O et al (1994) Autoimmune thyroid disorders and coeliac disease. *European Journal of Endocrinology* **130:** 137–140.

Eade OE, Lloyd RS, Lang C & Wright R (1977) IgA and IgG reticulin antibodies in coeliac and non-coeliac patients. *Gut* **18:** 991–993.

Fälth-Magnusson K, Jansson G, Stenhammar L & Magnusson KER (1994) Serum food antibodies analyzed by enzyme-linked immunosorbent assay (ELISA) and diffusion-in-gel (DIG)-ELISA methods in children with and without celiac disease. *Journal of Pediatric Gastroenterology and Nutrition* **18:** 56–62.

Ferguson A, Arranz E & O'Mahoney O (1993) Clinical and pathological spectrum of coeliac disease—active, silent, latent, potential. *Gut* **34:** 150–151.

Ferreira M, Lloyd Davies S, Butler M et al (1992) Endomysial antibody: is it the best screening test for coeliac disease? *Gut* **33:** 1633–1637.

Finn R, Harvey MM, Johnson PM et al (1985) Serum IgG antibodies to gliadin and other dietary antigens in adults with atopic eczema. *Clinical and Experimental Dermatology* **10:** 222–228.

Forrest BD (1988) Identification of an intestinal immune response using peripheral blood lymphocytes. *Lancet* **i:** 81–83.

Friis SU & Gudmand-Hoyer E (1986) Screening for coeliac disease in adults by simultaneous determination of IgA and IgG gliadin antibodies. *Scandinavian Journal of Gastroenterology* **21:** 1058–1062.

Garrote JA, Blanco A, Alonso M et al (1991) Usefulness of antiendomysial antibodies as a serological marker in coeliac children. *Pediatric Allergy and Immunology* **4:** 199–208.

Grodzinsky E, Hed J, Lieden G et al (1990) Presence of IgA and IgG antigliadin antibodies in healthy adults as measured by micro-ELISA. Effect of various cutoff levels of specificity and sensitivity when diagnosing coeliac disease. *International Archives of Allergy and Applied Immunology* **92:** 119–123.

Hällström O (1989a) Comparison of IgA-class reticulin and endomysium antibodies in coeliac disease and dermatitis herpetiformis. *Gut* **30:** 1225–1232.

Hällström O (1989b) IgA-class reticulin antibody test in coeliac disease and dermatitis herpetiformis. *Acta Universitatis Tamperensis Series A* **281:** 1–98.

Halstensen TS, Hvatum M, Scott H et al (1992) Association of subepithelial deposition of activated complement and immunoglobulin G and M response to gluten in celiac disease. *Gastroenterology* **102:** 751–759.

Holm K (1993) Latent and silent coeliac disease. A family study. *Acta Universitatis Tamperensis Series A* **371:** 1–90.

Hvatum M, Scott H & Brandtzaeg P (1992) Serum subclass antibodies to a variety of food antigens in patients with coeliac disease. *Gut* **33:** 632–638.

Janeway CA & Golstein P (1991) Lymphocyte activation and effector functions. *Current Opinion in Immunology* **3**: 283–286.

Kagnoff MF (1993) Immunology of the intestinal tract. *Gastroenterology* **105**: 1275–1280.

Kapuscinska A, Zalewski T, Chorzelski TP et al (1987) Disease specificity and dynamics of changes in IgA class anti-endomysial antibodies in celiac disease. *Journal of Pediatric Gastroenterology and Nutrition* **6**: 529–534.

Kárpáti S, Török E & Kosnai I (1986) IgA class antibody against human jejunum in sera of children with dermatitis herpetiformis. *Journal of Investigative Dermatology* **87**: 703–706.

Kárpáti S, Kósnai I, Török É & Kovács JB (1988) Immunoglobulin A deposition in jejunal mucosa of children with dermatitis herpetiformis. *Journal of Investigative Dermatology* **91**: 336–339.

Kárpáti S, Burgin-Wolff A, Krieg T et al (1990) Binding to human jejunum of serum IgA antibody from children with coeliac disease. *Lancet* **336**: 1335–1338.

Kárpáti S, Stolz W, Meurer M et al (1991) Extracellular binding sites of IgA anti-jejunal antibodies on normal small bowel detected by indirect immunoelectron microscopy. *Journal of Investigative Dermatology* **96**: 228–233.

Kárpáti S, Meurer M, Stolz W et al (1992) Ultrastructural binding sites of endomysium antibodies from sera of patients with dermatitis herpetiformis and coeliac disease. *Gut* **33**: 191–193.

Kemp M, Husby S, Larsen ML & Svehag SE (1988) ELISA analysis of IgA subclass antibodies to dietary antigens. Elevated IgA$_1$ antibodies in childen with coeliac disease. *International Archives of Allergy and Applied Immunology* **87**: 247–253.

Kett K, Scott H, Fausa O & Brandtzaeg P (1990) Secretory immunity in celiac disease: cellular expression of immunoglobulin A subclass and joining chain. *Gastroenterology* **99**: 386–392.

Kieffer M & Barnetson RStC (1983) Increased gliadin antibodies in dermatitis herpetiformis and pemphigoid. *British Journal of Dermatology* **108**: 673–678.

Kilander AF, Nilsson LÅ & Gillberg L (1987) Serum antibodies to gliadin in coeliac disease after gluten withdrawal. *Scandinavian Journal of Gastroenterology* **22**: 29–34.

Kilander AF, Dotevall G, Fällström SP et al (1983) Evaluation of gliadin antibodies for detection of coeliac disease. *Scandinavian Journal of Gastroenterology* **18**: 377–383.

Kumar V, Hemedinger E, Chorzelski TP et al (1987) Reticulin and endomysial antibodies in bullous disease. *Archives of Dermatology* **123**: 1179–1182.

Lancaster-Smith M, Joyce S & Kumar P (1977) Immunoglobulins in the jejunal mucosa in adult coeliac disease and dermatitis herpetiformis after the reintroduction of dietary gluten. *Gut* **18**: 887–890.

Lazzari R, Volta U, Bianchi BF et al (1984) R1 reticulin antibodies: markers of celiac disease in children on a normal diet and on gluten challenge. *Journal of Pediatric Gastroenterology and Nutrition* **3**: 516–522.

Levenson SD, Austin RK, Dietler MD et al (1985) Specificity of anti-gliadin antibody in celiac disease. *Gastroenterology* **89**: 1–5.

McMillan SA, Haughton DJ, Biggart JD et al (1991) Predictive value for coeliac disease of antibodies to gliadin, endomysium, and jejunum in patients attending for jejunal biopsy. *British Medical Journal* **303**: 1163–1165.

Magalhaes AFN, Peters TJ & Doe WF (1974) Studies on the nature and significance of connective tissue antibodies in adult coeliac disease and Crohn's disease. *Gut* **15**: 284–288.

Mäki M (1992) Use of serological antibody tests in celiac disease. In Branski D, Rozen P & Kagnoff MF (eds) *Gluten-sensitive Enteropathy. Frontiers of Gastrointestinal Research*, vol. 19, pp 108–129. Basel: Karger.

Mäki M, Hällström O, Vesikari T & Visakorpi JK (1984a) Evaluation of a serum IgA-class reticulin antibody test for the detection of childhood celiac disease. *Journal of Pediatrics* **105**: 901–905.

Mäki M, Hällström O, Huupponen T et al (1984b) Increased prevalence of coeliac disease in diabetes. *Archives of Disease in Childhood* **59**: 739–742.

Mäki M, Hällström O, Verronen P et al (1988) Reticulin antibody, arthritis, and coeliac disease in children. *Lancet* **i**: 479–480.

Mäki M, Lähdeaho ML, Hällström O et al (1989) Postpubertal gluten challenge in coeliac disease. *Archives of Disease in Childhood* **64**: 1604–1607.

Mäki M, Holm K, Koskimies S et al (1990) Normal small bowel biopsy followed by coeliac disease. *Archives of Disease in Childhood* **65**: 1137–1141.

Mäki M, Hällström O & Marttinen A (1991a) Reaction of human non-collagenous polypeptides with coeliac disease autoantibodies. *Lancet* **338**: 724–725.

Mäki M, Holm K, Collin P & Savilahti E (1991b) Increase in gamma/delta T cell receptor bearing lymphocytes in normal small bowel mucosa in latent coeliac disease. *Gut* **32**: 1412–1414.

Mäki M, Holm K, Lipsanen V et al (1991c) Serological markers and HLA genes among healthy first-degree relatives of patients with coeliac disease. *Lancet* **338**: 1350–1353.

Mäki M, Hällström O, Marttinen A et al (1992) Screening tools for use in coeliac disease. In Auricchio S & Visakorpi JK (eds) *Common Food Intolerances 1: Epidemiology of Coeliac Disease, Dynamic Nutrition Research*, vol. 2, pp 93–104. Basel: Karger.

Marsh MN (1992) Gluten, major histocompatibility complex, and the small intestine. A molecular and immunobiologic approach to the spectrum of gluten sensitivity ('celiac sprue'). *Gastroenterology* **102**: 330–354.

Marsh MN, Ensari A & Morgan S (1993) Evidence that gluten sensitivity is an immunologic disease. *Current Opinion in Gastroenterology* **9**: 994–1000.

Marttinen A & Mäki M (1993) Purification of fibroblast-derived celiac disease autoantigen molecules. *Pediatric Research* **34**: 420–423.

Mascart-Lemone F, Cadranel S, Van den Broeck J et al (1988) IgA immune response patterns to gliadin in serum. *International Archives of Allergy and Applied Immunology* **86**: 412–419.

Mawhinney H & Love AHG (1975) Anti-reticulin antibody in jejunal juice in coeliac disease. *Clinical and Experimental Immunology* **21**: 394–398.

Mayer L (1991) Antigen presentation in the intestine. *Current Opinion in Gastroenterology* **7**: 446–449.

Mayer M, Greco L, Troncone R et al (1989) Early prediction of relapse during gluten challenge in childhood celiac disease. *Journal of Pediatric Gastroenterology and Nutrition* **8**: 474–479.

Not T, Ventura A, Peticarari S et al (1993) A new, rapid, noninvasive screening test for celiac disease. *Journal of Pediatrics* **123**: 425–427.

O'Farrelly C, Kelly J, Hekkens W et al (1983) Gliadin antibody levels: a serological test for coeliac disease. *British Medical Journal* **286**: 2007–2010.

O'Farrelly C, Marten D, Melcher D et al (1988) Association between villous atrophy in rheumatoid arthritis and a rheumatoid factor and gliadin-specific IgG. *Lancet* **ii**: 819–822.

O'Mahoney S, Vestey JP & Ferguson A (1990) Similarities in intestinal humoral immunity in dermatitis herpetiformis without enteropathy and in coeliac disease. *Lancet* **335**: 1487–1490.

O'Mahoney S, Arranz E, Barton JR & Ferguson A (1991) Dissociation between systemic and mucosal humoral immune responses in coeliac disease. *Gut* **32**: 29–35.

Parker DC (1993) T cell-dependent B cell activation. *Annual Review of Immunology* **11**: 331–360.

Pettersson A, Sjöberg K, Lernmark Å Eriksson S (1993) HLA genotypes in coeliac disease and healthy individuals carrying gliadin antibodies. *European Journal of Gastroenterology and Hepatology* **5**: 445–450.

Pras M & Glynn LE (1973) Isolation of a non-collagenous reticulin component and its primary characterization. *British Journal of Experimental Pathology* **54**: 449–456.

Pras M, Johnson GD, Holborow EJ & Glynn LE (1974) Antigenic properties of a non-collagenous reticulin component of normal connective tissue. *Immunology* **27**: 469–478.

Rantala I, Mäki M, Laasonen A & Visakorpi JK (1985) Periodate–lysine–paraphormaldehyde as a fixative for the study of duodenal mucosa. Morphologic and immunohistochemical results at light and electron microscopic levels. *Acta Pathologica Microbiologica Scandinavica Section A* **93**: 165–173.

Rizzetto M & Doniach D (1973) Types of 'reticulin' antibodies detected in human sera by immunofluorescence. *Journal of Clinical Pathology* **26**: 841–851.

Rossi TM, Kumar V, Lerner A et al (1988) Relationship of endomysial antibodies to jejunal mucosal pathology: specificity towards both symptomatic and asymptomatic coeliacs. *Journal of Pediatric Gastroenterology and Nutrition* **7**: 858–863.

Salmi M & Jalkanen S (1991) Regulation of lymphocyte traffic to mucosa-associated lymphatic tissues. *Gastroenterology Clinics of North America* **20:** 495–510.

Sategna-Guidetti C, Pulitano R, Grosso S & Ferfoglia G (1993) Serum IgA entiendomysium antibody titers as a marker of intestinal involvement and diet compliance in adult celiac sprue. *Journal of Clinical Gastroenterology* **17:** 123–127.

Savilahti E, Viander M, Perkkiö M et al (1983) IgA antigliadin antibodies: a marker of mucosal damage in childhood coeliac disease. *Lancet* **i:** 320–322.

Schroeder P (1990) Upper gastrointestinal endoscopy at a student health centre. *Scandinavian Journal of Primary Health Care* **8:** 191–195.

Scott H, Fausa O, Ek J et al (1990) Measurements of serum IgA and IgG activities to dietary antigens. A prospective study of the diagnostic usefulness in adult coeliac disease. *Scandinavian Journal of Gastroenterology* **25:** 287–292.

Scott H, Kett K, Halstensen TS et al (1992) The humoral immune system in coeliac disease. In Marsh MN (ed.) *Coeliac Disease*, pp 239–282. Oxford: Blackwell Scientific Publications.

Seah PP, Fry L, Hoffbrand AV & Holborow EJ (1971a) Tissue antibodies in dermatitis herpetiformis and adult coeliac disease. *Lancet* **i:** 834–836.

Seah PP, Fry LL, Rossiter MA et al (1971b) Anti-reticulin antibodies in childhood coeliac disease. *Lancet* **ii:** 681–682.

Shiner M & Ballard J (1972) Antigen–antibody reactions in jejunal mucosa in childhood coeliac disease after gluten challenge. *Lancet* **i:** 1202–1205.

Ståhlberg MR, Savilahti E & Viander M (1986) Antibodies to gliadin by ELISA as a screening test for childhood coeliac disease. *Journal of Pediatric Gastroenterology and Nutrition* **5:** 726–729.

Stern M, Fisher K & Gruttner R (1979) Immunofluorescent serum gliadin antibodies in children with coeliac disease and various malabsorptive disorders. *European Journal of Pediatrics* **130:** 155–164.

Suomalainen H, Isolauri E, Kaila M et al (1992) Cow's milk provocation induces an immune response to unrelated dietary antigens. *Gut* **33:** 1179–1183.

Troncone R & Ferguson A (1991) Anti-gliadin antibodies. *Journal of Pediatric Gastroenterology and Nutrition* **12:** 150–158.

Uibo O, Uibo R, Kleimola V et al (1993) Serum IgA anti-gliadin antibodies in an adult population sample. High prevalence without celiac disease. *Digestive Diseases and Sciences* **38:** 2034–2037.

Unsworth DJ & Brown DI (1994) Serological screening suggests that adult coeliac disease is underdiagnosed in the UK and increases the incidence by up to 12%. *Gut* **35:** 61–64.

Unsworth DJ, Scott DL, Almond TJ et al (1982) Studies on reticulin. I: Serological and immunohistological investigation of the occurrence of collagen type III, fibronectin and the non-collagenous glycoprotein of Pras and Glynn in reticulin. *British Journal of Experimental Pathology* **63:** 154–166.

Unsworth DJ, Walker-Smith JA & Holborow EJ (1983) Gliadin and reticulin antibodies in childhood coeliac disease. *Lancet* **i:** 874–875.

Unsworth DJ, Scott DL, Walton KW et al (1984) Failure of R1 type antireticulin antibody to react with fibronectin, collagen type III or the non-collagenous reticulin component (NCRC). *Clinical and Experimental Immunology* **57:** 609–613.

Unsworth DJ, Leonard JN, Hobday CM et al (1987) Gliadin binds to reticulin in a lectin-like manner. *Archives of Dermatological Research* **279:** 232–235.

Vainio E, Kalimo K, Reunala T et al (1983) Circulating IgA- and IgC-class antigliadin antibodies in dermatitis herpetiformis detected by enzyme-linked immunosorbent assay. *Archives of Dermatological Research* **275:** 15–18.

Valeski JE, Kumar V, Beutner EH et al (1990) Immunology of celiac disease: tissue and species specificity of endomysial and reticulin antibodies. *International Archives of Allergy and Applied Immunology* **93:** 1–7.

Volta U, Lenzi R & Cassani F (1985) Antibodies to gluten detected by immunofluorescence and a micro-ELISA method: markers of active childhood and adult coeliac disease. *Gut* **26:** 667–671.

Volta U, Bonazzi C, Lazzari R et al (1988) Immunoglobulin A antigliadin antibodies in jejunal juice: markers of severe intestinal damage in coeliac children. *Digestion* **39:** 35–39.

Volta U, Molinaro M, Fratangelo D & Bianchi FB (1990) IgA subclass antibodies to gliadin in serum and intestinal juice of patients with coeliac disease. *Clinical and Experimental Immunology* **80:** 192–195.

Weiss JB, Austin RK, Schanfield MS et al (1983) Gluten-sensitive enteropathy: immunoglobulin G heavy-chain (Gm) allotypes and the immune response to wheat gliadins. *Journal of Clinical Investigation* **72:** 96–99.

4

T-cell responses and cellular immunity in coeliac disease

LUDWIK K. TREJDOSIEWICZ
PETER D. HOWDLE

The need to understand the immunopathology of coeliac disease has been a stimulus to the study of mucosal immunity in general, and reports relating to coeliac disease provide data about the mucosal immune system of the human gastrointestinal tract. In this chapter, current understanding of the mucosal cellular immune system is discussed in terms of organization and function, as well as the changes observed in coeliac disease. The way in which such changes can relate to the pathogenesis of the condition is also considered.

ANATOMICAL ASPECTS

Interest in cellular immunity in coeliac disease has revolved mainly around lymphocytes in the gastrointestinal mucosa, especially in the small bowel. Because intestinal immunocytes (i.e. lymphocytes, mononuclear phago-cytes and polymorphonuclear cells) are segregated into epithelial and lamina propria compartments, investigators have considered these two compartments separately. Although these compartments are populated by distinct immunocyte populations, it has long been recognized that there are changes in lymphocyte numbers in both compartments in patients with coeliac disease.

Intraepithelial lymphocytes

Human intraepithelial lymphocytes (IELs) have excited interest amongst anatomists and immunologists for many years (Ferguson, 1977; Dobbins, 1986; Brandtzaeg, 1989; Brandtzaeg et al, 1989a) and have been reviewed recently (Cerf-Bensussan and Guy-Grand, 1991; Brandtzaeg et al, 1992, 1993; Cerf-Bensussan et al, 1993; Trejdosiewicz, 1992, 1993). In the intestinal mucosa, IELs are located within the epithelial layer between the enterocytes. IELs display considerable heterogeneity in size, shape and structural detail, varying in morphology from small lymphocytes to large blasts, and in size from 3 to 11 μm (Marsh, 1980), although the majority are of medium size with darkly staining nuclei. The cells are rounded or ovoid, and where active inflammation is present they often have elongated cytoplasmic processes which make intimate contact with adjacent epithelial cell membranes (Dobbins, 1986). Whereas lymphoblasts ($\geqslant 9\,\mu$m in diameter) form a minority population of 2.5% is of the normal mucosal IELs, in coeliac disease the percentage increases to about 8%, together with an increase in mitotic activity (Marsh, 1980).

Enumeration of IELs

During the 1970s and 1980s there was controversy concerning the enumeration of IELs. In 1971 Ferguson and Murray related the number of IELs to the number of enterocytes, and this criterion was generally accepted by most investigators of coeliac disease and other enteropathies (Fry et al, 1972). However, Marsh proposed in 1980 that the number of IELs should be related to a specific volume of mucosa, thus producing an 'areal' density for lymphocytes, not related to the number of enterocytes, which may vary in a particular disease state. The example most quoted was that of coeliac disease where the number of IELs increased on a 'per 100 enterocytes' basis, but decreased on the basis of mucosal volume.

It is simplistic to believe that the number of lymphocytes is increased simply because the number of enterocytes may be decreased. Indeed Corazza et al (1984) showed that both parameters changed with treatment in coeliac disease. The modern consensus view is that cell density is a more accurate means of determining 'absolute' numbers of IELs but that the relative number (i.e. assessed on a per enterocyte basis) is a useful means of detecting minor changes. Evidence in support of the independent variability of IELs and enterocyte numbers comes from Marsh et al (1990), who showed an increase in the number of IELs in first-degree relatives of coeliac patients, with no change in mucosal morphology. Marsh has since shown that IEL infiltration in a variety of clinical situations in response to varying doses of gluten is an indication of gluten sensitivity in particular individuals without there necessarily being any change in intestinal morphology (for a full discussion see Chapter 5).

Phenotypic analysis of intraepithelial lymphocytes

Numerous phenotypic studies of tissue sections and cell isolates have established that human IELs are predominantly (>95%) CD3$^+$ CD2$^+$ T cells. There is little doubt that IELs are a distinct and distinctive population of T cells, and differ in many ways from T cells of the periphery and non-mucosal lymphoid organs. Indeed, animal studies suggest that many IELs mature extrathymically (reviewed by Rocha et al, 1992).

The 70–90% majority of IEL T cells are CD8$^+$, suggestive of a cytotoxic–suppressor cell function, the remainder being largely CD4$^+$ (helper) cells and a <5% minority population of CD4$^-$ CD8$^-$ 'double-negative' cells. In both humans and the mouse, at least some of the CD8$^+$ IELs express CD8 in an $\alpha\alpha$ homodimeric form, rather than the usual CD8 $\alpha\beta$ heterodimer expressed by peripheral blood lymphocyte (PBL) T cells (Guy-Grand et al,

1991; Rocha et al, 1991; Rust et al, 1992). The $CD8^+$ subset of IELs also tends to express CD5, although at reduced density (Malizia et al, 1985; Ebert, 1989; Smart et al, 1989; Jarry et al, 1990; Trejdosiewicz et al, 1989), reminiscent of the $CD8^+$ $CD5^{low}$ phenotype of graft-versus-host disease infiltrating lymphocytes and suggestive of cytolytic activity. Low expression of CD5 (and CD6) also implies little involvement with B cells, as CD5 is the counter-receptor for CD72 on B cells known to be important for T–B cell interactions. IELs also express reduced amounts of leukocyte (β_2) integrins, the heterodimeric adhesion receptors involved in cell–cell and cell–matrix interactions. In particular, IELs are characterized by reduced expression of lymphocyte function-associated antigen 1 (LFA-1: CD11a/CD18, the $\alpha^L\beta_2$ integrin) (Smart et al, 1991) and very late activation antigen 4 (VLA-4: CDw49d/CD29, the $\alpha^4\beta_1$ integrin) (Trejdosiewicz, 1992). IELs also express little or no detectable CD11b, CD16, CD56 or other markers associated with cytotoxicity, with the possible exception of TIA-1 (Russell et al, 1993). It should also be mentioned that a number of minority cell populations of IELs of unusual phenotype have now been described by flow cytometry (Jarry et al, 1990) and that analysis of T-cell antigen receptor (TCR) V_β gene usage suggests that IELs (as well as lamina propria lymphocytes (LPLs)) are oligoclonal (Balk et al, 1991; Van Kerckhove et al, 1992; Blumberg et al, 1993) as they do not express the full TCR repertoire of PBLs.

IELs are characterized by high expression of the HML-1-defined β_7 integrin, an antigen expressed by almost all IELs, up to 50% of LPLs, but not by peripheral T cells (Cerf-Bensussan et al, 1987, 1992; Micklem et al, 1991; Parker et al, 1992). As β_7 expression is inducible in peripheral T cells in vitro (Schieferdecker et al, 1990), this provides further weight to the suggestion that IELs are semi-activated cells (Malizia et al, 1985). As yet, the role of the 'mucosal' β_7 integrin has not been identified. There is increasing evidence that β_7 mediates IEL recognition of intestinal as well as other epithelial cells (Ebert and Roberts, 1993; Cepek et al, 1993; Roberts et al, 1993a,b) and hence the as-yet unidentified α-chain has been dubbed α^E (Parker et al, 1992). There is also evidence that β_7 may function as an alternative accessory molecule for IELs, necessary for IEL activation (Sarnacki et al, 1992) as discussed below.

Unlike in mice, the majority of human IELs express the 'conventional' ($\alpha\beta$) form of the TCR and only a minority of 1–10% express the variant TCR $\gamma\delta^+$ type (Halstensen et al, 1989; Spencer et al, 1989; Trejdosiewicz et al, 1989, 1991), although, unlike peripheral blood TCR $\gamma\delta^+$ T cells, IEL TCR $\gamma\delta^+$ cells are usually $CD8^+$ and use the V_{δ_1} chain rather than V_{δ_2}. A striking feature of coeliac disease is the increase in abundance and percentage of TCR $\gamma\delta^+$ IELs (Halstensen et al, 1989; Spencer et al, 1989; Trejdosiewicz et al, 1991), irrespective of gluten challenge (Savilahti et al, 1990) and even in well-treated patients with normal or near-normal morphology (Trejdosiewicz et al, 1991). The tendency to increased TCR $\gamma\delta^+$ IELs is also a feature of latent disease (Mäki et al, 1991), dermatitis herpetiformis (Savilahti et al, 1992) and even in individuals thought to be genetically predisposed to coeliac disease (Holm et al, 1992). Furthermore, the increased numbers of TCR $\gamma\delta^+$ IELs maintain the 'intestinal' $V_{\delta_1}^+ V_{\gamma_9}^-$ phenotype, although the majority become CD4⁻ CD8⁻ double negatives (Halstensen et al, 1989; Trejdosiewicz et al, 1991). However, the increase in TcR $\gamma\delta^+$ is not specific for coeliac disease and increases have been described in other small bowel enteropathies (Spencer et al, 1991).

As yet, the significance of increased TCR $\gamma\delta^+$ IEL numbers is unknown. It seems unlikely that they represent 'immune surveillance' cells that eliminate damaged autologous epithelial cells by virtue of cross-reactivity with heat-shock proteins, as was originally postulated (see discussion by Trejdosiewicz et al, 1991). However, in transgenic mice, alloreactive TCR $\gamma\delta^+$ cells are eliminated in the thymus, but persist in the intestinal epithelium, albeit in an anergic or 'tolerized' form (Barrett et al, 1992). Thus, alloreactive murine TCR $\gamma\delta^+$ IELs have the potential to mediate autoimmune disease (Barrett et al, 1993) and it is possible that they might 'break tolerance' and mediate some of the enterocytic damage that is a feature of coeliac disease.

In addition to the increase in TCR $\gamma\delta^+$ IELs, earlier studies described other, more subtle, changes in IEL phenotypes in patients with coeliac disease. Although normally low, CD5 expression is upregulated by the CD8⁺ subset of IELs (Selby et al, 1981), particularly in untreated disease (Malizia et al, 1985). As CD5 expression is upregulated during T-lymphocyte activation, this may be taken as evidence of increasing IEL activity. Increased expression of the CD7 receptor characteristic of lymphoblasts by the minority CD4⁺ helper IEL subset has also been shown to correlate with mucosal pathology (Malizia et al, 1985), adding further weight to this hypothesis. The demonstration in coeliac mucosa that a higher proportion of IELs express CD45 isoforms associated with antigen-primed or memory function (Brandtzaeg et al, 1989b; Halstensen et al, 1990a,b) suggests that immune activation has occurred. Against this must be set the suggestion that CD8⁺ CD45R0⁺ IELs may not, in fact, be memory cells in the accepted sense (Ebert, 1993).

Although we did not observe an increase in Ki67⁺ mitotic IELs in coeliac disease (Malizia et al, 1985), Halstensen and Brandtzaeg (1993) subsequently showed that there is in fact an increase. It has also been demonstrated that there is an increase in expression of the LFA-1 (CD11a/CD18; $\alpha^L\beta_2$) leucointegrin by IELs in coeliac disease, particularly by the CD4⁺ helper cell subset (Smart et al, 1991). Although affinity was not measured, this increase in density is additional evidence for increased activation.

Lamina propria lymphocytes

In the lamina propria, T cells account for some 25–40% of all leukocytes, as there are numerous immunoglobulin-containing cells (B cells and plasma cells) as well as cells of the mononuclear phagocyte lineage (monocytes, histiocytes and dendritic cells), eosinophils and mast cells. In untreated coeliac disease, the leukocyte population is more dense than normal, although few authors have attempted to enumerate LPL cell types. Several older studies suggested that, in coeliac patients taking a normal diet, there were significant increases in total and plasma cell counts and a significant reduction in small lymphocyte numbers (Holmes et al, 1974; Lancaster-Smith et al, 1975). Following treatment with a gluten-free diet, lymphocyte numbers returned to normal, although the number of plasma cells remained raised. Later studies, however, showed increases in all white cell populations in untreated coeliac mucosa, including lymphocytes (Dhesi et al, 1984).

Numerous phenotypic studies have revealed substantial similarities between normal LPL and PBL T cells; insofar as the CD4$^+$ helper subset predominates, the T cells are almost exclusively of the TCR $\alpha\beta^+$ type and express the leukocyte VLA-4 ($\alpha^4\beta_1$) and LFA-1 ($\alpha^L\beta_2$) integrins at high density. However, unlike T cells in the periphery, where at least half express the CD45R0$^-$ CD45RA$^+$ phenotype of 'naive' or virgin cells, virtually all LPL T cells express the CD45R0 isoform of the leukocyte common antigen, indicative of antigen-primed or memory cells (Smart et al, 1989). LPL T cells are also almost invariably negative for L-selectin (also known as lecin-like cell adhesion molecule, LECAM-1 or Leu-8 antigen) (Kanof et al, 1988; Smart et al, 1988; Berg et al, 1991) but up to 50% express the HML-1 β_7 integrin (Cerf-Bensussan et al, 1987, 1992).

In untreated coeliac disease there are few reports of changes in LPL T-cell markers. Malizia et al (1985) noted an accumulation of semi-activated (CD7$^+$) CD4$^+$ cells in the subepithelial region, and subsequent authors have shown increased expression of CD25 (interleukin (IL) 2 receptor) in LPLs, particularly in the subepithelial region, with an increase in CD25$^+$ CD4$^+$ from <2% to some 15% (Halstensen and Brandtzaeg, 1993). However, this upregulation of CD25 by LPL CD4$^+$ cells is probably modest, since previous authors, using less sensitive techniques, did not observe any marked changes in CD25 expression (Selby et al, 1981; Malizia et al, 1985). We have looked for expression of IL-6 by LPLs, but found that the principal IL-6-containing cells are the enterocytes and that expression did not markedly alter in coeliac disease (Jones et al, 1993). Although the increased TCR $\gamma\delta^+$ cells remain largely in the epithelial compartment, occasional TCR $\gamma\delta^+$ cells have also been observed in the lamina propria (Trejdosiewicz et al, 1991).

Summary

Extensive immunophenotypic studies have shown that IELs are predominantly CD8$^+$ TCR $\alpha\beta^+$ cells expressing the HML-1-defined β_7 integrin, whereas mucosal LPL T cells are mainly CD4$^+$ of the antigen-committed (CD45R0$^+$) phenotype. In coeliac disease there is an increase in the number of IEL blasts, variant TCR $\gamma\delta^+$ types and mitotic IELs. These findings are indicative that the cells have undergone mitotic stimulation. There are also indications of increased IEL activation insofar as the dominant CD8$^+$ subset shows increased expression of CD5, whereas the minority CD4$^+$ subset has upregulated expression of the LFA-1 integrin. Although LPL T-cell populations do not undergo marked changes in numbers, there is an increase in CD7 and CD25 expression by the majority CD4$^+$ subset, both indicative of immune activation.

FUNCTIONAL STUDIES OF MUCOSAL T CELLS

For at least a decade, investigators have attempted to isolate lymphocytes from the intestinal mucosa in order to study their characteristics and functions (e.g. Greenwood et al, 1983; Cerf-Bensussan et al, 1985; Gibson et al, 1985; Smart et al, 1988). In all such studies, the results must be interpreted with caution as the isolation techniques can deplete certain populations (Selby et al, 1984). There may also be problems in the isolation of pure populations of IELs and LPLs. For example, given the subepithelial accumulation of activated CD4$^+$ cells in untreated disease (Malizia et al, 1985), it is likely that IEL populations from coeliac mucosa may be contaminated with LPL-derived CD4$^+$ cells. It must also be remembered that lymphoid aggregates of >90% CD4$^+$ cells are a feature of coeliac, but not normal, small bowel lamina propria (Malizia et al, 1985), which could distort the phenotype of isolated LPLs.

Intraepithelial lymphocytes

It is now well accepted that IELs respond poorly to conventional lectin mitogens or to anti-CD3 antibodies which are mitogenic by virtue of cross-linking the TCR/CD3 complex (reviewed by Trejdosiewicz, 1993). However, culture with sheep erythrocytes does result in efficient stimulation of IELs of colonic origin (Ebert et al, 1986; Ebert, 1989, 1990) and small bowel origin of both TCR $\alpha\beta^+$ and TCR $\gamma\delta^+$ type (Smart et al, 1990; C. J. Smart et al, unpublished results), presumably acting via the CD2 (LFA-2) 'alternate pathway' of T-cell activation. This would accord with the expression of CD58 (LFA-3), a counter-receptor for CD2, by enterocytes (see Trejdosiewicz, 1993). Although the implications of this are that IELs do not respond to antigens presented to the TCR, recent evidence suggests that this is not necessarily so, since IELs have been reported to respond to anti-CD3 cross-linking in the presence of HML-1 antibody (Sarnacki et al, 1992). This would suggest that IELs are not anergic, but rather that they have different accessory molecule requirements from peripheral T cells.

Suppressor cell activity by IELs

The expression of CD8 by the majority of IELs would suggest that they are either suppressor or cytotoxic cells (or both). There is some evidence that colonic IELs can act as suppressor or pro-suppressor cells (reviewed by Trejdosiewicz, 1993), and there is some murine evidence that IELs may exert a non-antigen-specific suppressive effect to dietary antigens at first presentation (Sugita-Konishi et al, 1992). Unlike PBL CD8$^+$ T suppressor–inducer cells, which recognize antigens in the context of MHC class I (HLA-A, B, C), it has been suggested that colonic CD8$^+$ IELs recognize antigens in the context of MHC class II (HLA-D region) antigens, which are expressed constitutively by small bowel enterocytes (see Mayer et al, 1992). Although suppressor effects have been described by some workers (e.g. Hoang et al, 1991), others have found either no immunoregulatory (helper or suppressor) effects (Smart et al, 1988) or at best feeble (Ebert, 1990) suppressor cell activity by human IELs.

Cytotoxicity by IELs

Human IELs display little spontaneous natural killer (NK) activity, although they can be induced to exhibit some cytotoxicity after CD2 or CD3 ligation (Ruthlein et al, 1992). Some lymphokine-activated killer (Ebert and Roberts, 1993) and allogeneic cytolytic activity has also been demonstrated, but not antibody-dependent cellular cytotoxicity (Roberts et al, 1993a). Colonic IELs have been shown to be capable of spontaneously lysing NK-resistant enterocytic cells of colonic carcinoma origin (Taunk et al, 1992), this cytolysis being dependent on the $\alpha^E \beta_7$ integrin (Roberts et al, 1993a). Furthermore, it has been reported that IELs can exert a strong cytotoxic effect on enterotoxin-coated target cells (Cerf-Bensussan et al, 1993). Rust et al (1992) have isolated IEL cell clones of both TCR $\alpha\beta^+$ and TCR $\gamma\delta^+$ type and of CD8$^+$ and CD4$^-$ CD8$^-$ phenotype from coeliac mucosa. Of the CD8$^+$ clones, some expressed CD8 as an $\alpha\beta$ heterodimer, whereas other expressed the CD8 $\alpha\alpha$ homodimer characteristic of some IELs. Functionally, TCR $\gamma\delta^+$ clones were shown to be cytotoxic against a variety of target cells. Thus, the possibility certainly cannot be excluded that some of the pathology of coeliac disease could be due to IEL-mediated damage to enterocytes by TCR $\gamma\delta^+$ cells, perhaps following inappropriate activation, or even due to enterotoxin coating. It is also worth noting that IELs can secrete pleitrophic cytokines, notably interferon-γ and tumour necrosis factor (TNF) (Deem et al, 1991), which are known mediators of cytolytic activity. Furthermore, murine studies suggest that TCR $\gamma\delta^+$ IELs may be alloreactive cytotoxic cells capable of mediating autoimmune phenomena (Barrett et al, 1993). This has interesting implications in view of the increase in TCR $\gamma\delta^+$ IELs in patients with coeliac disease.

Antigen presentation and antigenic specificity of IELs

Given the considerable evidence that IELs are activated in coeliac disease, it may seem paradoxical that antigenic specificity has yet to be demonstrated. We have been unable to detect specific responses to Fraser's gluten fraction III by long-term IEL cell lines isolated from coeliac patients using either antigen alone, or in conjunction with phytohaemagglutinin (PHA) or sheep erythrocytes as a co-mitogen (unpublished results). This apparent inability to detect gluten peptides may reflect unusual accessory molecule requirements for IELs. As noted above, it has been suggested that CD8$^+$ IELs may recognize MHC class II, rather than class I, molecules. More compelling is the evidence that IELs may recognize 'non-conventional' MHC molecules such as the CD1 family (Balk et al, 1991; Panja et al, 1993) or the 'thymus–leukaemia' specificities (Teitell et al, 1991; Wu et al, 1991), perhaps by means of the CD8 $\alpha\alpha$ homodimer exhibited by some IELs. However, there is no evidence as yet that antigenic peptides might be presented by such 'unconventional' MHC-like molecules (discussed by Trejdosiewicz, 1993).

For activation of peripheral T cells, 'professional' antigen-presenting cells are needed to secrete IL-1 and interact with the T cell via 'classical' MHC molecules and via the following additional receptors: (a) LFA-1 (CD11a/CD18) and its counter-receptor ICAM-1 (CD54); and (b) BB1/B7 and/or B70 with counter-receptors CD28 and/or CTLA-4 (see Travers, 1993). Without these interactions, anergy rather than responsiveness occurs. It has been suggested that human enterocytes are unlikely to act as 'professional' antigen-presenting cells (Brandtzaeg et al, 1992) as murine studies would tend to suggest (Barrett et al, 1993). Enterocytes express no detectable mRNA for IL-1, although both IL-6 mRNA (Mayer et al, 1992) and IL-6 protein are readily demonstrable (Jones et al, 1993). Second, as noted above, IELs express low amounts of LFA-1 (Smart et al, 1991). ICAM-1 is also not expressed by normal enterocytes or by enterocytes in treated or untreated coeliac disease (Sturgess et al, 1990; Smart et al, 1991), or indeed even in inflammatory bowel disease, despite the massive upregulation of ICAM-1 in the lamina propria (Malizia et al, 1991). Finally, there is little evidence for CD28 expression by IELs (see Trejdosiewicz, 1993) and BB1/B7 or B70 has not yet been demonstrated on enterocytes. Thus, it seems most unlikely that enterocytes present gluten-derived antigens to IELs by the conventional route. However, the evidence reviewed above strongly suggests that IELs can be activated via CD2 and the TCR in conjunction with β_7, perhaps in the context of 'non-classical' MHC molecules of the CD1 and/or thymus–leukaemia type.

Thus, there are virtually no data on the functional activity of IELs from coeliac mucosa. Clearly, it will be very important to determine whether IELs can recognize gliadin antigen(s) and whether IELs are cytotoxic effector cells that contribute to mucosal damage, or suppressor cells that perhaps fail adequately to downregulate a pro-inflammatory immune response mediated by LPLs in the coeliac lesion (see below).

Lamina propria lymphocytes

Most in vitro studies of intestinal LPLs have concentrated on the colon and few authors have studied small bowel LPLs *per se*. An interesting parallel with IELs is that LPLs are also poor proliferative responders to CD3, but respond well to CD2 stimulation (Pirzer et al, 1990; Qiao et al, 1991a). However, this is thought to be due to mucosal factors, rather than any innate anergy of the LPL, as peripheral blood T cells become similarly unresponsive after culture with intestinal mucosa (Qiao et al, 1991b, 1993). Nevertheless, LPLs do respond to antigen stimulation by secreting cytokines (Zeitz et al, 1988; Strober and Ehrhardt, 1993). It has also been shown that LPLs can exert helper functions (Ming et al, 1989), particularly for the secretion of immunoglobulins of the IgA isotype (Smart et al, 1988).

Recently, Lundin et al (1993) isolated activated T cells and established polyclonal T-cell lines after culture of coeliac biopsy tissue with gluten. These cells recognized wheat proteins, but not proteins from other cereals, when presented by cells expressing the coeliac-associated HLA-DQ heterodimer $\alpha 1*0501$-$\beta 1*0201$ (see Chapter 2). These gluten-reactive T cells were of the $CD4^+$ $CD8^-$ phenotype of lamina propria cells and used diverse combinations of TCR V_α and V_β chains. Such data demonstrate that antigen-specific T-helper cells exist in the coeliac mucosa and, furthermore, that they are MHC class II restricted. This concords with the immunohistological observation of greater CD25 expression by LPL T cells in coeliac disease (Halstensen et al, 1993). The secretion of cytokines by gluten-activated T cells in the coeliac mucosa may therefore be an important factor in the aetiology of mucosal damage.

It has not yet been determined whether $CD4^+$ helper LPLs in either normal or coeliac mucosa are predominantly of the Th_1 ('inflammatory mediator') helper subtype, secreting IL-2, interferon γ and lymphotoxin (TNF-β), the Th_2 helper subtype secreting cytokines involved in promotion of B-cell growth, differentiation and immunoglobulin secretion (IL-4, IL-5, IL-6 and IL-10), or the Th_0 subtype capable of secreting virtually all lymphokines. In humans, Th_0 cells predominate in the periphery but not necessarily in tissues, and the situation with respect to the small intestinal mucosa has not been determined. There are data to suggest that cytokines associated with both Th_1 (IL-2, interferon γ) the Th_2 cells (IL-4) are produced by LPL T cells in the colon after mitogen stimulation or CD2 cross-linking (Zeitz et al, 1988; Strober and Ehrhardt, 1993). As the cytokine milieu is likely to influence local immune responses profoundly, the cytokine secretions in the intestinal mucosa will clearly be a key issue to address.

Organ culture and cellular immunity

Several groups have studied biopsies in organ culture (Howdle et al, 1981), in some cases with the aim of studying cellular immune mechanisms. Ferguson et al (1975) showed that coeliac mucosa challenged in organ culture with α-gliadin secretes a putative cytokine into the supernatant, results subsequently confirmed by Howdle et al (1982), where the cytokine activity was detected by a migration inhibition assay. Non-specific T-cell activation using polyclonal activation has also been investigated in organ culture. In fetal bowel organ culture, pokeweed mitogen and anti-CD3 increases the mitotic rate of enterocytes (MacDonald and Spencer, 1988; Ferreira et al, 1990; Evans et al, 1992) and, furthermore, results in the activation of LPL $CD4^+$ TCR $\alpha\beta^+$ T cells which secrete IL-2 and inter-feron γ, mediating a coeliac-like lesion (MacDonald, 1992). In normal adult small bowel organ cultures, pokewood mitogen and anti-CD3 increased mucus synthesis and secretion in a cyclosporin-dependent manner (Crabtree et al, 1990). Moreover, increased mucus production was also demonstrated in treated but not untreated coeliac disease. These data suggest that T cells may act on enterocytes, perhaps by a cytokine-mediated mechanism, and further suggest that T cells are already highly activated in untreated disease, being incapable of further stimulation.

Recently, it has been shown that organ culture of jejunal biopsies with a peptic–trypic gluten digest resulted in activation of lamina propria T cells of the $CD4^+$ (helper) phenotype within 48 h. The effect occurred only in coeliac biopsies and, interestingly, no increase in IEL activation, numbers of Ki67$^+$ mitotic cells or crypt hyperplasia was observed within this time period (Halstensen et al, 1993). The activation of T helper cells is likely to result in the production of inflammatory cytokines, which would accord with the results obtained in fetal organ culture (MacDonald, 1992). These data also provide further evidence for the hypothesis that antigen-specific responses in the coeliac mucosa are a feature of the lamina propria T helper cell subset (Lundin et al, 1990, 1993).

PERIPHERAL CELLULAR IMMUNITY

Responses in peripheral blood

There have been many attempts over the years to study cellular immune responses in coeliac disease using peripheral blood lymphocytes. The position as regards lymphocyte transformation was summarized by Asquith and Haeney in 1979 and, although there were no consistent findings, they concluded that in untreated coeliac disease there is probably impairment of PHA-stimulated lymphocyte transformation, but stimulation of lymphocyte transformation by gluten subfractions. Investigators have also sought evidence of lymphokine secretion, as demonstrated by significant inhibition of leukocyte migration in response to gluten (Bullen and Losowsky, 1978a; Haeney and Asquith, 1978). However, leukocyte migration inhibition is not exclusively mediated by T-cell factors (Corazza et al, 1989; Simpson et al, 1983a) and could be due to antibody or immune complexes, both of which are present in the circulation in patients with coeliac disease. Because of this potential caveat, leukocyte migration is not now commonly used, although Karagiannis et al (1987) and Mantzaris et al (1990) adopted this approach in the assessment of synthetic gluten-related peptides. Similar to previous studies (Bullen and Losowsky, 1978a), they found increased inhibition by leukocytes from treated rather than untreated coeliac patients. There is evidence, however, that such responses are not specific for gluten but rather represent an increased T-cell reactivity to food antigens (Simpson et al, 1982), presumably as part of the 'oral tolerance' phenomenon.

The macrophage procoagulant assay has been suggested as a more specific test of cell-mediated immunity (Geczy and Hopper, 1981). Using this assay, Devery and colleagues (1990, 1991) showed responses to gluten-derived peptides in the peripheral blood of coeliac but not control donors. A related observation from our laboratory is that an increase in serum-soluble IL-2 receptor in coeliac patients is related to the gluten content of the diet (Crabtree et al, 1989). As soluble IL-2 receptor is principally shed by activated T cells, this is *prima facie* evidence of gluten-related T-cell activation, although it has not yet been determined whether these activated cells are mucosal, in the draining lymph nodes or peripheral T cells stimulated by residual circulating gluten peptides.

Some studies have shown that total circulating lymphocyte numbers are reduced (O'Donoghue et al, 1976; Bullen and Losowsky, 1978b), although the CD4:CD8 balance is not altered (Corazza et al, 1983). Several groups have examined peripheral suppressor cell activity, reporting both increases (Robertson et al, 1982; O'Farrelly et al, 1984a,b) and reductions (Pignata et al, 1985; Corazza et al, 1986; Sollid et al, 1986). O'Farrelly and colleagues (1984a) have suggested that increased helper cell numbers in the small intestine (Malizia et al, 1985) together with increased peripheral suppressor cell activity may reflect a redistribution of T-cell subsets in coeliac disease. Such observations were supported by our findings of an inverse relationship between peripheral and mucosal leukocyte migration inhibition factor production, this being related to the gluten content of the diet, suggesting that in the untreated state gluten-sensitive lymphocytes are more likely to be in the mucosa, at the site of gluten presentation, rather than in the periphery (Howdle et al, 1986).

Skin reactions to gluten

Several groups have attempted to demonstrate peripheral cell-mediated immunity to gluten by skin testing for type IV delayed-type hypersensitivity responses. Asquith and Haeney (1979) reported a positive reaction in only one coeliac patient. Positive reactions were observed by Baker and Read (1978), but the kinetics of the response and histological examination were suggestive of a type III antibody-mediated Arthus reaction. Approximately 50% of coeliac patients were positive in this test. Another study found positive skin reactions in all coeliac patients, although 50% of those with Crohn's disease and 27% of those with ulcerative colitis were also positive (Rawcliffe et al, 1978). There is therefore no evidence of specific T cell-mediated reactions to skin testing with gluten in coeliac patients.

GASTRIC AND RECTAL MUCOSA IN COELIAC DISEASE

The gastric mucosa

There are several old studies of gastric function in coeliac disease which suggest that there is an approximately 40% prevalance of achlorhydria with associated chronic gastritis (reviewed by Marsh, 1992). There are no formal immunohistological studies of the type(s) of infiltrating leukocytes in coeliac disease-associated gastritis. There has been some recent interest in lymphocytic gastritis, which was said to be present in about 50% of patients with 'sprue and sprue-like intestinal lesions' (Wolber et al, 1990). However, this was a poorly controlled retrospective study. Other workers have suggested that lymphocytic gastritis is related to *Helicobacter pylori* infection (Dixon et al, 1988), and we have demonstrated serologically that coeliac patients had a similar prevalence of *H. pylori* colonization as a control population (Crabtree et al, 1992), suggesting that some of the lymphocytic gastritis was probably related to the bacterial infection rather than to coeliac disease *per se*. This is an area requiring further research.

The rectal mucosa

Early studies suggested that some 5% of coeliac patients had an abnormal rectal mucosa (Flick et al, 1962; Dobbins and Rubin, 1964). Breen and colleagues (1987) reported 'procititis' in 11 of 42 coeliac patients who presented with diarrhoea, and Dubois et al (1989) found evidence of 'microscopic lymphocytic colitis' in five of 21 coeliac patients. However, these studies were mainly retrospective and uncontrolled. By contrast, Marsh and colleagues have examined the rectal mucosa in coeliac disease in a formal and systematic way (Loft et al, 1989, 1990). They showed that in untreated coeliac disease there is a mild chronic inflammatory cell infiltrate in the rectal mucosa which resolves following treatment with a gluten-free diet. They also found no alterations from normal in LPLs after rectal challenge with gluten, although there was an increase in the number of IELs, peaking at 6 h. This type of response was predictive of gluten sensitivity in an individual patient and was even more specific when TCR $\gamma\delta^+$ IELs were assessed after challenge (Marsh et al, 1993). Although gliadin specificity for IELs has not been formally demonstrated in vitro, these rectal challenge experiments demonstrate that gliadin sensitivity is not confined to T cells of the small bowel, but rather is mediated by T cells that home to the gut in response to the presence of gluten.

SUMMARY OF T-CELL PERTURBATIONS IN COELIAC DISEASE

The above summarizes a large amount of data demonstrating changes in the cellular immune system occurring in response to dietary gluten.

In the small intestinal mucosa the epithelium becomes infiltrated with T lymphocytes, with a progressive increase in numbers of lymphoblasts. These are $CD8^+$ TCR $\alpha\beta^+$ cells of a mitotic and activated phenotype showing characteristics of memory cells, as well as cells of the variant TCR $\gamma\delta^+$ type. The increase in TCR $\gamma\delta^+$ IELs remains, even in well-treated disease. In the lamina propria there is probably an increase in total T-cell numbers in untreated disease, but the predominant type remains $CD4^+$ memory cells, almost exclusively expressing TCR $\alpha\beta$. There is evidence of $CD4^+$ cell activation and accumulation beneath the epithelium.

The function of intestinal $CD8^+$ cells, predominantly from the epithelium, remains elusive, although there is increasing, albeit indirect, evidence for a cytotoxic role. There is a consensus that IELs respond poorly to mitogenic stimulation via conventional pathways, but increasing evidence pointing to their requirement for unusual accessory co-stimulatory molecules. As yet, no antigenic specificity has been determined for IELs.

The $CD4^+$ population of LPL T helper cells is presumed to be involved in cytokine secretion, although it remains to be determined whether they are inflammatory-mediator, B-cell helper, or intermediate cells according to cytokine secretion profile(s). The demonstration of gluten-specific $CD4^+$ cells suggests a fundamental role for local cytokine-mediated phenomena in coeliac disease, and organ cultures have demonstrated the secretion of lymphokines on gluten challenge.

Rectal challenge studies suggest that gluten-sensitive cells are found throughout the gut in coeliac disease and can rapidly recirculate to sites of antigenic challenge.

PATHOGENESIS OF THE COELIAC LESION

Despite the large body of evidence discussed above, all of which points to T-cell activity and stimulation of the cellular immune system in coeliac disease, this does not necessarily mean that T-cell activity is a primary event in the production of the mucosal lesion. Indeed, it can be argued that most, if not all, of the changes described above are secondary to the exposure of genetically susceptible individuals to dietary gluten. However, some of the data would seem to be of fundamental importance to the pathogenesis of coeliac disease, an example being the gluten-driven lymphocyte infiltration described by Marsh (see Chapter 5) and the gluten-specific MHC-restricted mucosal lymphocytes described by Lundin et al (1990, 1993). The question thus arises that, if cell-mediated immune mechanisms are activated in coeliac disease, are they responsible for the typical lesion and what are the mechanisms involved?

It is known from animal studies that cellular immune responses in the mucosa can mediate villous atrophy and crypt hyperplasia. These studies have used either graft-versus-host disease (MacDonald and Ferguson, 1977; Guy-Grand and Vassalli, 1986; Mowat et al, 1987; Felstein and Mowat, 1988) or a phenomenon thought to be mediated by the same mechanisms, allograft rejection (Holmes et al, 1971; MacDonald and Ferguson, 1976), as the model for cell-mediated immunity (CMI). Both graft rejection and graft versus host disease are thought to be mediated by class II incompatibilities involving activation of $CD4^+$ cells, which in turn recruit cytolytic $CD8^+$ effector cells. Thus, it is interesting to note that in patients with graft versus host disease, there is an infiltration of $CD4^+$ TCR $\alpha\beta^+$ T cells in the intestinal mucosa (Cerf-Bensussan et al, 1993; Kutlu et al, 1993), whereas there is one case report of a patient whose intestinal transplant rejection with villous atrophy and crypt hyperplasia was associated with a heavy infiltrate of TCR $\alpha\beta^+$ $CD8^+$ lymphocytes (Brousse et al, 1992).

As noted above, mitogen activation of T cells in fetal organ cultures can also induce $CD4^+$ T-cell activation, lymphokine secretion and villous atrophy with crypt hyperplasia (MacDonald, 1992). The effect was observed only in tissues obtained after T cells have appeared in the intestine (usually 17–20 weeks of gestation), providing further evidence for a T-cell-mediated pathogenesis. Although this model shows striking similarities with coeliac disease, it should be noted that the characteristic damage to enterocytes does not occur in this fetal in-vitro system. However, these studies have shown that enterocyte proliferation is induced before villous flattening occurs (Ferreira et al, 1990). This would support the work of Marsh (see Chapter 5), who has suggested that lymphocytic infiltration followed by crypt hyperplasia proceed the villous atrophy classically associated with the coeliac lesion.

There are several further observations that have a bearing on the question of CMI involvement in the aetiology of the coeliac lesion. Recent experiments with transgenic 'gene knockout' mice have shown that disruption of certain key cytokines, namely IL-2 (Sadlack et al, 1993) and IL-10 (Kuhn et al, 1993), or disruption of the TCR itself (Mombaerts et al, 1993) all result in spontaneous chronic inflammatory enteropathies, although the lesions resemble those of inflammatory bowel disease rather than coeliac disease. It has been suggested that this type of disruption of cellular immunity leads to reduced suppressor cell activity and hence overproduction of mucosal immunoglobulins (Strober and Ehrhardt, 1993). However, coeliac disease can occur in patients with IgA deficiency and, importantly, there is a well-documented case of a patient with coeliac disease and hypogammaglobulinaemia (Webster et al, 1981). This would suggest that humoral immunity is not important to the development of the mucosal pathology even though most coeliac patients have high titres of mucosal and systemic anti-gliadin antibodies in coeliac disease (see Chapter 3). Furthermore, we have shown that an anti-gliadin monoclonal antibody capable of mediating footpad responses to gliadin challenge in mice did not produce an enteropathy in gliadin-fed animals despite the fact that gliadin feeding produced a reduction in circulating antibody titre (Smart et al, 1992). Although humoral responses have been implicated in the pathogenesis of the coeliac lesion (Brandtzaeg et al, 1993), it is probable that these are secondary to T-cell activation and helper-cell recruitment, although they may be important in the amplification of the immune response and proliferation of mucosa-damaging mechanisms.

Several years ago, we attempted to show that T-cell products could produce an effect on coeliac mucosa in organ culture after 24 h with and without gluten and with and without autologous peripheral blood cells. Culture with both gluten and peripheral leukocytes resulted in a significantly greater reduction in enterocyte height than culture with either gliadin or leukocytes alone (Simpson et al, 1983b). These results were interpreted as suggestive that gluten-specific responses of peripheral leukocytes were capable of provoking damage to autologous jejunal mucosa, possibly as a result of the cytokines that such leukocytes had previously been shown to secrete (Bullen and Losowsky, 1978a). Although this was thought to be a T-cell-mediated phenomenon, further work was obviously necessary to elucidate these intriguing results.

CONCLUSIONS

There is abundant evidence of T-cell activation and involvement in coeliac disease and considerable circumstantial evidence that T cells can produce mucosal changes in a variety of experimental situations. An important question remains as to the mechanisms of production of mucosal lesions. There is little information about this, but the data do suggest that IELs may be involved in enterocytolytic mechanisms and that lamina propria CD4[+] cells can produce inflammation-mediating cytokines, such as IL-2 and interferon γ, as well as helper cytokines, such as IL-4. Pro-inflammatory cytokines enhance T-cell cytolytic activity and it is possible that LPLs thus contribute to IEL activation, and perhaps even induce an autocrine loop, resulting in IEL-mediated enterocyte damage. In addition to their effects on immunocyte function, local cytokines can have effects on other cell types. Thus, interferon γ is a known upregulator of MHC class II expression, and pro-inflammatory cytokines can affect tight junctions and epithelial cell barrier functions (Madara and Stafford, 1989) as well as directly producing epithelial damage (Deem et al, 1991). A scheme of such cellular immunopathogenetic mechanisms, which could be involved in the intestinal mucosa, is outlined in Figure 1.

SUMMARY

Increasing evidence points to a direct role for T cells in the mediation of the coeliac intestinal lesion. There is good evidence for increased local T-cell reactivity, manifest as increased in T-cell activation in the lamina propria

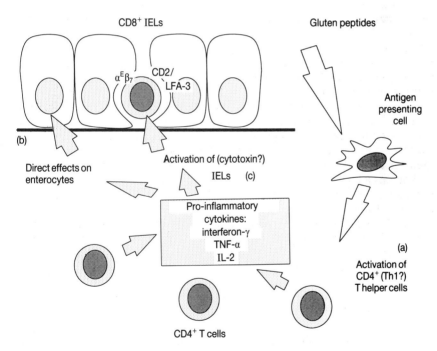

Figure 1. A simplified model for T cell-mediated tissue damage in coeliac disease: (a) Gluten-derived antigenic peptides are presented to sensitized CD4⁺ T helper cells, probably of the T^H1 (inflammatory mediator) subtype, which do not proliferate but activate and respond by secretion of proinflammatory cytokines. (b) Proinflammatory cytokines can act directly on enterocytes, exerting toxic effects and/or modifying their phenotype. (c) Proinflammatory cytokines also help activate the CD8⁺ TcR αβ⁺ and TCR γδ⁺ IELs, which may be stimulated to allocytotoxicity to enterocytes via interactions of CD2 (LFA-2, the sheep erythrocyte receptor on T cells) with CD54 (LFA-3) and the α^Eβ₇ (HML-1) integrin.

and T-cell proliferation in the epithelial compartment. A likely scenario is that gluten elicits antigen-specific responses by lamina propria T helper cells, probably of the *Th1* (inflammatory-mediator) subtype, leading to secretion of pro-inflammatory cytokines. Such cytokines may have direct effects on intestinal enterocytes, as well as mediating indirect effects by upregulation of MHC antigens and by enhancing the activity of cytolytic T cells. Although gluten-specific IEL responses have not been demonstrated by intraepithelial T lymphocytes (IELs), increasing evidence suggests that IELs can act as cytolytic effector cells and hence are likely to exert enteropathic effects under the influence of pro-inflammatory cytokines.

REFERENCES

Asquith P & Haeney MR (1979) Coeliac disease. In Asquith P (ed.) *Immunology of the Gastrointestinal Tract*, pp 66–94. Edinburgh: Churchill Livingstone.

Baker PG & Read AE (1978) Positive skin reactions to wheat, barley and oats in coeliac disease. In McNicholl B, McCarthy CF & Fottrell PF (eds) *Perspectives in Coeliac Disease*, pp 351–363. Lancaster: MTP Press.

Balk SP, Ebert EC, Blumenthal RL et al (1991) Oligoclonal expansion and CD1 recognition by human intestinal intraepithelial lymphocytes. *Science* 253: 1411–1415.

Barrett TA, Delvy ML, Kennedy DM et al (1992) Mechanism of self-tolerance of γ/δ T cells in epithelial tissue. *Journal of Experimental Medicine* 175: 65–70.

Barrett TA, Tatsumi Y & Bluestone JA (1993) Tolerance of T cell receptor γ/δ cells in the intestine. *Journal of Experimental Medicine* 177: 1755–1762.

Berg M, Murakawa Y, Camerini D & James SP (1991) Lamina propria lymphocytes are derived from circulating cells that lack the Leu-8 lymph node homing receptor. *Gastroenterology* 101: 90–99.

Blumberg RS, Yockey CE, Gross GG, Ebert EC & Balk SP (1993) Human intestinal intraepithelial lymphocytes are derived from a limited number of T cell clones that utilize multiple V_β T cell receptor genes. *Journal of Immunology* 150: 5144–5153.

Brandtzaeg P (1989) Overview of the mucosal immune system. *Current Topics in Microbiology and Immunology* 146: 13–25.

Brandtzaeg P, Halstensen TS, Kett K et al (1989a) Immunobiology and immunopathology of human gut mucosa: humoral immunity and intraepithelial lymphocytes. *Gastroenterology* 97: 1562–1584.

Brandtzaeg P, Bosnes V, Halstensen TS et al (1989b) T lymphocytes in human gut epithelium preferentially express the α/β antigen receptor and are often CD45/UCHL1-positive. *Scandinavian Journal of Immunology* 30: 123–128.

Brandtzaeg P, Halstensen TS, Huitfeldt HS et al (1992) Epithelial expression of HLA, secretory component (poly-Ig receptor), and adhesion molecules in the human alimentary tract. *Annals of the New York Academy of Sciences* 664: 157–179.

Brandtzaeg P, Halstensen TS, Hvaturn M et al (1993) The serologic and mucosal immunologic basis of celiac disease. In Walker WA (ed.) *Immunology of the Gut*, pp 295–333. New York: Academic Press.

Breen EG, Coughlan G, Connolly EC et al (1987) Coeliac proctitis. *Scandinavian Journal of Gastroenterology* 22: 471–477.

Brousse N, Sarnacki S, Canioni D & Cerf-Bensussan N (1992) Immunology of intestinal transplantation in man and animal. In MacDonald TT (ed.) *Immunology of Gastrointestinal Diseases*, pp 87–103. London: Kluwer Academic Publishers.

Bullen AW & Losowsky MS (1978a) Cell mediated immunity to gluten fraction III in adult coeliac disease. *Gut* 19: 126–131.

Bullen AW & Losowsky MS (1978b) Lymphocyte subpopulations in adult coeliac disease. *Gut* 19: 892–897.

Cepek KL, Parker CM, Madara JL & Brenner MB (1993) Integrin $\alpha^E\beta_7$ mediates adhesion of T lymphocytes to epithelial cells. *Journal of Immunology* 150: 3459–3470.

Cerf-Bensussan N & Guy-Grand D (1991) Intestinal intraepithelial lymphocytes. *Gastro-enterology Clinics of North America* **20;** 549–576.

Cerf-Bensussan N, Guy-Grand D & Griscelli C (1985) Intraepithelial lymphocytes of human gut: isolation, characterisation and study of natural killer activity. *Gut* **26:** 81–88.

Cerf-Bensussan N, Jarry A, Brousse N et al (1987) A monoclonal antibody (HML-1) defining a novel membrane molecule present on human intestinal lymphocytes. *European Journal of Immunology* **17:** 1279–1285.

Cerf-Bensussan N, Begue B, Gagnon J & Meo T (1992) The human intraepithelial lymphocyte marker HML-1 is an integrin consisting of a β_7 subunit associated with a distinctive α chain. *European Journal of Immunology* **22:** 273–277.

Cerf-Bensussan N, Cerf M & Guy-Grand D (1993) Gut intraepithelial lymphocytes and gastrointestinal diseases. *Current Opinion in Gastroenterology* **9:** 953–961.

Corazza GR, Tabacchi P, Frisoni M et al (1983) T-lymphocyte subsets in adult coeliac disease. *Clinical Science* **65:** 89–90.

Corazza GR, Frisoni M & Gasbarrini G (1984) Jejunal intraepithelial lymphocytes in coeliac disease: are they increased or decreased? *Gut* **25:** 158–162.

Corazza GR, Sardinelli P, Londei M et al (1986) Gluten specific suppressor T cell dysfunction in coeliac disease. *Gut* **27:** 392–398.

Corazza GR, Frisoni M, Mule P et al (1989) Cytophilic antibodies cause leucocyte migration inhibition in coeliac disease. *Journal of Laboratory and Clinical Medicine* **28:** 79–83.

Crabtree JE, Heatley RV, Juby LD et al (1989) Serum interleukin 2 receptor in coeliac disease: response to treatment and gluten challenge. *Clinical and Experimental Immunology* **77:** 345–348.

Crabtree JE, Heatley RV, Trejdosiewicz LK & Losowsky MS (1990) T lymphocyte stimu-lation of small intestinal glycoprotein biosynthesis: effects of anti-CD3 antibody on normal and coeliac mucosa. *International Archives of Allergy and Applied Immunology* **93:** 35–40.

Crabtree JE, O'Mahoney S, Wyatt JI et al (1992) *H. pylori* serology in patients with coeliac disease and dermatitis herpetiformis. *Journal of Clinical Pathology* **45:** 597–600.

Deem RL, Shanahan F & Targan SR (1991) Triggered human mucosal T cells release tumour necrosis factor-alpha and interferon-gamma which kill human colonic epithelial cells. *Clinical and Experimental Immunology* **83:** 79–84.

Devery JM, Geczy CL, de Carle DJ et al (1990) Macrophage procoagulant activity as an assay of cellular hypersensitivy to gluten peptides in coeliac disease. *Clinical and Experimental Immunology* **82:** 333–337.

Devery JM, Bender V, Pentilla I & Skerritt JH (1991) Identification of reactive synthetic gliadin peptides specific for coeliac disease. *International Archives of Allergy and Applied Immunology* **95:** 356–362.

Dhesi I, Marsh MN, Kelly C & Crowe PT (1984) Morphometric analysis of small intestinal mucosa. II: Detemination of lamina propria volumes, plasma cells and neutrophil populations within control and coeliac disease mucosae. *Virchows Archiv* **403:** 173–180.

Dixon M, Wyatt J, Burke D & Rathbone B (1988) Lymphocytic gastritis—relationship with *Campylobacter pylori* infection. *Journal of Pathology* **154:** 125–132.

Dobbins WO (1986) Human intestinal intraepithelial lymphocytes. *Gut* **27:** 972–985.

Dobbins WO & Rubin CE (1964) Studies of the rectal mucosa in coeliac sprue. *Gastro-enterology* **47:** 471–479.

Dubois RN, Lazenby AJ, Yardley JH et al (1989) Lymphocytic enterocolitis in patients with 'refractory sprue'. *Journal of the American Medical Association* **262:** 935–937.

Ebert EC (1989) Proliferative responses of human intraepithelial lymphocytes to various T-cell stimuli. *Gastroenterology* **97:** 1372–1381.

Ebert EC (1990) Intra-epithelial lymphocytes: interferon-gamma production and suppressor/cytotoxic activities. *Clinical and Experimental Immunology* **82:** 81–85.

Ebert EC (1993) Do the CD45RO$^+$CD8$^+$ intestinal intraepithelial T lymphocytes have the characteristics of memory cells? *Cellular Immunology* **147:** 331–340.

Ebert EC & Roberts AI (1993) Lymphokine-activated killing by human intestinal lymphocytes. *Cellular Immunology* **146:** 107–116.

Ebert EC, Roberts AI, Brokin RE & Raska K (1986) Examination of the low proliferative capacity of human jejunal intraepithelial lymphocytes. *Clinical and Experimental Immunology* **65:** 148–157.

Evans CM, Phillips AD, Walker-Smith JA & MacDonald TT (1992) Activation of lamina propria T cells induces crypt epithelial proliferation and goblet cell depletion in cultured human fetal colon. *Gut* **33**: 230–235.

Felstein MV & Mowat AM (1988) Experimental studies of immunologically mediated entero-pathy. IV. Correlation between immune effector mechanisms and type of enteropathy during a GVHR in neonatal mice of different ages. *Clinical and Experimental Immunology* **72**: 108–112.

Ferguson A (1977) Intraepithelial lymphocytes of the small intestine. *Gut* **18**: 921–937.

Ferguson A & Murray D (1971) Quantification of intraepithelial lymphocytes in human jejunum. *Gut* **12**: 988–994.

Ferguson A, MacDonald TT, McClure JP & Holden RJ (1975) Cell mediated immunity to gliadin within the small intestinal mucosa in coeliac disease. *Lancet* **i**: 895–901.

Ferreira RC, Forsyth LE, Richman PI et al (1990) Changes in the rate of crypt epithelial cell proliferation and mucosal morphology induced by a T-cell-mediated response in human small intestine. *Gastroenterology* **98**: 1255–1263.

Flick AL, Vaergthin KF & Rubin CE (1962) Clinical experience with suction biopsy of the rectal mucosa. *Gastroenterology* **42**: 691–705.

Fry L, Seah PP, McMinn RMH & Hoffbrand AV (1972) Lymphocytic infiltration of epithelium in diagnosis of gluten-sensitive enteropathy. *British Medical Journal* **3**: 371–374.

Geczy CL & Hopper KE (1981) A mechanism of migration inhibition in delayed-type hyper-sensitivity reactions. II. Lymphokines promote procoagulant activity of macrophages in vivo. *Journal of Immunology* **126**: 1059–1065.

Gibson PR, Hermanowicz A, Verhaar HJJ et al (1985) Isolation of intestinal mononuclear cells: factors released which affect lymphocyte viability and function. *Gut* **26**: 60–68.

Greenwood JH, Austin LL & Dobbins WO (1983) In vitro characterisation of human intestinal intraepithelial lymphocytes. *Gastroenterology* **85**: 1023–1035.

Guy-Grand D & Vassalli P (1986) Gut injury in mouse graft–versus–host disease. *Journal of Clinical Investigation* **77**: 1584–1595.

Guy-Grand D, Cerf-Bensussan N, Malissen B et al (1991) Two gut intraepithelial CD8[+] lymphocyte populations with different T cell receptors: a role for the gut epithelium in T cell differentiation. *Journal of Experimental Medicine* **173**: 471–481.

Haeney MR & Asquith P (1978) Inhibition of leucocyte migration by α-gliadin in patients with gastrointestinal disease: its specificity with respect to α-gliadin and coeliac disease. In McNicholl B, McCarthy CF & Fottrell PF (eds) *Perspectives in Coeliac Disease*, pp 229–242. Lancaster: MTP Press.

Halstensen TS & Brandtzaeg P (1993) Activated T lymphocytes in the celiac lesion: non-proliferative activation (CD25) of CD4[+] α/β cells in the lamina propria but proliferation (Ki-67) of α/β and γ/δ cells in the epithelium. *European Journal of Immunology* **23**: 505–510.

Halstensen TS, Scott H & Brandtzaeg P (1989) Intraepithelial T cells of the TcR γ/δ[+] CD8[−] $V_{\delta 1}/J_{\delta 1}{}^{+}$ phenotypes are increased in coeliac disease. *Scandinavian Journal of Immunology* **30**: 665–672.

Halstensen TS, Farstad IN, Scott H et al (1990a) Intraepithelial TcR α/β[+] lymphocytes express CD45R0 more often than the TcR γ/δ[+] counterparts in coeliac disease. *Immunology* **71**: 460–466.

Halstensen TS, Scott H & Brandtzaeg P (1990b) Human CD8[+] intraepithelial T lymphocytes are mainly CD45RA[−]RB[+] and show increased co-expression of CD45R0 in celiac disease. *European Journal of Immunology* **20**: 1825–1830.

Halstensen TS, Scott H, Fausa O & Brandtzaeg P (1993) Gluten stimulation of coeliac mucosa in vitro induces activation (CD25) of lamina propria CD4[+] T cells and macrophages but no crypt-cell hyperplasia. *Scandinavian Journal of Immunology* **38**: 581–590.

Hoang P, Dalton HR & Jewell DP (1991) Human colonic intra-epithelial lymphocytes are suppressor cells. *Clinical and Experimental Immunology* **85**: 498–503.

Holm K, Maki M, Savilahti E et al (1992) Intraepithelial γ-δ T-cell-receptor lymphocytes and genetic susceptibility to coeliac disease. *Lancet* **339**: 1500–1503.

Holmes GKT, Asquith P, Stokes PL & Cooke WT (1974) Cellular infiltrate of jejunal biopsies in adult coeliac disease in relation to gluten withdrawal. *Gut* **15**: 278–283.

Holmes JT, Klein MS, Winawer SJ & Fortner JG (1971) Morphological studies of rejection in canine jejunal allografts. *Gastroenterology* **61**: 693–706.

Howdle PD, Corazza GR, Bullen AW & Losowsky MS (1981) Gluten sensitivity of small intestinal mucosa in vitro: quantitative assessment of histologic change. *Gastroenterology* **80:** 442–450.

Howdle PD, Bullen AW & Losowsky MS (1982) Cell-mediated immunity to gluten within the small intestinal mucosa in coeliac disease. *Gut* **23:** 115–122.

Howdle PD, Simpson FG & Losowsky MS (1986) The distribution of gluten-sensitive lymphocytes in coeliac patients—is it related to dietary gluten. *Clinical and Experimental Immunology* **66:** 393–398.

Jarry A, Cerf-Bensussan N, Brousse N et al (1990) Subsets of CD3$^+$ (T cell receptor α/β or γ/δ and CD3$^-$ lymphocytes isolated from normal human gut epithelium display phenotypical features different from their counterparts in peripheral blood. *European Journal of Immunology* **20:** 1097–1103.

Jones SC, Trejdosiewicz LK, Banks RE et al (1993) Expression of interleukin-6 by intestinal enterocytes. *Journal of Clinical Pathology* **46:** 1097–1100.

Kanof ME, Strober W, Fiocchi C et al (1988) CD4 positive Leu-8 negative helper-inducer T cells predominate in the human intestinal lamina propria. *Journal of Immunology* **141:** 3029–3036.

Karagiannis JA, Priddle JD & Jewell DP (1987) Cell mediated immunity to a synthetic gliadin peptide resembling a sequence from adenovirus 12. *Lancet* **i:** 884–886.

Kuhn R, Lohler J, Rennick D et al (1993) Interleukin-10-deficient mice develop chronic enterocolitis. *Cell* **75:** 263–274.

Kutlu T, Brousse N, Rambaud C et al (1993) Numbers of T cell receptor (TcR) $\alpha\beta^+$ but not of TcR $\gamma\delta^+$ intraepithelial lymphocytes correlate with the grade of villous atrophy in coeliac patients on a long term normal diet. *Gut* **34:** 208–214.

Lancaster-Smith M, Kumar PJ & Dawson AM (1975) The cellular infiltrate of the jejunum in adult coeliac disease and dermatitis herpetiformis following the reintroduction of dietary gluten. *Gut* **16:** 683–688.

Loft DE, Marsh MN, Crowe PT et al (1989) Studies of intestinal lymphoid tissue. XII: Epithelial lymphocyte and mucosal response to rectal gluten challenge on celiac sprue. *Gastroenterology* **97:** 29–37.

Loft DE, Marsh MN & Crowe PT (1990) A prospective study of rectal gluten challenge: a new diagnostic test for coeliac disease. *Lancet* **335:** 1293–1295.

Lundin KEA, Sollid LM, Qvigstad E et al (1990) T lymphocyte recognition of a celiac disease-associated *cis-* or *trans-*encoded HLA-DQ α/β heterodimer. *Journal of Immunology* **145:** 136–139.

Lundin KEA, Scott H, Hansen T et al (1993) Gliadin-specific HLA-DQ(α1*0501, β1*0201) restricted T cells isolated from the small intestinal mucosa of celiac disease patients. *Journal of Experimental Medicine* **178:** 187–196.

MacDonald TT (1992) T cell mediated intestinal injury. In Marsh MN (ed.) *Coeliac Disease*, pp 283–304. Oxford: Blackwell Scientific Publications.

MacDonald TT & Ferguson A (1976) Hypersensitivity reactions in the small intestine. II. The effect of allograft rejection on mucosal architecture and lymphoid cell infiltrate. *Gut* **17:** 81–91.

MacDonald TT & Ferguson A (1977) Hypersensitivity reaction in the small intestine. III. The effect of allograft rejection and graft-versus-host disease as epithelial cell kinetics. *Cell and Tissue Kinetics* **10:** 301–312.

MacDonald TT & Spencer J (1988) Evidence that activated mucosal T cells play a role in the pathogenesis of enteropathy in human small intestine. *Journal of Experimental Medicine* **167:** 1341–1349.

Madara JL & Stafford J (1989) Interferon-gamma directly affects barrier function of cultured intestinal epithelial monolayers. *Journal of Clinical Investigation* **83:** 724–727.

Mäki M, Holm K, Collin P & Savilahti E (1991) Increase in γ/δ T cell receptor bearing lymphocytes in normal small bowel mucosa in latent coeliac disease. *Gut* **32:** 1412–1414.

Malizia G, Trejdosiewicz LK, Wood GM et al (1985) The microenvironment of coeliac disease: T cell phenotypes and expression of the T2 'T blast' antigen by small bowel lymphocytes. *Clinical and Experimental Immunology* **60:** 437–446.

Malizia G, Calabrese A, Cottone M et al (1991) Expression of leukocyte adhesion molecules by mucosal mononuclear phagocytes in inflammatory bowel disease. *Gastroenterology* **100:** 150–159.

Mantzaris GJ, Karagiannis JA, Priddle JD & Jewell DP (1990) Cellular hypersensitivity to a synthetic dodecapeptide derived from human adenovirus 12 which resembles a sequence of A-gliadin in patients with coeliac disease. *Gut* **31**: 668–673.

Marsh MN (1980) Studies of intestinal lymphoid tissue. III: Quantitative analyses of epithelial lymphocytes in the small intestine of human control subjects and of patients with celiac sprue. *Gastroenterology* **79**: 481–492.

Marsh MN (1992) Mucosal pathology in gluten sensitivity. In Marsh MN (ed.) *Coeliac Disease*, pp 136–191. Oxford: Blackwell Scientific Publications.

Marsh MN, Bjarnasson I, Shaw J et al (1990) Studies of intestinal lymphoid tissue. XIV: HLA status, mucosal morphology, permeability and epithelial lymphocyte populations in first degree relatives of patients with coeliac disease. *Gut* **31**: 32–36.

Marsh MN, Ensari A & Morgan S (1993) Evidence that gluten sensitivity is an immunologic disease. *Current Opinion in Gastroenterology* **9**: 994–1000.

Mayer L, Panja A, Li Y et al (1992) Unique features of antigen presentation in the intestine. *Annals of the New York Academy of Sciences* **664**: 39–46.

Micklem KJ, Dong Y, Willis A et al (1991) HML-1 antigen on mucosa-associated T cells, activated cells, and hairy leukemic cells is a new integrin containing the β_7 subunit. *American Journal of Pathology* **139**: 1297–1301.

Ming RH, Stickland RG, Listron M & Fengoglio-Preiser C (1989) The CD4 Leu8⁻ T helper cell in colonic mucosa: a quantitative and functional analysis. *Clinical and Experimental Immunology* **75**: 297–300.

Mombaerts P, Mizoguchi E, Grusby M et al (1993) Spontaneous development of inflammatory bowel disease in T cell receptor mutant mice. *Cell* **75**: 275–282.

Mowat AM, Felstein MV & Baca ME (1987) Experimental studies of immunologically mediated enteropathy III. Severe and progressive enteropathy during a graft-versus-host reaction in athymic mice. *Immunology* **61**: 185–188.

O'Donoghue DP, Lancaster-Smith M, Laviniere P & Kumar PJ (1976) T cell depletion in untreated adult coeliac disease. *Gut* **17**: 328–331.

O'Farrelly C, Feighery CF, Whelan CA & Weir DG (1984a) Suppressor cell activity in coeliac disease induced by α-gliadin, a dietary antigen. *Lancet* **ii**: 1305–1307.

O'Farrelly C, McKeever V, Feighery CF & Weir DG (1984b) Increased concanavalin A-induced suppression in treated and untreated coeliac disease. *Gut* **25**: 644–648.

Panja A, Blumberg RS, Balk SP & Mayer L (1993) CD1d is involved in T cell-intestinal epithelial cell interactions. *Journal of Experimental Medicine* **178**: 1115–1119.

Parker CM, Cepek KL, Russell GJ et al (1992) A family of β_7 integrins on human mucosal lymphocytes. *Proceedings of the National Academy of Sciences of the USA* **89**: 1924–1928.

Pignata C, Troncone R, Monaco G et al (1985) Impaired suppressor activity in children affected by coeliac disease. *Gut* **26**: 285–290.

Pirzer UC, Schurmann G, Post S et al (1990) Differential responsiveness to CD3-Ti vs CD2-dependent activation of human intestinal T lymphocytes. *European Journal of Immunology* **20**: 2239–2342.

Qiao L, Schurmann G, Betzler M & Meuer SC (1991a) Activation and signaling status of human lamina propria T lymphocytes. *Gastroenterology* **101**: 1529–1536.

Qiao L, Schurmann G, Betzler M & Meuer S (1991b) Down-regulation of protein kinase C activation in human lamina propria T lymphocytes: influence of intestinal mucosa on T cell reactivity. *European Journal of Immunology* **21**: 2385–2389.

Qiao L, Schurmann G, Autschbach F et al (1993) Human intestinal mucosa regulates T cell activities. *Gastroenterology* **105**: 814–819.

Rawcliffe PM, Anand BS, Offord RE et al (1978) A skin test for coeliac diseae. In McNicholl B, McCarthy CF & Fottrell (eds) *Perspectives in Coeliac Disease*, pp 347–349. Lancaster: MTP Press.

Roberts AI, O'Connell SM, Baincone L et al (1993a) Spontaneous cytotoxicity of intestinal intraepithelial lymphocytes: clues to the mechanism. *Clinical and Experimental Immunology* **94**: 527–532.

Roberts AI, O'Connell SM & Ebert EC (1993b) Intestinal intraepithelial lymphocytes bind to colon cancer cells by HML-1 and CD11a. *Cancer Research* **53**: 1608–1611.

Robertson DAF, Bullen AW, Field HP et al (1982) Suppressor cell activity, splenic function and HLA-B8 status in man. *Journal of Clinical and Laboratory Immunology* **9**: 133–138.

Rocha B, Vassalli P & Guy-Grand D (1991) The Vβ repertoire of mouse gut homodimeric α CD8$^+$ intraepithelial T cell receptor α/β$^+$ lymphocytes reveals a major extrathymic pathway of T cell differentiation. *Journal of Experimental Medicine* 173: 483–486.

Rocha B, Vassalli P & Guy-Grand D (1992) The extrathymic T-cell development pathway. *Immunology Today* 13: 449–454.

Russell GJ, Nagler-Anderson C, Anderson P & Bhan A (1993) Cytotoxic potential of intra-epithelial lymphocytes (IELs): presence of TIA-1, the cytolytic granule-associated protein, in human IELs in normal and diseased intestine. *American Journal of Pathology* 143: 350–354.

Rust C, Kooy Y, Pena S et al (1992) Phenotypical and functional characterisation of small intestinal TcR γδ$^+$ T cells in coeliac disease. *Scandinavian Journal of Immunology* 35: 459–468.

Ruthlein J, Heinze G & Auer IO (1992) Anti-CD2 and anti-CD3 induced T cell cytotoxicity of human intraepithelial and lamina propria lymphocytes. *Gut* 33: 1626–1632.

Sadlack B, Merz H, Schorle H et al (1993) Ulcerative colitis-like disease in mice with a disrupted interleukin-2 gene. *Cell* 75: 253–261.

Sarnacki S, Begue B, Buc H et al (1992) Enhancement of CD3-induced activation of human intestinal intraepithelial lymphocytes by stimulation of the β$_7$-containing integrin defined by HML-1 monoclonal antibody. *European Journal of Immunology* 22: 2887–2892.

Savilahti E, Arato A & Verkasalo M (1990) Intestinal γ/δ receptor-bearing T lymphocytes in celiac disease and inflammatory bowel diseases in children. Constant increase in celiac disease. *Pediatric Research* 28: 579–581.

Savilahti E, Reunala T & Maki M (1992) Increase of lymphocytes bearing the γ/δ T cell receptor in the jejunum of patients with dermatitis herpetiformis. *Gut* 33: 206–211.

Schieferdecker HL, Ullrich R, Weiss-Breckwoldt AN et al (1990) The HML-1 antigen of intestinal lymphocytes is an activation antigen. *Journal of Immunology* 144: 2541–2549.

Selby WS, Janossy G, Bofill M & Jewell DP (1981) Lymphocyte subpopulations in the human intestine. The findings in normal mucosa and in the mucosa of patients with adult coeliac disease. *Clinical and Experimental Immunology* 52: 219–228.

Selby WS, Janossay G, Bofill M & Jewell DP (1984) Intestinal lymphocyte subpopulations in inflammatory bowel disease: an analysis by immunohistological and cell isolation tech-niques. *Gut* 25: 32–40.

Simpson FG, Robertson DAF, Howdle PD & Losowsky MS (1982) Cell mediated immunity to dietary antigens in coeliac disease. *Scandinavian Journal of Gastroenterology* 17: 671–676.

Simpson FG, Field HP, Howdle PD et al (1983a) Leucocyte migration inhibition test in coeliac disease—a reappraisal. *Gut* 24: 311–317.

Simpson FG, Howdle PD, Robertson DAF & Losowsky MS (1983b) Jejunal biopsy and lymphocyte co-culture in coeliac disease. *Scandinavian Journal of Gastroenterology* 18: 749–754.

Smart CJ, Trejdosiewicz LK, Badr-el-Din S & Heatley RV (1988) T lymphocytes of the human colonic mucosa: functional and phenotypic analysis. *Clinical and Experimental Immunology* 73: 63–69.

Smart CJ, Heatley RV & Trejdosiewicz LK (1989) Expression of CD6 and the UCHL1-defined CD45 (p180) antigen by human colonic T lymphocytes. *Immunology* 66: 90–65.

Smart CJ, Howdle PD, Boylston AW & Trejdosiewicz LK (1990) Intraepithelial T cell clones from the small intestinal mucosa of coeliac patients. *Gut* 31: A1193.

Smart CJ, Calabrese A, Oakes DJ et al (1991) Expression of the LFA-1 β$_2$ integrin (CD11a/CD18) and ICAM-1 (CD54) expression in normal and coeliac small bowel mucosa. *Scandinavian Journal of Immunology* 34: 229–305.

Smart CJ, Trejdosiewicz LK & Howdle PD (1992) Specific circulating anti-gliadin IgG-class antibody does not mediate intestinal enteropathy in gliadin-fed mice. *International Archives of Allergy and Applied Immunology* 97: 160–166.

Sollid LM, Brusend O, Gauderneck G & Thorsby E (1986) The role of the CD8-positive subset of T cells in proliferative responses to soluble antigens. *Scandinavian Journal of Immunology* 23: 461–467.

Spencer J, Isaacson PG, Diss TC & MacDonald TT (1989) Expression of disulfide-linked and non-disulfide-linked forms of the T cell receptor γ/δ heterodimer in human intestinal intraepithelial lymphocytes. *European Journal of Immunology* 19: 1335–1338.

Spencer J, Isaacson PG, MacDonald TT et al (1991) γ/δ T cells and the diagnosis of coeliac disease. *Clinical and Experimental Immunology* **85**: 109–113.

Strober W & Ehrhardt RO (1993) Chronic intestinal inflammation: an unexpected outcome in cytokine or T cell receptor mutant mice. *Cell* **75**: 203–205.

Sturgess RP, Macartney JC, Makgoba MW et al (1990) Differential upregulation of inter-cellular adhesion molecule-1 in coeliac disease. *Clinical and Experimental Immunology* **82**: 489–492.

Sugita-Konishi Y, Smart CJ & Trejdosiewicz LK (1992) Regulation of intestinal immuno-globulin production in response to dietary ovalbumin. *International Archives of Allergy and Applied Immunology* **98**: 64–69.

Taunk J, Roberts AI & Ebert EC (1992) Spontaneous cytotoxicity of human intraepithelial lymphocytes against epithelial cell tumors. *Gastroenterology* **102**: 69–75.

Teitell M, Mescher MF, Olson CA et al (1991) The thymus leukemia antigen binds human and mouse CD8. *Journal of Experimental Medicine* **174**: 1131–1138.

Travers P (1993) Immunological agnosia. *Nature* **363**: 117–118.

Trejdosiewicz LK (1992) Intestinal intraepithelial lymphocytes and lymphoepithelial inter-actions in the human gastrointestinal mucosa. *Immunology Letters* **32**: 13–19.

Trejdosiewicz LK (1993) What is the role of human intestinal intraepithelial lymphocytes? *Clinical and Experimental Immunology* **94**: 395–397.

Trejdosiewicz LK, Smart CJ, Oakes DJ et al (1989) Expression of T-cell receptors TcR1 (γ/δ) and TcR2 (α/β) in the human intestinal mucosa. *Immunology* **68**: 7–12.

Trejdosiewicz LK, Calabrese A, Smart CJ et al (1991) γδ T cell receptor-positive cells of the human gastrointestinal mucosa: occurrence and V region gene expression in *Helicobacter pylori*-associated gastritis, coeliac disease and inflammatory bowel disease. *Clinical and Experimental Immunology* **84**: 440–444.

Van Kerckhove C, Russell GJ, Deusch K et al (1992) Oligoclonality of human intestinal intraepithelial T cells. *Journal of Experimental Medicine* **175**: 57–63.

Webster ADB, Slavin G, Shiner M et al (1981) Coeliac disease with severe hypogamma-globulinaemia. *Gut* **22**: 153–157.

Wolber R, Owen D, DelBuono L et al (1990) Lymphocytic gastritis in patients with celiac sprue or spruelike intestinal disease. *Gastroenterology* **98**: 310–315.

Wu M, van Kaer L, Itohara S & Tonegawa S (1991) Highly restricted expression of the thymus leukemia antigens on intestinal epithelial cells. *Journal of Experimental Medicine* **174**: 213–218.

Zeitz M, Quinn TC, Graeff AS & James SP (1988) Mucosal T cells provide helper function but do not proliferate when stimulated by specific antigen in lymphogranuloma venereum proctitis in nonhuman primates. *Gastroenterology* **94**: 353–366.

5

Morphology of the mucosal lesion in gluten sensitivity

MICHAEL N. MARSH
PETER T. CROWE

The introduction of the peroral jejunal biopsy technique in the late 1950s provided a highly specific test for distinguishing gluten-induced, from non-gluten-associated, forms of intestinal malabsorption. Thus, from 1960 onwards, the demonstration of a severe proximal mucosal lesion confirmed a clinical diagnosis of gluten sensitivity (or symptomatic 'coeliac disease') in any person presenting with steatorrhoea or weight loss, in addition to a severe nutritional impairment such as chronic iron deficiency (Rubin et al, 1960; Booth, 1970).

That position has now changed. In recent years it has become apparent that histological changes of lesser degrees are also consistent with a state of gluten sensitivity (Marsh 1992a,b, 1993a) (Figure 1) and that a considerable

Table 1. Family studies: latent individuals with flat–destructive lesions.

Region	Reference	Flat lesions in first-degree relatives (%)	Asymptomatic (latent) gluten-sensitive relatives with a flat mucosa (%)	Families affected with additional cases (%)
Seattle, Washington	MacDonald et al (1965)	10	50	35
Galway, Ireland	Mylotte et al (1974)	10	50	25
Birmingham, UK	Stokes et al (1976)	20	50	—
Melbourne, Australia	Shipman et al (1975)	10	45	25
Birmingham, UK	Rolles et al (1974)	6	55	20
Mean		11	50	26

In all series, approximately 11% of relatives were found to have a type 3 flat–destructive lesion of upper jejunal mucosa; of these, approximately 50% were latent or asymptomatic. Only one quarter of all families surveyed revealed additional cases of latent gluten sensitivity.

Baillière's Clinical Gastroenterology—
Vol. 9, No. 2, June 1995
ISBN 0–7020–1953–4

number of gluten-sensitized individuals are asymptomatic, to whom the term 'latent' should thus be applied. Several studies over the years have amply demonstrated that latent gluten sensitivity may be associated with any type of mucosal abnormality, ranging from a superficially normal appearance to the severe classical flat lesion (Table 1).

At this point, some definitions need to be advanced. Gluten sensitivity is defined as a state of heightened immunological responsiveness to gluten protein in a genetically predisposed (DQw2) individual. Within that framework will be encompassed asymptomatic (latent) individuals irrespective of degree of proximal mucosal involvement, and symptomatic patients who will either have classical features (coeliac disease) or certain atypical features (Table 2).

This chapter examines the architectural (histological) features of the varied mucosal responses in gluten sensitivity, their dynamic interrelationships and pathogenesis.

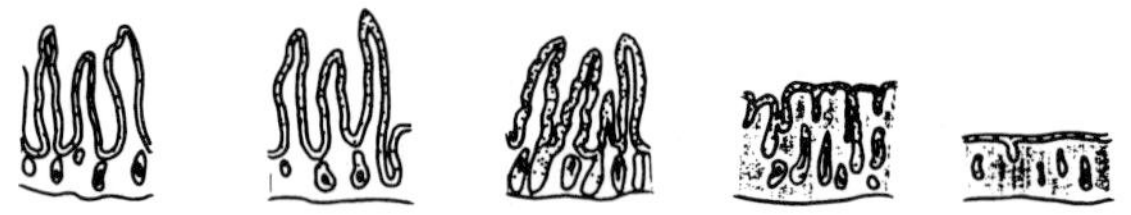

	"PRE-" INFILTRATIVE (TYPE 0)	"INFILTRATIVE" (TYPE 1)	"INFILTRATIVE - HYPERPLASTIC" (TYPE 3)	"FLAT DESTRUCTIVE" (TYPE 3)	"ATROPHIC - HYPOPLASTIC" (TYPE 4)
■ 1 PROLAMINE HYPERSENSITIVITIES : WHEAT, BARLEY, RYE, OATS	+	+	+	+	+
■ 2 INFECTIVE / PARASITIC : GIARDIASIS/CRYPTOSPORIDIOSIS INFECTIVE ENTERITIS AIDS ENTEROPATHY	+	+	+	+	
■ 3 TROPICAL DIARRHOEA - MALABSORPTION SYNDROME : ("TROPICAL SPRUE AND TROPICAL ENTEROPATHY")	+	+	+	+	
■ 4 GRAFT-VERSUS-HOST DISEASE :		+	+	+	
■ 5 TRANSIENT FOOD SENSITIVITIES : MILK PROTEINS, EGG, SOYA CHICKEN, FISH		+	+	+	

Figure 1. Representative drawings of the main five lesions associated with gluten sensitivity. In becoming flat, the mucosa passes through an initial phase in which hypertrophy of the crypts is a substantial architectural change before villous flattening, or increased enterocyte losses, occur. The so-called 'haemolytic' model is no longer able to account for mucosal flattening. A comparison is drawn with other conditions, in which one or more types of mucosal response have been described, such as giardiasis, tropical enteric diseases and various transient food protein sensitivities. In all of these, it is evident that the spectrum of responses is identical and typical of intestinal cell-mediated immune responses to the inciting antigen(s). Only with a synthesis of this kind can the various types of mucosal responses seen with these antigens be fully understood. However, the emergence of a truly atrophic, unresponsive mucosa (type 4) appears to occur with gluten sensitivity alone, usually as a result of lymphoma. The pre-infiltrative (type 0) lesion occurs with high-titre, local antigliadin antibody production. Reproduced from Marsh (1992c, *Gastroenterology* 102: 330–354) with permission.

Table 2. Gluten sensitivity: typical and atypical features.

Typical	Atypical
Weakness and fatigue	Pigmentation, hypotension (?Addison's
Weight loss	disease)
Diarrhoea	Rapid weight loss with or without diarrhoea
Abdominal distension	(hyperthyroidism, diabetes)
Nausea, vomiting and anorexia	Hair loss
Cramps, tetany	Unusual skin rashes
Skin bleeding	Arthropathy, 'rheumatism' (vitamin D
Oedema	deficiency)
Glossitis	Arthropathy (mono/poly) (small or large
	joint inflammation)
	Peripheral neuropathy
	Abdominal pain
	Dental hyperplasia
	Infertility
	Growth defect
	Abnormal liver function tests

THE CLASSICAL FLAT LESION

This is a very complicated lesion that involves all parts of the mucous membrane, i.e. surface epithelium, crypt epithelium and lamina propria. Because it has become so commonplace to examine biopsy specimens of the mucous membrane (or even more superficial tissue fragments obtained endoscopically), we have forgotten that the gluten-induced lesion also involves the submucosa. Thus the intestinal wall is more extensively inflamed than often realized, as is evident both from Paulley's original full-thickness laparotomy specimens (Paulley, 1954) and from Loft's gluten challenge work on rectal mucosa (Loft et al, 1989).

The major features of the flat lesion, critically evaluated by Rubin and colleagues (1960), comprise the vastly hypertrophied crypts and the characteristically flattened, or cuboidal, enterocytes that lie on the mucosal surface between the widened crypt wells (Marsh, 1972). In the past it was generally accepted that the surface enterocyte is directly damaged by gluten; however, there is no evidence to substantiate this view, and other possible causes for the presence of abnormal cells must be considered (Marsh, 1992b,c; see review by Crowe and Marsh, 1993). There is also a paradox in that while these 'damaged' cells manifest low brush-border membrane hydrolase activity, they nevertheless retain the ability to upregulate expression of secretory component and major histocompatibility (MHC) class 2 allo-antigen.

It has been widely assumed and concluded that because the surface enterocytes have a reduced cuboidal profile when observed in section, they are necessarily small cells. This conclusion, however, is not self-evident, as many experimental studies of the restitution and healing of surgically inflicted epithelial lesions readily show. The phenomenon of small surface cells is not, of course, exclusive to gluten sensitivity, but is a characteristic of most other flat lesions resulting from tropical diarrhoea–malabsorption syndrome, giardiasis, immunoproliferative small intestinal disease, immunodeficiency and so on. What is even more interesting is that the reason for such a curious cellular response to injury has, to our knowledge, never been questioned or investigated.

In our laboratory we have actually demonstrated by computerized image analysis (Marsh, 1988) that the mean volume of surface enterocytes in a

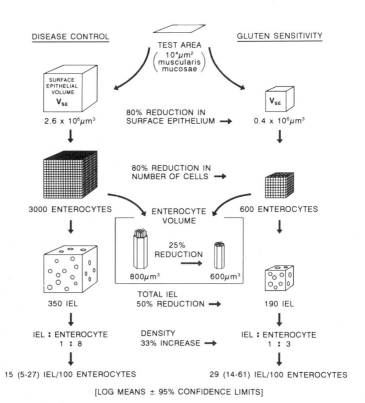

Figure 2. Morphometric analysis of small intestinal mucosa was performed by computerized image analysis, based on a reference test area ($10^4\ \mu m^2$) of muscularis mucosa; the latter acts as a third-party invariant structure for all other variables measured, or derived by calculation. The overlying volume of surface epithelium (V_{SE}) is reduced by a mean of 80% in a severe, flat, gluten-induced lesion. Likewise, the total number of enterocytes within V_{SE} is reduced by 80%, from 3000 to 600, while their mean volume is reduced by 25% from 800 to 600 μm^3. Likewise, V_{SE} contains an absolute population of IELs, reduced by 50% in flat mucosa, although their density is increased from 1 IEL per 8 enterocytes (control) to 1 IEL per 3 enterocytes (or 13, and 33 IEL per 100 enterocytes, respectively). However, profile density counts (Ferguson and Murray, 1971) performed on the same groups of patients yield values of 24 and 61 IEL per 100 enterocytes, respectively, which are clearly inaccurate, since they are twice the absolute value. For an explanation of this anomaly and the errors that lead to this two-fold error in IEL populations, see Crowe and Marsh (1993, 1994). New revised log-transformed ranges ($\pm 95\%$ confidence limits) for IELs, based on controlled morphometric analysis for disease control and untreated gluten sensitivity, are 15 (5–27) and 29 (14–61), respectively.

severe flat–destructive (type 3) lesion is reduced by 25%, from approximately 800 μm^3 to 600 μm^3 (Figure 2) (Crowe and Marsh, 1993). Since the mean volume of the flattened surface epithelium is reduced by 80% (from 2.6 to $0.4 \times 10^6 \mu m^3$), the mean overall reduction in enterocyte populations between control (3000) and flat gluten-sensitive (600) mucosa is 80% (Crowe and Marsh, 1993).

From these data, the absolute relationship of intraepithelial lymphocytes (IELs) to enterocytes is 1 in 8 for disease-control mucosa, and 1 in 3 for flat gluten-induced lesions. The actual numerical values (and ranges) for IELs given here are lower, by a factor of two, than conventional profile-density counts (Figure 2). The reasons for this discrepancy and their overestimation have been detailed in a series of 'proofs' elsewhere (Crowe and Marsh, 1993, 1994).

The actual density of IELs is increased in flat mucosa by 1 in 5, representing a rise in percentage epithelial volume occupancy of 2.5, compared with a control value of 0.65. Furthermore, it must always be borne in mind that, in gluten sensitivity, the crypts carry a considerably greater increase in IELs than surface epithelium (Marsh and Hinde, 1986), yet their capacity to increase the size, rate of cell division and migration, to upregulate expression of MHC class 2 surface alloantigen and to maintain production of differentiated cells (Paneth, endocrine, goblet) is clearly unimpaired.

IELs (both $CD3^+$ and $\gamma\delta^+$) display an increased rate of mitotic activity (Marsh, 1982; Marsh and Haeney, 1983), which is more accurately quantifiable immunohistochemically with Ki-67 monoclonal antibody (Halstensen et al, 1990). IELs are also increased in size but this is not directly related to the presence of antigen (gluten), since in milder lesions IELs are of normal size and virtually non-mitotic. It may be that proliferation maintains the size of a subpopulation of resident IELs when the mucosa is most severely damaged, although speculative views of this type require further detailed critical examination.

Immunocytochemistry has revealed that IEL populations are extremely heterogeneous and, despite considerable investigation over several decades, their real function is still unknown. Moreover, their relevance to the immunopathology of gluten sensitivity is equally uncertain. The only reality is that gluten evokes dose-dependent rises in the IEL population (both $CD3^+$ and $\gamma\delta^+$).

THE INFILTRATIVE–HYPOPLASTIC LESIONS OF GLUTEN SENSITIVITY

The infiltrative lesion of gluten sensitivity was first identified by Fry and colleagues (1972, 1974) who, in proximal biopsies taken from patients with dermatitis herpetiformis, noted marked infiltrations of IELs within a structurally normal mucosa which were sensitive to gluten withdrawal. The significance of such infiltrates has, perhaps, become interpretable only in the light of studies on graft-versus-host reactions in experimental animals (MacDonald, 1992; Ferguson, 1987), which indicate that this kind of host response, with accompanying crypt hypertrophy (Mowat and Ferguson, 1982), is a local T-cell-dependent response of intestinal mucosa to foreign antigen.

Although these lesions have sporadically been observed in gluten-sensitive subjects (Mäki et al, 1990), and in studies of family relatives of known coeliac malabsorption cases (Marsh et al, 1990), they have best been

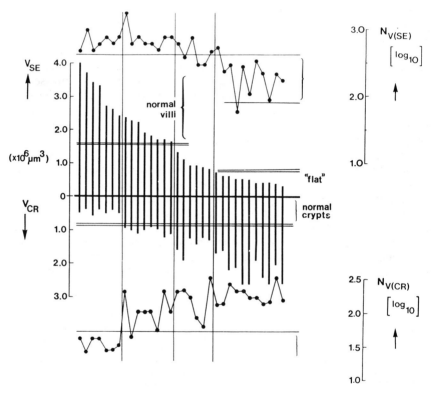

Figure 3. Mucosa from 32 patients with untreated dermatitis herpetiformis DH are displayed (left to right) in terms of surface epithelial volumes ($\times 10^6\,\mu m^3$) (V_{SE} vertical axis) and, below zero, corresponding crypt epithelial volumes (V_{CR}). Horizontal paired lines represent lower range for control villi (V_{SE}), upper range for 'flat' untreated coeliac sprue mucosa (V_{SE}) and upper range for control crypts (V_{CR}). Values for lymphoid populations within surface ($N_{v,SE}$) and crypt ($N_{v,CR}$) epithelium are displayed on right-hand axes, and expressed logarithmically; horizontal lines on these axes represent the lower and upper range for IEL populations in villi and the upper range for crypts, respectively. The first seven mucosae (up to the first vertical line) are normal except for lymphocytic infiltration of villous epithelium (infiltrative lesions). The next eight mucosae (up to the second vertical line) reveal crypt hypertrophy exceeding the upper reference range, and are now infiltrated with small lymphocytes (infiltrative-hypertrophic lesions). Flat mucosae (beyond the third vertical line) reveal marked crypt hypertrophy and sustained lymphoid infiltration; however, the flattened surface epithelium now contains a reduced number of lymphocytes (flat–destructive lesions) that, numerically, lie within the control reference range (bracketed). Reproduced from Marsh (1989, *Virchows Archiv. A, Pathological Anatomy and Histopathology* **416:** 125–132, © Springer-Verlag) with permission.

categorized in large series of patients with dermatitis herpetiformis, many of whom illustrate the infiltrative–hyperplastic lesion (Marsh, 1989a). Here, there is crypt hypertrophy, often with accompanying lymphocytic infiltrates, in addition to infiltration of villous epithelium (Figure 3).

Certain statements and conclusions about these lesser forms of mucosal change in gluten-sensitive patients need to be made. As observed above, it is difficult to envisage that these lymphocytic infiltrates damage either mucosa or enterocytes, because there is no evidence for structural or functional impairment, and because the crypts themselves remain unscathed. Although the lymphoid infiltrate in these cases is gluten-driven, the phenomenon is a non-specific event and its other causes (Table 3) need to be considered when the histological differential diagnosis is considered. It therefore seems the most plausible explanation that receptors, expressed on the enterocyte membrane, display luminal antigen (food derived, microbial elements, etc.) that leads to infiltration either via the basement membrane (and this probably applies to $CD3^+$, $CD8^+$, $\alpha\beta^+$ cells arriving from lamina propria) or by interepithelial proliferation of resident IEL subsets (as, for example, T-cell receptor (TCR) $\gamma\delta^+$ cells). The slower rise in $\gamma\delta^+$ TCR cells, compared with $CD8^+$ $\alpha\beta^+$ cells, following antigen challenge may, in fact, reflect a differential in mitotic activity and hence their potential to expand in response to the appropriate local antigenic signal.

Given that, the disposition of lymphocytes within epithelium does provide a reference point for the identification and conceptual representation ('pattern recognition') of the spectrum of mucosal change and injury characteristic of gluten-sensitized individuals. The non-specificity of these responses, however, is also emphasized when it is noted that similar tissue

Table 3. Causes of flat, and infiltrative, mucosal lesions.

Flat–destructive mucosa (type 3)	Lymphocyte-infiltrated mucosa (types 1 and 2)
Tropical bowel disease	Gluten sensitivity
Immunodeficiency	Tropical bowel disease
Immunoproliferative disease of small intestine	Infective or parasitic
	Giardiasis
Intestinal lymphoma	Cryptosporidiosis
Drug-induced	Acute infection (Norwalk etc.)
Infestation (parasitic)	Acquired immune deficiency syndrome
Giardiasis	enteropathy
Cryptosporidiosis	Graft-versus-host disease
Food protein hypersensitivity	
Milk	
Eggs	
Fish	
Rice	
Chicken	
Trauma or damage	
Acid (Zollinger–Ellison syndrome)	
Transplantation	
Exteriorization	

(?host) responses occur with other food sensitivities, as well as infections and infestations of the gastrointestinal tract (see Figure 1).

Curiously, the truly unresponsive atrophic–hypoplastic lesion seen occasionally in moribund coeliac patients with unremitting malabsorption may represent a graft-versus-host response to multifocal areas of tumour development, akin to lesions seen in experimental animals with chronic graft-versus-host disease (Mowat and Felstein, 1991).

DYNAMIC INTERRELATIONSHIPS OF TYPES 1–3 LESIONS

The static display of representative gluten-induced mucosal lesions (Figure 3) provides no proof of their interrelationships (Marsh, 1989a). There are in the literature sporadic case reports that indicate progression of change, from mild to more severe lesions (in the absence of induced gluten challenge) (Egan-Mitchell et al, 1981; Marsh, 1989b; Mäki et al, 1990).

To provide a more factual basis for these data, groups of treated gluten-sensitive patients were challenged orally with a single dose of a peptic–tryptic digest of gliadin, in a range of doses from 0.1 to 12.0 g (Leigh et al, 1985; Marsh et al, 1992).

These extensive time-course studies provide clear evidence for a dose-dependent accumulation of ($CD8^+$) lymphocytes into surface and crypt epithelium during the lower-dose challenges (0.1–3 g). It is noteworthy that the IEL response in surface epithelium occurs earlier than that of crypt epithelium, although the latter response is greater, both quantitatively and temporally (Figure 4).

Second, it is important to note (as with the static analysis of dermatitis herpetiformis mucosa; see Marsh, 1989a) that crypt hypertrophy is the first architectural change to be observed in the absence of any marked loss of villous volume (epithelial volume is not a measure of villous height) (Figure 5). This is exactly analogous to the T-cell-mediated effects in mild enteropathies described by Mowat and Ferguson (1982) and in organ culture of fetal mucosa stimulated by anti-CD3 monoclonal antibody (MacDonald, 1992). All these data indicate a direct effect of the (?activated) T cell on crypt size. Clearly, this is strong evidence against that view that crypt hypertrophy is a sole response to villous loss, or even enterocyte damage, a theory (haemolytic) that was highly favoured by earlier workers to explain the 'small' enterocytes. Such an isolated view fails to take account of the remaining transmural immuno-inflammatory response.

The terminal phase in the immunological evaluation of local T-cell activity at the mucosal level is villous effacement, developing progressively from the infiltrative (type 1) and infiltrative–hyperplastic (type 2) lesions. At this stage, because of the greatly heightened loss of surface enterocytes (six- to tenfold), part of the crypt response may be directed towards maintaining equilibration and, in particular, ensuring that the surface epithelium remains covered with cells. Thus, rapid turnover and, perhaps, partial

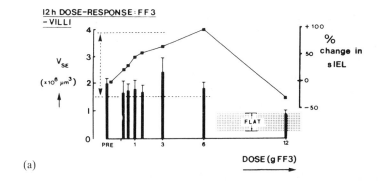

(a)

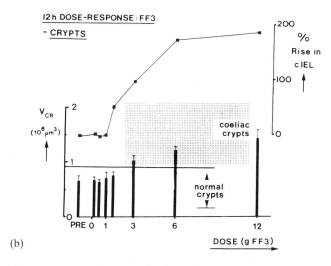

(b)

Figure 4. These two panels illustrate cumulative dose–response data at 12 hours for: (a) villi; and (b) crypts. For villi there is no alteration in surface epithelial volume (V_{SE}) for doses of Frazer's fraction III (FF-III) up to 6 g. With 12 g FF-III there is mucosal flattening, at which time there is a concurrent reduction in surface lymphocytes (sIELs). The rise in crypt IELs (cIELs) first occurred with 1.5 g FF-III challenge and thus was slower than the response in sIELs, but preceded the initial increase in crypt size (with 3 g). Note that the maximal plateau reached by cIELs is + 200% over control values, whereas that for sIELs is only approximately 100%. Reproduced from Marsh et al (1992, *European Journal of Gastroenterology & Hepatology* 4: 667–673) with permission.

ischaemia (Aho et al, 1973) resulting from changes in the microcirculation as a result of vascular inflammation and remodelling of the mucosa (Marsh, 1992b,c) could provide an explanation for the small-volume cuboidal enterocytes that typify this lesion. Viewed in this light, it is apparent that a direct 'noxious' effect of gluten on the enterocyte utterly fails to explain any of the features of the fully established lesion (Figure 5).

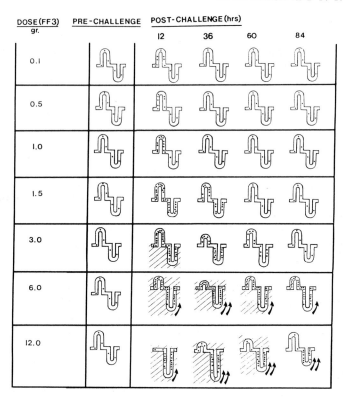

Figure 5. Representation in chequerboard format of complete dose–time responses of coeliac mucosa to challenge with increasing doses of Frazer's fraction III (FF-III). Cross-hatching indicates architectural changes to crypts of villi. Arrows indicate increases in crypt cell mitotic activity.

THE LAMINA PROPRIA

Few investigators in the past have concentrated on the mucosal lamina propria and yet it is here, and not in the epithelium or the IEL, that the central immunological activity in the gluten-induced lesion must occur. Such a view was proposed over 10 years ago (Marsh, 1983), so it is now reassuring to see a wider interest in this part of the mucosa beginning to develop and assuming an air of scientific credibility.

In the flat–destructive lesion, the volume of lamina propria is increased twofold compared with that in control mucosa, an alteration that can be perceived only with properly controlled measurement (Dhesi et al, 1984). This swelling is dependent, in part, on efflux of plasma proteins as a result of microvascular hyperpermeability and to an increase in the size of lamina propria cell populations, including lymphocytes, plasma cells, mast cells, basophils, eosinophils and neutrophils (Dhesi et al, 1984; Marsh and Hinde, 1985). Biochemically, there is evidence for activation of neutrophils, eosinophils and complement; degranulation of mast cells; elaboration of lipoxygenase-derived products; and prostaglandin secretion (Krilis et al, 1986; Wingren et al, 1986; Griffiths et al, 1988; Hallgren et al, 1989; Horvath et al, 1989; Lavö et al, 1990; Desreumaux et al, 1992; Colombel et al, 1992; Talley et al, 1992). There is evidence of widespread expression of inter-leukin IL2-R (CD25) throughout the lamina, both on CD4$^+$ lymphocytes and subepithelial macrophage-like cells, and of its presence within the circulation (Crabtree et al, 1989; Penttilla et al, 1990; Halstensen et al, 1990). Clearly it is here that the gluten-induced immune response is initiated, followed by secondary recruitment of inflammatory cells, production of modulatory cytokines and progressive reorganization of mucosal architecture.

In the dermatitis herpetiformis specimens (Marsh, 1989a) progressive swelling of the lamina propria occurs with infiltration of neutrophils and basophils, as mucosal architectural (and IEL population) changes move through type 1, 2 and 3 stages to become flat (Figure 6(a)). Indeed, lamina swelling and neutrophil influx occur early when only crypt hypertrophy is the sole evidence (type 2 infiltrative–hyperplastic) of any architectural change. Because it is so difficult to observe these changes casually through the microscope, it is not surprising that claims of increased permeability are said to persist even in putatively 'normal' mucosae (Bjarnason et al, 1983); much care, therefore, needs to be exercised before such conclusions are judged to be accurate.

The disadvantage of a static display of multiple individual biopsies is that each depicts an event in the corresponding patient's illness, and therefore lacks a cohesive relationship in terms of either a time– or dose–response. However, the sequence of changes observed is similar to that seen after a series of graded challenges with oral gluten (enzyme digested) (Marsh et al, 1992), thus indicating a sequential pattern common to both.

The first changes in lamina propria volume occur with 3 g gluten digest (Figure 7), at the time when crypt epithelial volumes have extended beyond the upper reference range for control mucosa. A more pronounced lamina propria response is observed with the 6- or 12-g challenge. Infiltration of the lamina by neutrophils is moderate with the 3-g challenge (at 10 neutrophils per 10^4 μm^2 muscularis mucosa), rising to approximately 20 neutrophils with the 12-g challenge. These values are higher than those in DH patients for comparative changes in lamina propria volume. Scanty basophilic infiltration (2–8 cells per 10^4 μm^2 muscularis mucosa) occurs later (60–84 hours) in each of the challenge series with 3, 6 and 12 g peptide digest. There is no discernible alteration in either eosinophil or mast cell populations.

Although dose-responsive alterations in surface and crypt IEL populations in these experiments were observed before measurable alterations in lamina propria volume took place, reductions in enterocyte cell height and morphological evidence of IEL activation (increases in mitotic activity and mean nuclear diameter) occurred after the lamina propria became inflamed and were, in fact, features pertinent to the flattening of mucosae (12-g challenge). This is entirely consistent with the static data on 35 patients with untreated dermatitis herpetiformis, whose mucosae are arranged in descending order according to successive reductions in surface epithelial volume (V_{SE}) (Marsh, 1989a) (Figures 3 and 6(b)).

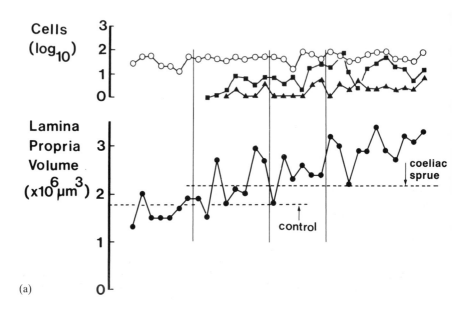

(a)

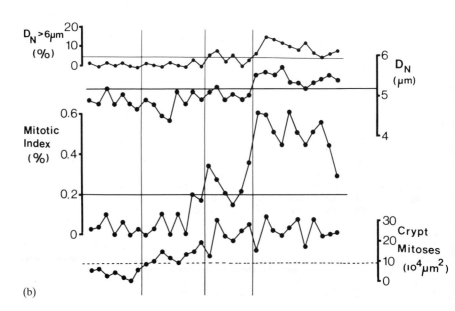

(b)

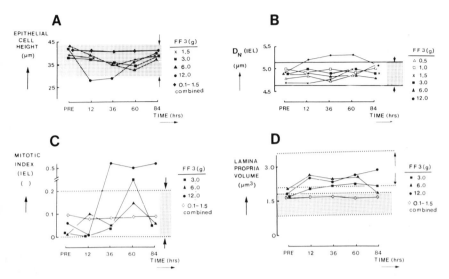

Figure 7. (A) Epithelial cell (profile) heights fell below the control reference range (30–42 μm, dotted area) during the period of marked flattening (12–36 hours) following 12 g Frazer's fraction III (FF-III) challenge. Although there were later, smaller, falls with 3–6-g challenges, the reductions were not significantly different from prechallenge control values. (B) The size of surface lymphocytes (sIELs), denoted by alterations in mean nuclear profile diameter (D_N : IEL) were significantly raised above the upper reference range of 5.2 μm (upper arrow, dotted area) only with a 12-g FF-III challenge. (C) The mitotic activity of IELs (% metaphases per 3000 sIELs per specimen), similar to levels (>0.2%) seen in untreated coeliac sprue disease (upper dotted line), occurred only with the 12-g challenge. (D) Alterations in lamina propria volume (V_{LP}) during various dose challenges. Note the control reference range (dotted area) and horizontal lines (arrowed) for untreated coeliac mucosal range. An increase into the untreated coeliac range occurred transiently with 3 g (36–84 hours), and more markedly with the 6-g and 12-g; challenges. These responses were also commensurate with the inflammatory cell infiltrates documented for each group of specimens analysed per challenge. Reproduced from Marsh et al (1992, *European Journal of Gastroenterology & Hepatology* **4**: 667–673) with permission.

Figure 6. (a) Lamina propria volumes ($\times 10^6$ μm^3 per 10^4 μm^2 muscularis mucosa) on lower vertical axis, together with mast cells (O), neutrophils (■) and basophils (▲) expressed in absolute population sizes (logarithmic) on upper vertical axis, corresponding to the 32 mucosal samples displayed in Figure 3. The infiltrative–hyperplastic mucosa (between the first and second vertical lines) demonstrates an increase in lamina propria volumes exceeding the upper control range and, in some instances, the lower range for flat coeliac sprue mucosa (horizontal dotted lines), together with the presence of neutrophils and some basophils indicating the occurrence of an inflammatory reaction within this region of these mucosae. As flattening progresses, there are further rises in the level of neutrophils, and a slower rise in basophils, while lamina propria volumes also increase, reaching a maximum as the mucosa becomes flat (to the right of the third vertical line). Mast cell content rises slowly throughout. (b) This diagram shows that, in terms of mean IEL nuclear diameter (D_N), the percentage of nuclei greater than 6 μm ('blast-like IEL': $D_N > 6$ μm) and the mitotic index, major changes are seen only in mucosa of the flat–destructive type (to the right of the third vertical line; see Figure 3). On the other hand, crypt cell mitotic activity, expressed as the number of mitoses per 10^4 μm^2 muscularis mucosae, shows an increasingly upward trend, exceeding the upper reference range (dotted line) at the point (Figure 3) where infiltrative–hyperplastic mucosa is identified. Reproduced from Marsh (1989a, *Virchows Archiv. A, Pathological Anatomy and Histopathology* **416**: 125–132, © Springer-Verlag) with permission.

THE PROXIMAL MUCOSAL LESION AND SYMPTOMATOLOGY

The histological features of the proximal jejunal mucosa are the yardstick for clinical diagnostic purposes. Although inevitable, this is unfortunate, since the presence of symptoms does not relate at all to the histological features of the proximal biopsy (MacDonald et al, 1964) but, approximately, to the length of jejunum involved. Moreover, for ease of comprehension of the physiopathology of gluten sensitivity, it is preferable to think in terms of residual unaffected bowel which, with proximal colon, may undergo functional hypertrophy and thus hold the balance between clinical symptoms (coeliac disease) or latency (Marsh, 1993b). Clearly, a flat proximal mucosal lesion does not imply symptoms; indeed, as has been shown (see Table 1) in many studies, latency is frequently consistent with a severe proximal lesion.

Since gluten sensitivity often retards growth in young children, one should question whether some patients are symptomatic because of an associated anatomical 'short-bowel' syndrome (Marsh, 1993b). Although studies are scarce, Thompson (1974) found the total bowel length in gluten-sensitized patients at post mortem to be within normal limits (15 ± 5 feet). In another study of ileal function in gluten sensitivity (Stewart et al, 1967), lesional

Table 4. Common factors involved in unmasking latent gluten sensitivity (irrespective of proximal mucosal pathology).

Gastrointestinal infections
Enteric bacteria/toxins (*Escherichia coli, Salmonella, Yersinia, Campylobacter, Aeromonas*)
Viral (rotavirus, astrovirus, adenovirus)
Parasitic (*Giardia, Cryptosporidium*)

Coexisting nutritional deficiencies
Iron deficiency
    Poor dietary intake (low iron content in food)
    Excessive losses (pregnancy or menstruation)
Folate deficiency
    Poor dietary intake (vegetables)
    Increased utilization (pregnancy, skin disease, increased enterocyte turnover)
Vitamin D
    Diet low in fish, fish oil, dairy products
    Low exposure to sunlight

Metabolic stress
Surgery of stomach, gallbladder, appendix
Acute pancreatitis, trauma
Pregnancy, postpartum period
Acute febrile illness (influenza, pneumonia)

Malignancy
Diffuse lymphoma (unresponsive end-stage disease with or without inflammatory
    jejunoileitis)
Mass lesions (intestinal obstruction, pain, haemorrhage, perforation)
Oesophagus (dysphagia)
Stomach (anorexia)
Other?

---

pathology was shown to involve less than one half of the total length of small bowel, while the distance over which the abnormal mucosa reverted to normality was fairly small (50 cm). In Thompson's post-mortem study, the mean length of mucosal flattening in six untreated gluten-sensitive patients was approximately 30%. Clinical experience of patients with fairly extensive resections for either mesenteric occlusions or diffuse Crohn's jejunitis indicates, by comparison, that the average length of lesional pathology in gluten sensitivity would generally be insufficient for the inevitable occurrence of intestinal malabsorption. Thus, additional factors are obviously necessary to unmask the latent susceptibility (Table 4).

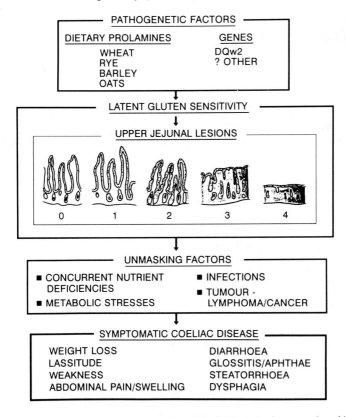

Figure 8. The ingestion of gluten proteins in DQw2 individuals leads to a series of immuno-pathologically based intestinal lesions and a latent state of gluten sensitivity. This latent form of gluten sensitivity may be awakened or unmasked by various environmental factors, resulting in multiple symptoms, signs or laboratory abnormalities which together are recognized as 'active coeliac disease'. The type of proximal jejunal lesion produced has no relationship to symptomatology. Conversely, the presence or absence of clinical disease bears no relationship to the proximal lesion; hence attempts to classify 'coeliac disease' as either symptomatic or latent, based on the appearance of the proximal lesion, are illogical. In practice, the medical attendant works the displayed algorithm in reverse, deciding first whether the symptoms merit a jejunal biopsy, and then considering which of the four groups of environmental factors (Table 4) has caused a symptomatic coeliac syndrome to appear. However, the presence of symptoms cannot foretell the type of lesion that may be present in any gluten-sensitized individual.

As defined at the outset, a heightened sensitivity to gluten protein occurs in DQw2 individuals, to result in a spectrum of mucosal lesions that are intrinsically latent (Figure 8). The unmasking of the latent state of gluten sensitivity (irrespective of proximal mucosal pathology) may be brought about by concurrent nutrient deficiencies (Marsh, 1993b). Thus, iron deficiency (which is still so unacceptably common, especially among females in the West), secondary to poor dietary intake, menstruation and childbirth coupled with the added malabsorptive defect, frequently yields clinical symptoms, with weakness, tiredness and loss of energy. Likewise, malabsorption of folate will be exaggerated both by concurrent poor intake and by increased losses incurred through increased cell production, and losses along the affected segment of bowel. The metabolic stresses of surgery, pregnancy or the puerperium, and severe systemic infections (like pneumonia), are further known precipitants of symptoms. Third, a person with latent sensitivity who is exposed to gluten for several decades is liable to develop lymphoma or, more rarely, cancer; these conditions may appear abruptly with abdominal pain and swelling, perhaps with features of either obstruction, perforation or haemorrhage. The proximal lesion may not always be severe (Freeman and Chin, 1986), so care must be taken to exclude gluten sensitivity as its underlying cause (Marsh, 1993a).

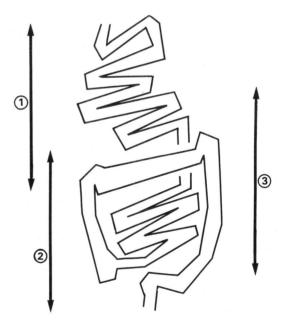

Figure 9. In gluten sensitivity the degree of malabsorption is determined by the length of functionally impaired bowel (1). The occurrence of symptoms (diarrhoea) depends largely on residual uninvolved jejunum, ileum and, in association with proximal colon, their combined functional reserve (2). Clearly, if the latter are suddenly impaired through infection, especially by organisms with tropism for distal bowel enterocytes, then colonic reserves will be acutely overwhelmed (3), resulting in a secretory diarrhoea.

Talley NJ, Gephart GM & McGovern TW (1992) Deposition of eosinophil granule major basic protein in eosinophilic gastroenteritis and celiac disease. *Gastroenterology* **103:** 137–145.
Thompson H (1974) The small intestine at autopsy. *Clinics in Gastroenterology* **3:** 171–181.
Wingren U, Hallert C, Norby K & Enerbäck L (1986) Histamine and mucosal mast cells in gluten enteropathy. *Agents and Actions* **18:** 266–268.

6

Coeliac disease in childhood

J. M. LITTLEWOOD

In his classical description of coeliac disease Samuel Gee noted that children between the age of 1 and 5 years were most commonly affected (Gee, 1888). He suggested that diet may be important in the causation of the condition but only relatively recently has the causative role of dietary gluten been identified (Dicke, 1950; Anderson et al, 1952; Dicke et al, 1953). The characteristic histological changes of subtotal villous atrophy (SVA) in the small bowel mucosa were first identified in specimens obtained at laparotomy from adults with idiopathic steatorrhoea (Paulley, 1954). In 1957 the characteristic SVA of small bowel mucosa was described in an intestinal biopsy specimen taken orally from a child with coeliac disease (Sakula and Shiner, 1957). The subsequent recovery of the intestinal mucosa, following withdrawal of gluten from the diet, was documented (Anderson, 1960).

Coeliac disease is currently defined as 'a disease of the small intestine characterised by an abnormal small intestinal mucosa associated with a persistent intolerance to gluten. Removal of gluten from the diet leads to a full clinical and histological remission' (Walker-Smith, 1988). Since the first descriptions of the characteristic small intestinal mucosal changes, the variability of the clinical features, diagnostic criteria, laboratory findings, association with other disorders and treatment have been well defined. The concept of trigger factor(s) inducing the coeliac reaction to occur in genetically predisposed individuals who are exposed to gluten is generally agreed. It has become apparent that there is a variable mucosal response to gluten both in severity and timing. Once the characteristic SVA of the mucosa has resolved, re-exposure to dietary gluten usually results, sooner or later, in recurrence of the intestinal mucosal abnormality in at least 95% of individuals (Schmitz et al, 1978, 1984; McNicholl et al, 1979; Littlewood and Losowsky, 1984; Mayer et al, 1989). The basic pathogenesis of coeliac disease is less well understood, although considerable progress has been made and is reviewed elsewhere in this volume.

CLINICAL SERIES OF COELIAC CHILDREN

There are relatively few large series reported where the diagnosis of coeliac disease is supported by histological evidence of mucosal damage (Hamilton et al, 1969; Young and Pringle, 1971; Littlewood et al, 1979; Mayer et al, 1989;

Walker-Smith, 1991; Ascher et al, 1993). The 108 children with coeliac disease described in this chapter attended the author's clinic; many had been referred by paediatric colleagues for jejunal biopsy. In all cases the diagnosis was supported by at least one abnormal jejunal biopsy and a favourable response to a gluten-free diet; the majority had a subsequent 'follow-up' biopsy whilst on a gluten-free diet, and many had a gluten challenge and third 'diagnostic biopsy' (Congdon et al, 1981; Littlewood and Losowsky, 1984).

MODE OF PRESENTATION, SYMPTOMS AND SIGNS

The classical picture of an unhappy blonde child with slender limbs, wasted buttocks and prominent abdomen is well known (Figure 1). The wide

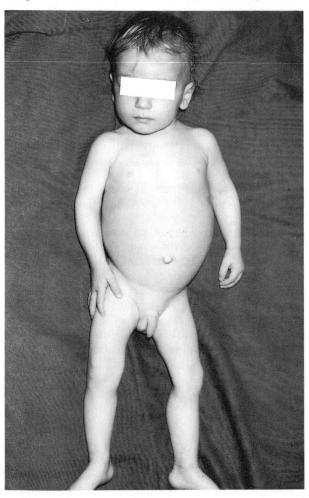

Figure 1. A child with coeliac disease.

forehead and narrower jaw characteristic of coeliac disease (Cooke et al, 1953) often contrasts with the severe degree of wasting of the limbs. The eye lashes are commonly long. Fortunately, with present-day community health supervision and the high standard of primary health care in the UK, children with coeliac disease are usually diagnosed before they become severely malnourished.

Age at onset

Fifty-two (48%) of our 108 children with coeliac disease were diagnosed during the first year of life (Figure 2(a)), a greater proportion than in earlier series including Gee's (Hamilton et al, 1969; Young and Pringle, 1971; Walker-Smith, 1988). The age of presentation may vary even in contemporary series in neighbouring countries, e.g. Sweden and Finland (Ascher et al, 1993). The earlier introduction of gluten-containing cereals as weaning foods is possibly relevant. Progress has usually been normal before the

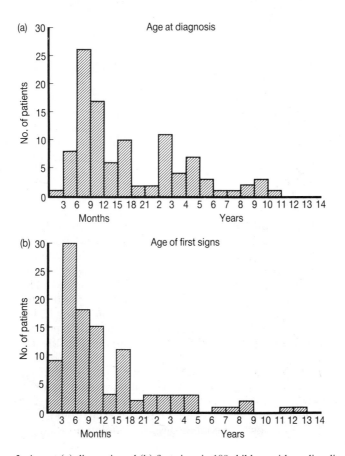

Figure 2. Age at (a) diagnosis and (b) first signs in 108 children with coeliac disease.

introduction of cereals into the diet. Some infants with coeliac disease have both gluten and cow's milk intolerance (Visakorpi and Immonen, 1967; Kuitunen et al, 1973; Kilby et al, 1975). These infants respond to a gluten- and cows' milk-free diet but it later becomes apparent that, although they develop tolerance to cows' milk, they remain intolerant of gluten. It has been suggested that cows' milk protein intolerance may precede and influence the development of coeliac disease in genetically predisposed individuals (Fallstrom et al, 1965).

Mode of presentation

In the present 108 coeliac children the main presenting complaints were as shown in Table 1.

Table 1. Main problem of 108 coeliac children at presentation.

	No. of children
Diarrhoea	50 (46)
Vomiting	20 (19)
Failure to thrive	14 (13)
Short stature	5 (5)
Abdominal pain	5 (5)
Abdominal distension	5 (5)
Weight loss	4 (4)
Anaemia	1 (1)
Constipation	1 (1)
General malaise	1 (1)
Mood disturbance	1 (1)

Values in parentheses are percentages.

Weight and height

In the majority of children the disturbed gastrointestinal function has an adverse effect on weight gain and growth. In infants and young children, who should be in a phase of rapid growth, there is usually significant interference with both weight and to a lesser extent height gain. At diagnosis 95.6% of all children and 98.2% of those less than 2 years old had a weight below the 50th centile. In fact, a weight centile over the 50th centile is strong evidence against the diagnosis of coeliac disease in young children (Figure 3). Although the height is usually less severely affected than weight, stunting with a normal weight for height may occasionally be the main growth abnormality (Figure 4).

Short stature and delayed onset of puberty may be the only outward evidence of coeliac disease, and the condition should be excluded in all children who are investigated for short stature or where there is delay in the onset of puberty (Groll et al, 1980; Knudtzon et al, 1991). A minority of older children, diagnosed in coeliac disease population or family screening studies, have entirely normal growth and are quite asymptomatic (Catassi et al, 1994).

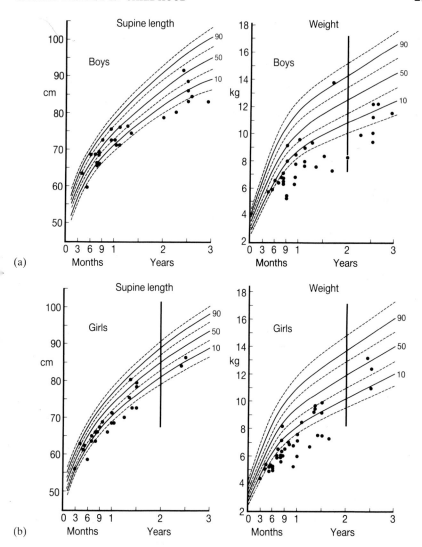

Figure 3. Weight and height centiles of 108 children with coeliac disease at the time of diagnosis before treatment. (a) Boys, (b) girls.

Bowel abnormalities

Stool abnormalities are not only the most common mode of presentation but are present in the majority of children with coeliac disease. Samuel Gee's generation looked more to the stools than the laboratory for diagnostic help, and his description of the stools is concise and to the point: 'Signs of the disease are yielded by the faeces; being loose, not formed, but not watery; more bulky than the food taken would seem to account for; pale in colour, as if devoid of bile; yeasty, frothy, an appearance probably due to fermentation; stinking, stench often great, the food having undergone putrefaction rather than concoction' (Gee, 1888).

Nowadays, the usual complaint is of diarrhoea: classical steatorrhoea is not usually reported by parents. In a minority there may be no complaint of any stool disorder and occasionally severe constipation may predominate (Egan-Mitchell and McNicholl, 1972).

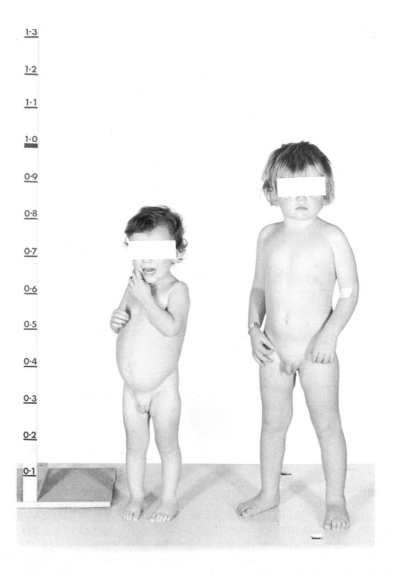

Figure 4. Boy with untreated coeliac disease compared with a child of the same age.

Abdominal pain

Coeliac disease may be diagnosed when children with recurrent abdominal pain are investigated. Recurrent abdominal pain was the main complaint in 36% of one recent series of coeliac children (Mäki, 1992). Thus, coeliac antibody tests should be included in the investigation of children with unexplained recurrent abdominal pain.

> Mary, aged 10 years, looked healthy and was well grown but had troublesome recurrent abdominal pain for 2 years, diagnosed as abdominal migraine by an experienced paediatrician. She was eventually referred for upper gastrointestinal endoscopy as the pain was so troublesome. This procedure included duodenal biopsies which suggested SVA, and this was confirmed on standard jejunal biopsy. Her pain settled completely and permanently on a gluten-free diet.

Abdominal distension

Fullness of the abdominal contour, which is dull rather than resonant to percussion, is an important and frequent sign of active coeliac disease in children, and was noted in 76% of our patients (Table 2). It was the main presenting complaint in 5% of the children. A flat or scaphoid abdomen is a useful sign, suggesting the child is unlikely to have coeliac disease.

Table 2. Frequency of signs and symptoms in 108 coeliac children.

	No. of children
Failure to thrive or growth problems	88 (81)
Abnormal stools	84 (78)
Abdominal distension	82 (76)
Weight loss	78 (72)
Diarrhoea	73 (68)
Vomiting	58 (54)
Pallor	53 (49)
Mood change	42 (39)
Preceding infection	29 (27)
Abdominal pain	16 (15)
Constipation	13 (12)
Slow development	10 (9)
Bleeding	5 (5)
Oedema	5 (5)
Rickets	3 (3)

Values in parentheses are percentages.

Vomiting

Fifty-four per cent of the children had a significant degree of vomiting. It was more common in younger patients and was the main presenting sign in 19%. When the vomiting is associated with a distended abdomen and fluid levels on erect abdominal radiography, unnecessary laparotomy may be undertaken for suspected intestinal obstruction. The investigation of intractable unexplained vomiting in an infant or young child should include a 2-week diagnostic trial on a basic elimination diet which, for an infant, consists of a milk substitute and baby rice and is thus gluten free (Litlewood and Mac-Donald, 1986).

Finger clubbing

This was present in 25% of one series of coeliac children at diagnosis, and improved with treatment (Hamilton et al, 1969). Koilonychia has also been described, and is reversible.

Aphthous ulceration

Although recurrent aphthous ulceration is cured following gluten withdrawal in some coeliac patients, the problem is less often due to coeliac disease than originally reported (Ferguson, 1980).

Neurological features

There is an association between bilateral occipital calcifications, epilepsy and coeliac disease, although the relationship between the conditions has not been clarified (Gobbi et al, 1992; Bye et al, 1993). Many children with coeliac disease have marked mood abnormalities, which often improve within days of starting a gluten-free diet. The marked hypotonia may at times suggest neuropathy or myopathy (Kaplan et al, 1988). In fact, a severe proximal myopathy was reported as the presenting feature of coeliac disease in an 8-year-old Moslem girl; the myopathy responded to a gluten-free diet (Hardoff et al, 1980). An isolated ocular myopathy in a 12-year-old girl with coeliac disease responded to a gluten-free diet (Sandyk and Brennan, 1983).

Specific nutritional deficiencies

The investigation of specific nutritional deficiencies may lead to the diagnosis of coeliac disease. The availability of coeliac antibody tests (see below) has identified previously undiagnosed coeliac disease as a likely cause in many of these clinical situations.

Iron-deficiency anaemia. The iron-deficiency anaemia associated with active coeliac disease responds temporarily to oral iron supplements but recurs when these are stopped. When coeliac disease is suspected, it is advisable to correct the iron deficiency before jejunal biopsy as mucosal abnormalities may be due to the iron deficiency (Naiman et al, 1964).

Rickets, hypocalcaemia, hypomagnesaemia and tetany. Vitamin D-deficient rickets occurs occasionally in active coeliac disease and is particularly likely to occur in Asian children (Nelson et al, 1973). Osteoporosis was significantly more common in 33 newly diagnosed coeliac children and adolescents than in controls, and improved whilst taking a gluten-free diet (Mora et al, 1993). The subject has been reviewed in detail (Walters, 1994).

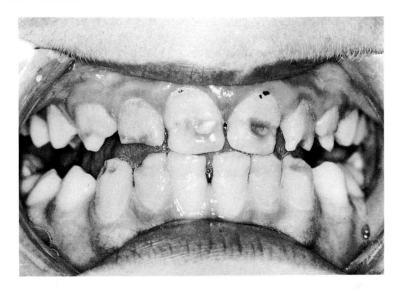

Figure 5. Severe example of dental lesions in a patient with coeliac disease.

Tooth enamel defects. Permanent characteristic dental enamel lesions are common in patients with coeliac disease (Figure 5). Twenty-five of 56 healthy first-degree relatives of coeliac patients had typical dental lesions. All underwent jejunal biopsy and seven had SVA, all of whom had typical dental lesions. The dental lesions were associated with HLA-DR3 (Aine et al, 1990; Mäki et al, 1991).

Pancreatic insufficiency. Ten of 44 children with untreated coeliac disease had significantly reduced pancreatic tryptic and lipolytic activity, which was reversible with treatment (Carroccio et al, 1991). Occasionally, more permanent pancreatic insufficiency may be the reason for lack of response to a gluten-free diet (Weizman et al, 1987).

COELIAC-RELATED DISEASES

A number of conditions are associated with coeliac disease more often than by chance.

Type 1 diabetes mellitus. These patients have an increased incidence of coeliac disease with a prevalence of 1.1–1.3% in Swiss and German patients (Koletzko et al, 1988). In Finland 1 (2.3%) of 43 child diabetics had coeliac disease (Mäki et al, 1984). It is wise to screen diabetic children for coeliac disease using antibody tests.

Immunoglobulin (Ig)A deficiency. IgA deficiency affects between 1 in 400 and 1 in 700 individuals (Koistinen, 1975). Those affected have a tenfold risk of coeliac disease compared with the general population (Collin et al, 1992b). IgA deficiency has practical implications when interpreting serum IgA antibody tests, but IgG anti-gliadin and endomysium antibody tests are usually positive. The coeliac disease of 25 IgA-deficient patients did not differ from that of other coeliac patients, although they more often had an associated autoimmune disorder (Collin et al, 1992b).

Other autoimmune diseases. Various connective tissue and collagen disorders have been reported in association with coeliac disease (Scott and Losowsky, 1975). Most of the patients with coeliac disease have been identified by screening for various gluten antibodies. In one series, Sjögren's syndrome was the most common disorder (Collin et al, 1992a).

Dermatitis herpetiformis. Typical dermatitis herpetiformis has been described in children but usually affects adults. Intestinal SVA, which responds to a gluten-free diet, is present in the majority of patients with this condition (Marks et al, 1966; Fry et al, 1968; Klaus, 1992). However, the onset of the SVA is variable in relation to the skin lesions; in monozygotic twins, where presentation of the dermatitis was synchronous, the SVA was delayed by 7 years in one twin (Anstey et al, 1991).

Pulmonary manifestations. Various pulmonary disorders, including fibrosing alveolitis, have been described in coeliac patients but are not documented in children, although bird-fancier's lung is associated with SVA (Berrill et al, 1975).

Down's syndrome. There is a clear relationship between coeliac disease and Down's syndrome, both conditions being associated with an altered immune system. Seven (4.5%) of 155 patients with Down's syndrome in one series (Castro et al, 1993) and 3 (4.3%) of 70 in another had coeliac disease (Zubillaga et al, 1993).

Liver disease. Abnormal liver function tests, which return to normal after starting a gluten-free diet, suggest some degree of subclinical and possibly unimportant liver involvement in untreated children with coeliac disease (Lindberg et al, 1978).

Cystic fibrosis. There are case reports of patients having both coeliac disease and cystic fibrosis; in one series 5 (0.5%) of 1100 patients with cystic fibrosis also had coeliac disease (Valletta and Mastella, 1989). A sweat test to exclude cystic fibrosis is mandatory in all coeliac children at the time of diagnosis, as is a jejunal biopsy in patients with cystic fibrosis who have significant unexplained persisting intestinal malabsorption despite reasonable enzyme replacement therapy (Littlewood, 1992).

GENETIC FEATURES

(In this section, *incidence* is the number of new cases occurring in a population during a given time period; *prevalence* is the number of cases in a population at any given time.)

Familial occurrence. Eleven (10.2%) of our 108 children with coeliac disease had a first-degree relative with symptomatic coeliac disease. A study that screened relatives of known coeliac patients revealed previously undiagnosed coeliac disease in 8.7% of relatives (Auricchio et al, 1988). In one large study the relatives of 115 patients with coeliac disease aged between 9 and 75 years were investigated. Of 689 relatives, 526 were alive and 324 underwent jejunal biopsy, of whom 41 had coeliac disease, i.e. 12.7% of those biopsied and 6% of all the relatives were affected (Stokes et al, 1976).

Sex. As in other series of patients with coeliac disease there was a slight female preponderance (57.8%) in our 108 children. There is no explanation for this female preponderance, which is even more pronounced in adults except in dermatitis herpetiformis which affects men slightly more than women (Klaus, 1992).

Concordance in monozygotic twins. Monozygotic twin studies show approximately 75% concordance for coeliac disease (Walker-Smith, 1973; Shale et al, 1982). Some discordant twins become concordant during follow-up (Walker-Smith, 1991). In monozygotic twins with dermatitis herpetiformis the onset of cutaneous lesions was identical but intestinal villous atrophy was delayed for 7 years in one (Anstey et al, 1991).

Blood groups and HLA typing. The association with human leukocyte antigens is now well established, particularly HLA-B8 (Falchuk et al, 1972; Stokes et al, 1972) and DR3 (Keuning et al, 1976). The antigen DQw2 is present in 98% of coeliac children (Tosi et al, 1983) and its absence has been suggested as a valid exclusion criterion in relatives suspected of having coeliac disease, particularly if the coeliac patient is DQw2 positive (Auricchio et al, 1988).

Racial trends. There are interesting differences in the prevalence of coeliac disease in various countries. The condition seems mainly to affect people of European origin, although it has been reported in others (Logan, 1992). A recent survey of the prevalence of coeliac disease reported rates as low as 0.078 per 1000 population in Greece to 3.52 per 1000 in Sweden. In Italy, rates varied between 0.63 per 1000 in the north and 1.06 per 1000 in the south (Greco et al, 1992). A recent population screening study from central Italy, using an initial antibody screen (IgG and IgA anti-gliadin, then IgA anti-gliadin, anti-endomysium antibody and immunoglobulins) followed by jejunal biopsy, revealed a surprisingly high prevalence of 3.87 per 1000 when known coeliac disease cases and the 11 new cases were combined (Catassi et al, 1994). There are areas of particularly high incidence, e.g.

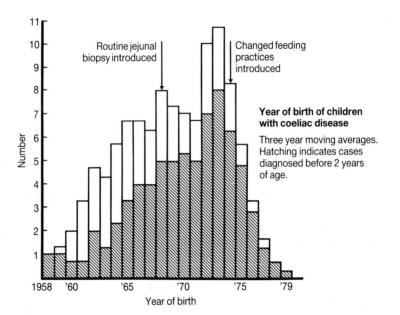

Figure 6. Changing incidence of coeliac disease in the north of England. Reproduced from Littlewood et al (1980, Childhood coeliac disease is disappearing. *Lancet* **ii:** 1359) © The Lancet Ltd. with permission.

County Galway, 1.94 per 1000 before and 0.73 per 1000 after 1976 (Stevens et al, 1987) and Gratz in Austria, 2.03 per 1000 before and 1.33 per 1000 after 1986 (Rossipal, 1991). Denmark has a particularly low incidence of coeliac disease (Weile and Krasilnikoff, 1993).

Changing incidence. A falling incidence of coeliac disease was reported by a number of clinics in the UK from the mid-1970s (Littlewood et al, 1980; Logan et al, 1986; Stevens et al, 1987; Logan, 1992) (Figure 6). Both the increase in the proportion of women breast-feeding (Greco et al, 1988) and the delay in the introduction of gluten-containing solids may have contributed to the fall in incidence. In Finland there was a significant decrease in the incidence in young children with coeliac disease from 1964 to 1988, but the total prevalence remained similar (Mäki and Holm, 1990). However, in neighbouring Sweden there has been an increase from 1.7 per 1000 before 1982 to 3.52 per 1000 in 1987. Changed environmental factors were considered responsible as the sudden increase was reported by many Swedish paediatric departments for births between 1983 and 1985 and then stabilized. From 1983, although the introduction of dietary gluten was delayed from 4 to 6 months, the gluten content of proprietary cereals was doubled by Swedish manufacturers. This was suggested as one of the important factors in the increased incidence (Cavell et al, 1992).

DIAGNOSIS

Although the diagnosis of coeliac disease may be suggested by clinical features, results of nutritional investigations, non-invasive tests of intestinal absorption and even gliadin antibody studies, *a jejunal biopsy is still required to establish the diagnosis.*

Over the past decade the use of the coeliac antibody tests (anti-gliadin IgA and anti-gliadin IgG, anti-reticulin IgA and anti-endomysium antibodies) has somewhat modified the use of jejunal biopsy and has largely superseded the non-invasive tests of intestinal absorption. Antibodies have proved useful in identifying particular groups of people who require jejunal biopsy, e.g. relatives of coeliac patients and children with short stature, diabetes mellitus and recurrent abdominal pain. They also provide support for a strong clinical suspicion of coeliac disease sufficient to justify proceeding directly to jejunal biopsy, thus avoiding tests of small bowel function, e.g. xylose absorption, differential sugar absorption and faecal fat absorption.

The possibility of coeliac disease should be investigated when the following are present:

- typical features of malabsorption and failure to thrive;
- unexplained recurrent abdominal pain in older children;
- small stature and/or delayed puberty;
- characteristic dental enamel defects;
- recurrent aphthous ulcers;
- specific nutritional problems, e.g. iron, vitamin D deficiency;
- conditions associated with coeliac disease: type 1 diabetes mellitus, IgA deficiency, dermatitis herpetiformis, Down's syndrome;
- first-degree relatives of coeliac patients;
- chronic illnesses where coeliac disease may be an additional problem, e.g. congenital heart disease (Congdon et al, 1982).

Investigations

The following investigations should be performed:

1. To obtain positive evidence of coeliac disease
   - (a) IgG anti-gliadin, IgA anti-gliadin, anti-reticulin and anti-endomysium antibodies;
   - (b) abnormal jejunal biopsy.
2. To identify the effects of the malabsorption:
   - (a) haemoglobin and full blood count;
   - (b) ferritin, red cell folate;
   - (c) urea and electrolytes;
   - (d) calcium, phosphorus, alkaline phosphatase;
   - (e) liver function tests;
   - (f) immunoglobulins;
   - (g) skeletal age from wrist radiography;
   - (h) faecal fat microscopy;
   - (i) faecal chymotrypsin.

3. To exclude other conditions:
   (a) sweat test;
   (b) faecal culture and microscopy;
   (c) giardiasis (faeces and jejunal biopsy).

Haematology

Iron-deficiency anaemia is common in coeliac disease. Seventy-two (70%) of 103 coeliac children for whom information was available had a haemoglobin concentration of less than 11 g/dl. In other reports iron-deficiency anaemia occurred in 72% (Young and Pringle, 1971) and 81% (Hamilton et al, 1969). Gluten ingestion in coeliac children rapidly induces iron deficiency as judged by ferritin levels (Stahlberg et al, 1991).

Folic acid

Folic acid deficiency is common in untreated coeliac disease but megaloblastic anaemia is rare (Dormandy et al, 1963). The serum folate level was reduced in 29 (60%) of 48 and the red cell folate in 15 (65%) of 23 of our series at diagnosis.

Vitamin B_{12}

Levels of vitamin B_{12} are usually normal (Hamilton et al, 1969), although B_{12} malabsorption occurs in active coeliac disease, possibly secondary to inadequate exocrine pancreatic stimulation (Hejlt and Krasilnikoff, 1990; Hjelt, 1991).

Immunological tests

Over the past decade anti-gliadin IgA (IgA AGA), anti-gliadin IgG (IgG AGA), anti-reticulin IgA (ARA) and anti-endomysium antibodies (EMA), referred to here as the 'coeliac antibodies', have been the subject of extensive investigation (Mäki, 1992). At the time of diagnosis IgA AGA and IgG AGA are present in virtually all patients with coeliac disease. However, IgG AGA is also found in some 25% of children with other gastrointestinal disorders (Burgin-Wolff et al, 1991). ARA has a high specificity for active coeliac disease of 96–100% and a sensitivity of 16–76% (Seah et al, 1971; Mäki et al, 1984). The disappearance of ARA correlates with mucosal healing and its reappearance with relapse (Mäki et al, 1989). EMA is also highly specific and positive in virtually all untreated coeliac patients, more commonly after the age of 2 years. It is also a sensitive indicator of silent relapse during re-exposure to gluten, and is not present in unaffected children. Of 340 untreated coeliac children, 338 (99.4%) had either IgG AGA and/or IgA AGA. The combined determination of IgA AGA and EMA, taking advantage of the high sensitivity of IgA AGA and the high specificity of EMA, gives an excellent prediction of the condition of the mucosa. Of 248 patients with a positive EMA and a positive IgA and IgG

AGA 247 (99.6%) had SVA on biopsy; 136 (99.3%) of 137 with neither EMA nor AGA had a normal mucosa (Burgin-Wolff et al, 1991).

Laboratory methods of performing tests for coeliac antibodies and their interpretation differ between centres. Tests for AGA are usually performed by enzyme-linked immunosorbent assay. At present there is no standard-reference positive antibody preparation and immunology laboratories establish their own normal ranges. ARA and EMA are detected by indirect immunofluorescence using a composite block of murine gastric, liver and kidney tissue, and monkey oesophagus, respectively. Again, there is no standard-reference positive antibody control.

These immunological investigations have had an increasing influence on the investigation and monitoring of coeliac patients. They are valuable and adequate both for screening tests in population studies and for long-term monitoring of patients with coeliac disease, as they are at least as useful and certainly more convenient than many of the previously used absorption tests, e.g. xylose absorption and differential sugar absorption tests (Rich and Christie, 1990). The latter tests are of limited value in predicting the state of the intestinal mucosa (Sanderson et al, 1975).

In the UK, where many coeliac children are commonly diagnosed and cared for by general paediatricians, it is important that an adequately evaluated coeliac antibody service is available; the serum can be sent to an appropriate laboratory. When children are considered to have coeliac disease, a negative antibody screen should prompt a careful review of the diagnosis. Although coeliac antibodies have not yet replaced the need for jejunal biopsy, it is difficult to appreciate the 'controversy' over the use of these tests, which are proving of such immense practical help (Lerner and Lebenthal, 1991).

We prefer to use all four tests (IgA AGA, IgG AGA, IgA ARA, EMA), and also estimate the plasma immunoglobulins to identify patients with IgA deficiency. The tests are particularly useful in excluding coeliac disease, for practical purposes, where the condition is possible yet improbable, e.g. in children with growth problems, delayed puberty, diabetes mellitus, recurrent abdominal pain and unexplained iron-deficiency anaemia.

After starting a gluten-free diet there is a gradual fall in the antibody levels over 3 months (Kilander et al, 1987); persistently positive antibody levels are valuable in indicating continuing gluten ingestion (Valletta et al, 1990). During a planned gluten challenge the re-appearance of antibodies has been used as an indication to perform the diagnostic biopsy; in one series, IgA AGA results were positive between the 15th and 35th day in 16 of 17 patients (Valletta et al, 1990). Although cellular and morphological changes of the intestinal mucosa can occur during gluten challenge without antibody response, when antibodies do become positive there will be diagnostic changes in the biopsy (Montgomery et al, 1988).

Intestinal fat malabsorption

The majority of children with coeliac disease have some degree of intestinal fat malabsorption (Shmerling et al, 1970), but in one series 8 (44%) of 18 and in another 14 (33%) of 43 did not have steatorrhoea. Fat absorption studies are not undertaken if jejunal biopsy is to be performed. Microscopy of the stool for split and neutral fat is a useful indication of malabsorption and has been compared with faecal fat studies (Walters et al, 1990).

Sweat test

It is important that a sweat test is performed to exclude cystic fibrosis in any child who is failing to thrive to a significant degree, particularly if there are gastrointestinal symptoms (Littlewood, 1986).

Giardiasis

A significant number of coeliac children have *Giardia* infection. It is important to examine the jejunal biopsy specifically for *Giardia lamblia* and to check the duodenal juice and faeces for this parasite (Carswell et al, 1973).

Radiology

Occasionally abdominal radiography shows dilated loops of small bowel and fluid levels suggesting intestinal obstruction. Contrast studies are abnormal in the majority of children with both coeliac disease and cystic fibrosis; there is dilatation of the small bowel and abnormalities of the mucosal folds (Howarth et al, 1968; Smith and Littlewood, 1977).

Skeletal age

Hypothyroidism and coeliac disease are the two major causes of severe retardation of skeletal development, evident by estimating the bone age from a wrist radiograph, which will also show rickets if present (Tanner et al, 1983).

> John, aged 10 years, was referred by the school doctor as his height reached only the 10th centile although his growth rate was normal and he had no symptoms. His skeletal age was only 5 years, which prompted a jejunal biopsy that revealed SVA. His growth accelerated after he started a gluten-free diet.

JEJUNAL BIOPSY

The demonstration of partial or SVA of the jejunal mucosa, with recovery after starting a gluten-free diet, remains an essential requirement for the diagnosis of coeliac disease (see below). Tissue obtained by small bowel biopsy can be examined with dissecting, light and electron microscopy. Histology and biochemical studies for disaccharidases should be performed on every specimen. Occasionally the unexpected absence of a disaccharidase will justify this policy; normal lactase levels support the impression from histological examination that the mucosa is normal. Also, various uptake and transport studies and in-vitro cultures are possible.

It is important that the interpretation of specimens obtained at biopsy is made by a pathologist familiar with the normal findings in children, i.e. under the dissecting microscope children have leaves rather than fingers, and slightly shorter villi than adults (Walker-Smith, 1967; Walker-Smith et al, 1991).

Technique of jejunal biopsy

On the evening before the biopsy, after applying local anaesthetic cream, a small cannula is inserted into an arm vein and flushed off for the night. The following morning, in the radiology department, intravenous diazepam is given until the child is well sedated. We use the twin-port Kilby (1976) modification of the Crosby capsule to obtain one specimen for histological purposes and the other for disaccharide estimation. The tube of the capsule is introduced, surrounded by a 12-Fr suction catheter with the tip removed and the capsule and catheter passed into the stomach. With the child in the right lateral position, the capsule is passed down the lesser curve into the antrum under fluoroscopy. The child is then placed supine, or supine with the right side raised, and metoclopramide is given. The capsule usually passes in 5–10 minutes to the duodenum, where the radiologist can assist its onward progress by pressure, with one hand under the left costal margin to prevent a loop forming and the other hand massaging the tube around the duodenal loop; a guide-wire also helps to stop loop formation. Most capsules are fired in the fourth part of the duodenum, the duodenojejunal loop being difficult to negotiate in children. Multiple forcible withdrawals of the plunger of a 20-ml syringe usually fire the capsule, success being monitored on the fluoroscopy screen (S.E.W. Smith, personal communication). The capsule is then slowly but firmly withdrawn. One biopsy specimen is placed in a plain bottle and deep frozen for estimation of disaccharidase levels; the other is spread on filter paper or plastic mesh and fixed in formal saline. If an immediate answer is required, the specimen is examined under the dissecting microscope; however, care should be taken not to damage the specimen and interfere with the quality of histological interpretation.

In the rare instance where biopsy fails with the standard capsule, a specimen can be obtained with the paediatric endoscope (Saverymuttu et al, 1991). Also, the endoscope is occasionally used to pass the standard biopsy capsule through the pylorus when this is not possible at radiological screening. The tube of the biopsy capsule is threaded up the suction channel of the endoscope from the tip; proximal traction is applied to the biopsy tube, which emerges from the proximal opening of the suction channel, pulling the biopsy capsule against the endoscope tip, which is then passed into the stomach. When the tip of the endoscope reaches the pylorus, the biopsy capsule is advanced into the duodenum and then on into the jejunum to be fired. After firing, the endoscope and capsule are withdrawn together. In very apprehensive children or where the standard procedure has failed, this technique is performed under general anaesthesia.

Contraindications to a small bowel biopsy are unavailability of a paediatric-size capsule or experienced staff, a bleeding diathesis, intercurrent illness and a severely debilitated infant. With experienced medical and nursing staff, the procedure rarely fails. With the technique described, using a stiffening tube and radiological assistance, failure to fire or obtain an adequate specimen can be corrected by immediate repeat of the procedure. In experienced hands, failure commonly results from failure of the capsule to pass through the pylorus, failure to fire, failure to separate the mucosal specimen from the bowel wall, and lack of a specimen in the capsule even though fired.

The most important complication is perforation of the bowel wall. Perforation will be avoided if a paediatric capsule is used by experienced personnel and the procedure is avoided in small, debilitated or distended infants. Problems of sedation and later emotional reactions to an unsatisfactory procedure may prove a deterrent if later follow-up biopsies are intended.

In our hospital, in excess of 1000 jejunal biopsies have been performed over the past 25 years in children as young as 3 months without serious complications. In ill and emaciated infants, where coeliac disease has been the probable explanation, the jejunal biopsy has been delayed for 2–3 weeks after starting a gluten-free (and frequently also a cow's milk-free) diet until the abdominal distension and general condition have improved.

We agree with others that infants and young children requiring small bowel biopsy should be referred to paediatric units undertaking the procedure on a regular basis (Walker-Smith et al, 1991).

CRITERIA FOR THE DIAGNOSIS OF COELIAC DISEASE IN CHILDREN

In 1969 criteria for the diagnosis of coeliac disease in children were proposed by members of the European Society for Paediatric Gastroenterology and Nutrition (ESPGAN). These original 'ESPGAN criteria' required that there should be a *structurally abnormal jejunal mucosa (usually the 'flat' mucosa with SVA) whilst on a gluten-containing diet, clear improvement in villous structure following removal of gluten from the diet, and subsequent mucosal deterioration following re-introduction of gluten into the diet* (Meeuwissse, 1970).

Although these guidelines were subsequently reviewed and considered to be satisfactory (Visakorpi, 1974), only two-thirds of the members of ESPGAN (paediatricians with an interest in gastroenterology) appeared to follow them and performed gluten challenges in patients with coeliac disease to confirm the diagnosis. Of 652 children considered to have coeliac disease by members of ESPGAN, the diagnosis was confirmed in 619 (95%) of those who subsequently had a gluten challenge (Shmerling, 1977; McNeish et al, 1979).

A recent report from Italy of further experience with the ESPGAN criteria in 3138 children with coeliac disease from 33 centres questioned the need for a gluten challenge in the majority. The need for gluten challenge unduly extended the time between the initial presentation and establishing a firm diagnosis (Guandalini et al, 1989). It was suggested that if children had clinically typical coeliac disease, a positive intestinal biopsy and a definite clinical response to the gluten-free diet, this permitted 'the definitive diagnosis of coeliac disease' to be made. Thereafter, the authors advised that 'gluten be permanently excluded from the diet'. However, it was recommended that the original ESPGAN diagnostic investigation of three biopsies, including a gluten challenge, should be used in doubtful or atypical cases (Guandalini et al, 1989). There has been some support for this approach (McNeish, 1989).

A further factor complicating the diagnosis has been the marked variability in mucosal susceptibility to gluten. Not only is there variability in the jejunal biopsy findings at presentation, but also in the speed of deterioration during subsequent gluten challenge after initial recovery of the mucosa (Egan-Mitchell et al, 1978; Schmitz et al, 1978; Littlewood and Losowsky, 1984). Also, the small bowel mucosa may be normal at the time of first biopsy yet the patient may subsequently develop SVA (Mäki et al, 1990).

The most recent review of the ESPGAN criteria followed a workshop in Budapest in 1989 (Walker-Smith et al, 1990). It was suggested that the finding of *an initial characteristic small intestinal mucosal biopsy abnormality should still be regarded as essential and that there should be a clear-cut clinical response to a strict gluten-free diet with relief of all symptoms within weeks.* However, in asymptomatic patients (e.g. relatives and screened patients), a second follow-up biopsy after starting the gluten-free diet was advised to demonstrate the histological recovery of the mucosa. *In contrast to the previous ESPGAN recommendations, a subsequent gluten challenge was not regarded as essential.* In children in whom doubt existed regarding the initial diagnosis, where an initial biopsy had not been performed, or when the diagnosis had been made before the age of 2 years, it was recommended that a second follow-up biopsy be performed to demonstrate recovery of the mucosa, followed by a standard gluten challenge. Thus, in practice, a substantial proportion of children do, in fact, qualify for a gluten challenge and a third diagnostic biopsy (Walker-Smith et al, 1990).

The useful supportive evidence provided by coeliac antibodies, which have been increasingly used since the first ESPGAN criteria were suggested in 1969, was emphasized but immunological investigations were still regarded as inadequate to establish the diagnosis; the false-negative results in coeliac patients with IgA deficiency were noted. It was suggested that it may be practical to recommend gluten provocation after not less than 2 years dietary treatment and preferably not before the age of 6 years or during the growth phase of puberty.

Problems with present ESPGAN recommendations

Many children with coeliac disease and their parents have difficulty in adhering to the gluten-free diet, and follow-up biopsies to demonstrate recovery of the mucosa reveal significant histological abnormalities (Congdon et al, 1981; Jackson et al, 1985; Colaco et al, 1987; Bardella et al, 1994). Continuing gluten ingestion is associated with variable histological abnormality of the intestinal mucosa. Although there may be few, if any, symptoms, a reduction in the patient's ultimate height may occur (Bardella et al, 1994). *Thus, the second 'follow-up biopsy' of the original 1969 ESP-GAN criteria is valuable in identifying the considerable number of children with coeliac disease who are not adhering to a gluten-free diet. We recommend a follow-up biopsy 2 years after starting the gluten-free diet in all coeliac patients to document the histological recovery of the jejunal mucosa* (Littlewood and Losowsky, 1984). Negative coeliac antibody test results before biopsy would suggest that gluten withdrawal had been achieved; if the antibody tests remain positive, the gluten-free diet should be reviewed by the dietitian and the biopsy postponed.

It is possible that increasing experience with coeliac antibodies may eventually reduce the need for these follow-up jejunal biopsies, although significant mucosal changes during gluten challenge may fail to elicit a measurable antibody response (Bardella et al, 1994). In patients with coeliac disease who regularly ingest 2.5–5 g gluten per day (one slice of bread), there was no significant change in IgA AGA or IgG AGA levels, but there was an increase in the level of intraepithelial lymphocytes (Montgomery et al, 1988).

Finally, some 5% of patients who have fulfilled both the original and most recent ESPGAN criteria for coeliac disease of having both intestinal SVA and an impressive clinical response to withdrawal of dietary gluten (and who may even have had histological relapse with a gluten challenge) may ulti-mately develop prolonged or even permanent tolerance to dietary gluten (Egan-Mitchell et al, 1978; Mäki et al, 1989). In some older children, the jejunal mucosa may even recover in the presence of continuing gluten ingestion (Schmitz et al, 1978, 1984). *As the gluten-free diet is a significant, life-long, social imposition on both the child and family, it is considered worthwhile and important to identify the 5% of individuals who appear to acquire permanent gluten tolerance.* This will involve either demonstrating a normal jejunal biopsy in those who have abandoned a gluten-free diet or following a planned gluten challenge if they have been adhering strictly to the diet. All patients, including the 5% who fail to relapse, should have long-term follow-up. If such patients have negative coeliac antibody tests, conversion from negative to positive would be an indication for a further jejunal biopsy.

In summary, it is recommended that all children with coeliac disease should have an initial jejunal biopsy within a few weeks of first presentation when their condition is improving. A follow-up biopsy is performed approximately 2 years after starting a gluten-free diet to ensure the mucosa has returned to normal. If the coeliac antibodies are positive, it is likely that the child has not been on a strict gluten-free diet. The diet should be reviewed and the biopsy delayed for 12 months; if the antibodies remain positive, biopsy should be performed. *All children diagnosed in the first 2 years of life, those in whom the diagnosis was doubtful and where there may have been other explanations for the jejunal mucosal abnormalities, and those who were asymptomatic at diagnosis should have a gluten challenge performed to confirm persisting gluten intolerance.* The challenge should not be performed in a child younger than 6 years, to avoid interference with tooth enamel formation, nor during puberty when growth may be compromised. *Eventually, all patients should*

be offered a gluten challenge, when growth has ceased, if they wish to know
whether they are among the 5% who have acquired tolerance to gluten.

GLUTEN CHALLENGE

Gluten challenge in a child may be regarded with severe apprehension by
parents who perceive the procedure as re-feeding the substance that caused
their child to have a serious and chronic illness. In such circumstances the
gluten challenge may be postponed until after puberty. Also, the gluten
challenge is usually delayed until catch-up growth has been completed,
which may be some years after starting the gluten-free diet. Gluten challenges are conveniently carried out by adding gluten powder (5–15 g daily,
depending on age) to the child's regular gluten-free diet. An alternative
method of challenge is to permit four slices of normal bread daily to be
added to the gluten-free diet (one slice of bread contains 2.5 g gluten).
Returning to a completely normal diet is unwise as the majority of children
will need to continue on a life-long gluten-free diet, which may then be more
difficult to adhere to.

A minority of patients develop severe symptoms, but most are asymptomatic for weeks or months. If gastrointestinal symptoms occur during the
challenge, the gluten is stopped and a biopsy performed within the next
week or two. If the child remains asymptomatic, a jejunal biopsy is performed after a 3-month gluten challenge—a duration that will provoke a
coeliac antibody response and histological change in the majority of children
with coeliac disease. A combination of coeliac antibodies (IgA AGA and
IgG AGA) and 1-hour blood xylose tests has been used to indicate the
appropriate time to perform the biopsy in 31 children (Mayer et al, 1989).
The median duration of challenge was 60 (range 14–205) days, and the

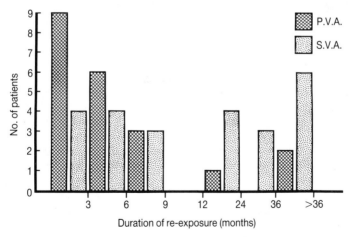

Figure 7. Response of the jejunal mucosa to gluten challenge in coeliac children. Reproduced
from Littlewood and Losowsky (1984, *Recent Advances in Paediatrics*. Edinburgh: Churchill
Livingstone) with permission.

asymptomatic relapse was predicted by raised AGA (37%), xylose malabsorption (7%) or both (57%). A discriminant coefficient using both rose sharply after 15 days. In another study IgA AGA became positive in 16 of 17 coeliac patients between the 15th and 35th day of the gluten challenge, which was concluded in all children after 20–45 days. The 1-hour xylose test was less reliable: in three patients with SVA it remained normal (Valletta et al, 1990).

Histological changes after gluten challenge are variable and correlate broadly with duration of exposure to gluten (Figure 7). Changes in the appearance of the villi and the increase in intraepithelial lymphocytes are evaluated, and usually show significant changes after the challenge. In most large series some 5% of patients considered to have coeliac disease will fail to relapse on re-exposure to normal quantities of dietary gluten (Egan-Mitchell et al, 1978; McNeish et al, 1979; Littlewood and Losowsky, 1984; Shmerling and Franckx, 1986).

DIFFERENTIAL DIAGNOSIS

In young infants there is a definite relationship between multiple food intolerance and coeliac disease. The malabsorption syndrome of infancy was reported as being due either to cow's milk protein or gluten intolerance (Visakorpi and Immonen, 1967). SVA of the small intestinal mucosa has been reported in association with a number of foods including cow's milk protein (Kuitunen et al, 1973; Kilby et al, 1975), soya protein (Ament and Rubin, 1972), and fish, chicken and rice (Vitoria et al, 1982). Transient intestinal damage is associated with gastroenteritis (Barnes and Townley, 1973) and may be followed by temporary cow's milk protein intolerance (Kilby et al, 1975). Some 10% of infants with mucosal histological abnormalities due to cow's milk protein will eventually develop coeliac disease (Visakorpi and Immonen, 1967). There are other conditions associated with significant enteropathy, some indistinguishable from that of coeliac disease, including pigeon-fancier's disease (Berrill et al, 1975), heavy infestation with *Giardia lamblia* (Carswell et al, 1973), autoimmune enteropathy (Mirakian et al, 1986), hypogammaglobulinaemia (Pelkonen et al, 1963) and acquired immunedeficiency syndrome (McLoughlin et al, 1987).

In practice, children found to have SVA on biopsy usually have coeliac disease. Some infants with cow's milk protein intolerance will have mucosal abnormalities, although these may be absent or minimal (Fontaine and Navarro, 1975; Kilby et al, 1975; Kuitunen et al, 1975). Follow-up challenge and biopsy of 116 children in Liverpool considered to have coeliac disease showed that 49% failed to relapse histologically following 10 g gluten per day for 3 months; only one other child had a late relapse. Cow's milk intolerance and post-enteritis syndrome were the likely explanations for their original illness (Taylor, 1988). Although in some series virtually all relapse (Packer et al, 1978), in some areas a routine gluten challenge spares many children from years of unnecessary dieting.

TREATMENT

Immediate treatment

Although weight gain has usually been poor before diagnosis, most children are not in a dehydrated condition and it is reasonable to start a gluten-free diet. In infants, where the nutritional state may be more compromised with diarrhoea, perhaps vomiting, considerable weight loss and even dehydration, it is reasonable to start with a gluten- and cow's milk-free diet. If a cow's milk-free diet is also started, a protein hydrolysate milk substitute will be required (Nutramigen, Pregestimil or Pepti-Junior). If the history and physical findings suggest that the diagnosis of coeliac disease is likely, and certainly if the infant's condition is poor and the abdomen distended, it is reasonable to start the diet and delay the jejunal biopsy for 2–3 weeks. *In such infants it is unwise to delay the start of treatment until after the biopsy has been performed. The risks of jejunal biopsy are reduced when the general condition has improved and the abdominal distension has lessened; the biopsy changes will still be present weeks or even months after starting the gluten-free diet.* Finally, such infants will eventually have a gluten challenge to confirm the diagnosis.

In severely ill and debilitated children in so-called 'coeliac crisis', the use of corticosteroids may cause a dramatic clinical improvement (Lloyd-Still et al, 1972). An improvement in the jejunal mucosal atrophy has been demonstrated in older patients following a short course of oral prednisolone (Wall et al, 1970); more recently, fluticasone has been used (Hutchinson et al, 1991).

It is important that the family start treatment with a good understanding of the aims and practical details of the gluten-free diet. The involvement of a paediatric dietitian (nutritionist) experienced in dealing with both children and coeliac disease is essential. The teaching and support of the patient and family in organizing the gluten-free diet is the single most important factor in achieving long-term compliance with the diet. Regular consultations with the dietitian are required in the early months after diagnosis, and the intervals may be increased gradually until there is an annual review. The importance of this regular follow-up to increase the success of long-term compliance with the diet is generally agreed (Bardella et al, 1994).

Wheat, rye, barley and oats are excluded initially, although there is some evidence that oats are tolerated by some patients (Dissanayake et al, 1974). Compliance with the diet may be enhanced by providing suggested meal plans, recipe ideas and information on the range of (and most palatable) gluten-free products available on prescription in the UK. The better the variety of choice in the diet, the higher the chance of compliance. Eventually, liaison with the school and advice on holidays will be required. Although uncommon, young women still attending the paediatric clinic may become pregnant and it is important to stress the importance of strict adherence to the gluten-free diet and adequate folic acid and vitamin supplementation in this event.

All families in the UK are advised to join the Coeliac Society (PO Box

220, High Wycombe, Buckinghamshire HP11 2HY) to obtain regular information, particularly the latest information on gluten-free foods. Many parents find it helpful to join their local branch. The Coeliac Society handbook of gluten-free foods is updated annually, with more frequent weekly information regarding changes to the list given on the national television (Ceefax). Manufacturers frequently change food ingredients, making it essential for families to update themselves regularly.

Clinical improvement follows removal of gluten from the diet within a few days. First, the mood improves, appetite increases and weight gain commences within 2 weeks or so. During this recovery phase of more rapid growth, general vitamin supplements, folic acid and iron are provided. More specific nutritional deficiencies, e.g. rickets or iron-deficiency anaemia, are treated appropriately. After catch-up growth is completed, the supplements are discontinued provided dietary compliance is assured by either experienced dietary evaluation, negative gluten antibodies or a recent normal follow-up jejunal biopsy. Catch-up growth may continue for months or even years (Prader et al, 1969). In our experience, as poor compliance with dietary treatment is relatively common, it is advisable to provide a multivitamin supplement throughout childhood while growth is occurring.

Monitoring of the gluten-free diet

In the present stage of knowledge, 95% of those diagnosed as having coeliac disease in childhood will require a permanent gluten-free diet to maintain a normal jejunal mucosa. This will reduce the risk of their developing local and general complications. Unfortunately there is a significant proportion of children and their families who are unable to keep to a strict gluten-free diet. In reports from specialized clinics in children's hospitals, where the patients are somewhat selected, follow-up jejunal biopsies taken whilst on a gluten-free diet are almost invariably normal, indicating compliance with the gluten-free diet (Packer et al, 1978). However, in unselected local populations where there are families of varied size and socio-economic status, there is evidence that keeping to a gluten-free diet presents major problems. Follow-up jejunal biopsies of many coeliac children, supposedly on gluten-free diets, show varying degrees of abnormality (Congdon et al, 1981; Jackson et al, 1985; Colaco et al, 1987; Kumar et al, 1988; Mäki et al, 1989; Bardella et al, 1994). The severity of the persisting abnormality correlates with the estimated degree of compliance with the diet (Congdon et al, 1981; Bardella et al, 1994).

Also, investigation of adults diagnosed as having coeliac disease in childhood who have returned to a normal diet reveals a significant number with villous atrophy. Although approximately half are asymptomatic, as a group those with mucosal abnormalities have poorer growth and more biochemical abnormalities than those on a gluten-free diet with normal mucosa (Bardella et al, 1994).

It is particularly important that gluten is permanently excluded from the diet of children with coeliac disease as there is increasing evidence that gluten avoidance reduces the incidence of subsequent gastrointestinal malignancy (Holmes et al, 1989; Holmes, 1992).

There is general agreement that the best chance of achieving compliance with the gluten-free diet is by regular monitoring of the patient at a paediatric clinic where there is not only an interested doctor but a paediatric dietitian. General progress is assessed by weight and height measurements, which are plotted on a growth chart appropriate for the child's local population. The doctor obtains the interval history and performs a physical examination. There follows a consultation with the paediatric dietitian to review the patient's and family's understanding of and compliance with the gluten-free diet. In our clinic the identification of continuing gluten ingestion whilst supposedly on a gluten-free diet is best achieved by the dietitian (Congdon et al, 1981). Once the gluten-free diet is established, the dietitian performs a full dietary assessment to ensure nutritional adequacy and determine the future need for vitamin and mineral supplements.

Coeliac antibody levels should be followed regularly, the frequency depending on previous knowledge of the family. They do provide useful, if not complete, information on the degree of gluten avoidance.

Even with skilled dietary assessment, good growth and normal coeliac antibody levels it is advisable to perform a follow-up jejunal biopsy 2 years or so after the start of the gluten-free diet to confirm that the mucosa has returned to normal. Persisting histological abnormalities at this stage are invariably the result of continuing gluten ingestion. The families are usually well aware of the dietary lapses; occasionally they are genuinely surprised and unaware of the source of the ingested gluten. The dietitian often helps to identify the source of the unrecognized dietary gluten.

If there have been specific nutritional deficiencies at the time of diagnosis, appropriate checks should be made on blood, vitamin levels or radiography.

Management of teenagers

Poor compliance is a particular problem in teenage patients (Kumar et al, 1988; Mayer et al, 1991). Growth and pubertal development will be normal in those following a gluten-free diet, although normal growth does not guarantee that the intestinal mucosa is normal. It is important to adhere to the diet and avoid planned gluten challenge through this period of rapid growth as the ultimate height may be compromised; this should be discussed with the patient. If final confirmation of persisting gluten intolerance is required, a planned gluten challenge should be undertaken after puberty is completed. The importance of adequate nutrition and vitamin supplementation in the crucial early weeks of pregnancy should be discussed with young women, who should perhaps be receiving regular vitamin supplementation if sexually active and at risk of becoming pregnant.

Long-term follow-up of coeliac children

Coeliac children should be followed by a hospital department indefinitely, their care being transferred from the paediatrician to a gastroenterologist at around 16 years when growth is completed. Investigation of adult patients who have been considered to have coeliac disease in childhood usually not only confirms the diagnosis but reveals a substantial proportion with jejunal biopsy abnormalities due to incomplete gluten exclusion (Paerregaard et al, 1988). Such a situation appears to be relatively common and represents an avoidable failure of management.

FUTURE DEVELOPMENTS

Although withdrawal of gluten-containing foods from the diet is associated with dramatic and sustained clinical improvement in the child's symptoms, emotional and nutritional state, this treatment is a permanent imposition on both the child's and the family's life-style. Obviously prevention would be better than a life-long diet. Coeliac patients have a variable reaction to gluten, both with time and between individuals. The development of coeliac disease in the genetically predisposed individual is not inevitable and indeed may not be permanent. Some 5% of those who have been diagnosed by acceptable criteria, even including gluten challenge, eventually maintain a normal jejunal morphology whilst ingesting gluten.

Perhaps we should be identifying susceptible children, e.g. HLA-typing the parents and infants where there is a family history of coeliac disease. The aim would be early avoidance of factors that may provoke the coeliac reaction. The early introduction of gluten in infancy and an excessive intake at any time would be avoided; breast-feeding rather than feeding a cow's milk-based formula would be encouraged. If breast-feeding was impossible, protein hydrolysate formula or similar preparation (Nutramigen, Pregestimil or Pepti-Junior) would be indicated to minimize the risk of cow's milk intolerance. Soya infant formula should be avoided as it is potentially allergenic. The temporary avoidance of gluten after gastroenteritis, when the mucosa is known to be temporarily damaged, may also be reasonable. If 10% of first-degree relatives of a patient with coeliac disease have the condition, as surveys seem to show, the preventive approach may be a reasonable alternative to a life-time of dieting.

There is a need for further evaluation and standardization of the various antibody tests. Although, by the very nature of the tests, there will never be complete agreement between laboratories, there is, nevertheless, a surprising diversity of opinion and methodology considering that the investigations have been available for over a decade. They do seem to be particularly needed where there are few cases of coeliac disease and limited experience with performance and interpretation of children's jejunal biopsies.

It is obvious that children who have coeliac disease require life-long supervision and are best followed up in clinics where there is a specialized interest in paediatric gastroenterology. Around the age of 16 years there should be formal transfer to a gastroenterologist rather than referral back to the family physician with the advice to 'keep to the gluten-free diet for life'. The inadequate arrangements for the long-term follow-up of many teenage coeliac patients results in much unnecessary suboptimal health and an increased risk of malignancy.

An incorrect initial diagnosis is not rare and inappropriate advice for a life-long gluten-free diet is relatively common in the UK, but such cases are rarely published. Inadequate or even a failure to obtain initial biopsy specimens, incorrect interpretation by pathologists more used to adult material, failure to distinguish a transient enteropathy that is recovering coincidentally with the onset of the gluten-free diet, and confusion with other food intolerance appear to be important areas of difficulty for general paediatricians.

However, recommendations from experience at large specialized paediatric gastroenterology units are not always appropriate for every child with coeliac disease. The new criteria of ESPGAN are probably suitable for the well-supervised socially advantaged child attending a department of paediatric gastroenterology, but are less appropriate for the socially disadvantaged child from a large family attending a busy general paediatric clinic in an industrial city. For this reason the suggestion that one jejunal biopsy and a clinical response to gluten-free diet are adequate for diagnosis is unacceptable as a general recommendation. In such children it is advisable to perform a second biopsy, not only to confirm recovery of the mucosa but also to identify the substantial number of children who are not keeping to a gluten-free diet.

Many children died from coeliac disease before Dicke's crucial observation of the harmful effect of wheat. Although death from coeliac disease is very rare nowadays, there is room for improvement in our present practice. More accurate diagnosis and more efficient follow-up, using all the presently available knowledge, would permit a greater proportion of coeliac children to be successful in excluding gluten from their diet. Fewer would have minimal but troublesome symptoms, subclinical nutritional deficiencies, suboptimal health and growth, and eventually fewer malignancies. Management along the lines suggested would also avoid unnecessary life-long gluten avoidance in the 5% of children considered to have coeliac disease but who appear to develop tolerance to gluten as they mature. They should be followed indefinitely, as should all coeliac patients, to ensure that the tolerance to gluten persists.

SUMMARY

Coeliac disease usually presents in infancy or early childhood with diarrhoea, vomiting and interference with weight gain and growth. Withdrawal of dietary gluten is followed by resolution of the symptoms and signs and restoration of normal weight gain and growth; the characteristic subtotal villous atrophy of the jejunal mucosa also recovers. Later re-introduction of dietary gluten will lead to a return of the jejunal mucosal abnormality in the majority and to clinical relapse in many but not all. The severity and timing of both are variable and 5% of children initially considered on clinical, biopsy and gluten response evidence to have coeliac disease appear to develop permanent tolerance to gluten, although mucosal relapse may occur years after the re-introduction of dietary gluten in a minority, emphasizing the need for long-term follow-up. Although a diagnostic and subsequent follow-up jejunal biopsy are necessary to confirm the diagnosis, anti-gliadin IgA and IgG, anti-reticulin and anti-endomysium antibodies are now almost totally reliable in identifying children who have coeliac disease and are valuable in monitoring the adequacy of gluten withdrawal. Dietary compliance is frequently poor and regular supervision by a paediatric dietitian is needed; indeed, lifelong supervision to ensure gluten withdrawal is essential to reduce the chance of developing later gastrointestinal malignancy.

Acknowledgements

The author thanks the medical, nursing and laboratory staff, too numerous to mention individually, who have helped with the investigation and management of our coeliac patients. Particular thanks are due to Sue Wolfe, Senior Paediatric Dietitian, and her colleagues past and present for their dedicated care and expertise.

REFERENCES

Aine L, Mäki M, Collin P & Keyrilainen O (1990) Dental enamel defects in celiac disease. *Journal of Oral Pathology and Medicine* 19: 241–245.
Ament ME & Rubin FE (1972) Soy protein—another cause of the flat intestinal lesion. *Gastroenterology* 62: 227–234.
Anderson CM (1960) Histological changes in the jejunal mucosa in coeliac disease. *Archives of Disease in Childhood* 35: 419–427.
Anderson CM, Frazer AC, French JM et al (1952) Coeliac disease gastrointestinal studies and the effect of dietary wheat flour. *Lancet* i: 836–842.
Anstey A, Wilkinson JD & Walshe MM (1991) Dermatitis herpetiformis in monozygous twins—concordance for dermatitis herpetiformis and gluten-sensitive enteropathy. *Clinical and Experimental Dermatology* 16: 51–52.
Ascher H, Holm K, Kristiansson B & Mäki M (1993) Different features of coeliac disease in two neighbouring countries. *Archives of Disease in Childhood* 69: 375–380.
Auricchio S, Mazzacca G, Tosi R et al (1988) Coeliac disease as a familial condition: identification of asymptomatic coeliac patients within family groups. *Gastroenterology International* 1: 25–31.
Bardella MT, Molteni N, Prampolini L et al (1994) Need for follow up in coeliac disease. *Archives of Disease in Childhood* 70: 211–213.
Barnes GL & Townley RRW (1973) Duodenal mucosal damage in 31 infants with gastroenteritis. *Archives of Disease in Childhood* 48: 343–349.
Berrill WT, Eade OE, Fitzpatrick PF et al (1975) Bird fancier's lung and jejunal villous atrophy. *Lancet* ii: 1006–1008.
Burgin-Wolff A, Gaze H, Hadziselimovic F et al (1991) Anti-gliadin and antiendomysium antibody determination for coeliac disease. *Archives of Disease in Childhood* 66: 941–947.
Bye AM, Andermann F, Robitaille Y et al (1993) Cortical vascular abnormalities in the syndrome of coeliac disease, epilepsy, bilateral occipital calcifications, and folate deficiency. *Annals of Neurology* 34(3): 399–403.
Carroccio A, Ianoco G, Montalto G et al (1991) Exocrine pancreatic function in children with coeliac disease before and after a gluten free diet. *Gut* 32: 796–799.
Carswell F, Gibson AAM & McAllister TA (1973) Giardiasis and coeliac disease. *Archives of Disease in Childhood* 45: 414.

Castro M, Crino A, Papadatou B et al (1993) Down's syndrome and celiac disease. *Journal of Pediatric Gastroenterology and Nutrition* **16:** 265–268.

Catassi C, Ratsch I-M, Fabiani E et al (1994) Coeliac disease in the year 2000: exploring the iceberg. *Lancet* **343:** 200–203.

Cavell B, Senhammar L, Ascher H et al (1992) Increasing incidence of childhood coeliac disease in Sweden. Results of a national study. *Acta Paediatrica Scandinavica* **81:** 589–592.

Colaco J, Egan-Mitchell B, Stevens FM et al (1987) Compliance with gluten free diet in coeliac disease. *Archives of Disease in Childhood* **62:** 706–708.

Collin P, Korpela M, Hallstrom O et al (1992a) Rheumatic complaints as a presenting symptom in patients with coeliac disease. *Scandinavian Journal of Rheumatology* **21:** 20–23.

Collin P, Mäki M, Keyrilainen O et al (1992b) Selective IGA deficiency and coeliac disease. *Scandinavian Journal of Gastroenterology* **27:** 367–371.

Congdon PJ, Mason MK, Smith SEW et al (1981) Small-bowel mucosa in asymptomatic children with celiac disease. *American Journal of Diseases of Children* **135:** 118–121.

Congdon PJ, Fiddler GI, Littlewood JM & Scott O (1982) Coeliac disease in children with congenital heart disease. *Archives of Disease in Childhood* **57:** 78–79.

Cooke WT, Peeney ALP & Hawkins CF (1953) Symptoms, signs and diagnostic features of idiopathic steatorrhoea. *Quarterly Journal of Medicine* **22:** 59–77.

Dicke WK (1950) *Coeliac disease. Investigation into the harmful effects of certain types of cereal on patients with coeliac disease.* MD thesis. University of Utrecht.

Dicke WK, Weijers HA & van de Kamer JH (1953) Coeliac disease, presence in wheat of a factor having deleterious effect in cases of coeliac disease. *Acta Paediatrica Scandinavica* **42:** 34–42.

Dissanayake AS, Truelove SC & Whitehead R (1974) Lack of harmful effect of oats on small intestinal mucosa in coeliac disease. *British Medical Journal* **4:** 189–191.

Dormandy KM, Waters AH & Mollifier DL (1963) Folic acid deficiency in coeliac disease. *Lancet* **i:** 632–635.

Egan-Mitchell B & McNicholl B (1972) Constipation in childhood coeliac disease. *Archives of Disease in Childhood* **47:** 238.

Egan-Mitchell B, Fottrell PF & McNicholl B (1978) Prolonged gluten intolerance in treated coeliac disease. In McNicholl B, McCarthy CF & Fottrell PF (eds) *Perspectives in Coeliac Disease,* pp 251–258. Lancaster: Kluwer Academic Publishers.

Falchuk ZM, Rogentine GN & Strober W (1972) Predominance of histocompatibility antigen HL-A8 in patients with gluten-sensitive enteropathy. *Journal of Clinical Investigation* **ii:** 1602.

Fallstrom SP, Winberg J & Andersen HJ (1965) Cow's milk induced malabsorption as a precursor of gluten intolerance. *Acta Paediatrica Scandinavica* **54:** 101.

Ferguson MM (1980) Coeliac disease with recurrent aphthae. *Gut* **21:** 223–226.

Fontaine JL & Navarro J (1975) Small intestinal biopsy in cow's milk protein allergy in infancy. *Archives of Disease in Childhood* **50:** 357–362.

Fry L, McMinn RMH, Cowan JD & Hoffbrand AV (1968) Effect of gluten free diet on dermatological, intestinal and haematological manifestations of dermatitis herpetiformis. *Lancet* **i:** 557–561.

Gee S (1888) On the coeliac affection. *St Bartholomew's Hospital Report* **24:** 17–20.

Gobbi G, Bouquet F, Greco L et al (1992) Coeliac disease, epilepsy, and cerebral calcifications. *Lancet* **ii:** 439–443.

Greco L, Auricchio S, Mayer M & Grimaldi M (1988) Case control study on nutritional risk factors in celiac disease. *Journal of Pediatric Gastroenterology and Nutrition* **7:** 395–399.

Greco L, Mäki M, Di Donato & Visakorpi JK (1992) Epidemiology of coeliac disease in Europe and the Mediterranean area. In: Auriccho S & Visakorpi JK (eds) *Common Food Intolerances 1: Epidemiology of Coeliac Disease,* pp 25–44. Basel: Karger.

Groll A, Candy DCA, Preece MA et al (1980) Short stature as the primary manifestation of coeliac disease. *Lancet* **ii:** 1097–1099.

Guandalini S, Ventura A, Ansaldi N et al (1989) Diagnosis of coeliac disease: time for a change? *Archives of Disease in Childhood* **64:** 1320–1325.

Hamilton JR, Lynch MJ & Reilly BJ (1969) Active coeliac disease in childhood. Clinical and laboratory findings in forty-two cases. *Quarterly Journal of Medicine* **38:** 135–158.

Hardoff D, Sharf B & Berger A (1980) Myopathy as a presentation of coeliac disease. *Developmental Medicine and Child Neurology* **22:** 781–783.

Hjelt K (1991) The role of the exocrine pancreas in early-onset vitamin B_{12} malabsorption in gluten challenged celiac children. *Journal of Pediatric Gastroenterology and Nutrition* **13:** 27–31.

Hjelt K & Krasilnikoff PA (1990) The impact of gluten on haematological status, dietary intakes of haematopoetic nutrients and vitamin B_{12} and folic acid absorption in children with coeliac disease. *Acta Paediatrica Scandinavica* **79:** 911–919.

Holmes GKT (1992) Long-term health risks of unrecognised coeliac patients. In Auricchio S & Visakorpi JK (eds) *Common Food Intolerances. 1: Epidemiology of Coeliac Disease*, pp 105–118. Basel: Karger.

Holmes GKT, Prior P, Lane MR et al (1989) Malignancy in coeliac disease—effect of a gluten free diet. *Gut* **30:** 333–338.

Howarth E, Hodson CJ, Pringle EM & Young WF (1968) The value of radiological investigations of the alimentary tract in children with coeliac syndrome. *Clinical Radiology* **19:** 65–76.

Hutchinson HC, al Mardini H, Gillespie S et al (1991) A pilot study of fluticasone propionate in untreated coeliac disease. *Gut* **32:** 260–265.

Jackson PT, Glasgow JFT & Thom R (1985) Parents' understanding of coeliac disease and diet. *Archives of Disease in Childhood* **60:** 672–674.

Kaplan JG, Pack D, Horoupian D et al (1988) Distal axonopathy associated with chronic gluten enteropathy. *Neurology* **38:** 642–645.

Keuning JJ, Pena AS, van Leeuwen A et al (1976) HLA-DW3 associated with coeliac disease. *Lancet* **i:** 506.

Kilander AF, Nilsson L-A & Gillberg R (1987) Serum antibodies to gliadin in coeliac disease after gluten withdrawal. *Scandinavian Journal of Gastroenterology* **22:** 29–34.

Kilby A (1976) Pediatric small intestinal biopsy capsule with two ports. *Gut* **17:** 158–159.

Kilby A, Walker-Smith JA & Wood CBS (1975) Small intestinal mucosa in cow's milk allergy. *Lancet* **i:** 531.

Klaus SN (1992) Dermatitis herpetiformis and celiac disease. *Frontiers of Gastrointestinal Research* **19:** 176–183.

Knudtzon J, Fluge G & Aksnes L (1991) Routine measurements of gluten antibodies in children of short stature. *Journal of Pediatric Gastroenterology and Nutrition* **12:** 190–194.

Koistinen J (1975) Selective IgA deficiency in blood donors. *Vox Sang* **29:** 192–202.

Koletzko S, Burgin-Wolff, Koletzko B et al (1988) Prevalence of coeliac disease in diabetic children and adolescents. *European Journal of Pediatrics* **148:** 113–117.

Kuitunen R, Rapola J, Savilahti E & Visakorpi JKV (1973) Response of the jejunal mucosa to cow's milk in the malabsorption syndrome with cow's milk intolerance. A light and electron microscopic study. *Acta Paediatrica Scandinavica* **62:** 585–595.

Kuitunen P, Visakorpi JK, Savilahti E & Pekonen P (1975) Malabsorption syndrome with cow's milk intolerance. Clinical findings and course in 54 cases. *Archives of Disease in Childhood* **50:** 351–356.

Kumar PJ, Walker-Smith JA, Milla P et al (1988) The teenage coeliac: follow up study of 102 patients. *Archives of Disease in Childhood* **63:** 916–920.

Lerner A & Lebenthal E (1991) The controversy of the use of anti-gluten antibody (AGA) as a diagnostic tool in celiac disease. *Journal of Pediatric Gastroenterology and Nutrition* **12:** 407–409.

Lindberg T, Berg NO, Borulf S & Jakobsson I (1978) Liver damage in coeliac disease or other food intolerance in childhood. *Lancet* **i:** 390–391.

Littlewood JM (1986) The sweat test. *Archives of Disease in Childhood* **61:** 1041–1043.

Littlewood JM (1992) Gastrointestinal complications in cystic fibrosis. *Journal of the Royal Society of Medicine* **85 (supplement 18):** 13–19.

Littlewood JM & Losowsky MS (1984) Modern investigation of gastrointestinal disease. In Meadow R (ed.) *Recent Advances in Paediatrics*, pp 77–101. Edinburgh: Churchill Livingstone.

Littlewood JM & MacDonald A (1986) Clinical aspects of food allergy and intolerance. In Heatley RV, Losowsky MS & Kelleher J (eds) *Clinical Nutrition in Gastroenterology*, pp 202–234. Edinburgh: Churchill Livingstone.

Littlewood JM, Crollick AJ, Smith SEW et al (1979) Coeliac disease in childhood. *Simposio Internanzionale, Bologna*, 1979, pp 21–37.

Littlewood JM, Crollick AJ & Richards IDG (1980) Childhood coeliac disease is disappearing. *Lancet* **ii:** 1359.

Lloyd-Still JD, Grand RJ, Kon-Taik Khaw MD & Schwachman H (1972) The use of corticosteroids in coeliac crisis. *Journal of Pediatrics* **81:** 1074–1081.

Logan RFA (1992) Descriptive epidemiology of celiac disease. *Frontiers of Gastrointestinal Research*, **19:** 1–14.

Logan RFA, Rifkind EA, Buttil A et al (1986) Prevalencce and 'incidence' of celiac disease in Edinburgh and the Lothian region of Scotland. *Gastroenterology* **90:** 334–342.

McLoughlin LC, Nord KS, Visay V & Connor EM (1987) Severe gastrointestinal involvement in children with acquired immunodeficiency syndrome. *Journal of Pediatric Gastroenterology and Nutrition* **4:** 517–525.

McNicholl B, Egan-Mitchell B & Fottrell PF (1979) Variability of gluten intolerance in treated childhood coeliac disease. *Gut* **20:** 126–132.

McNeish AS (1989) Diagnosis of coeliac disease: time for a change? Commentary. *Archives of Disease in Childhood* **64:** 1324–1325.

McNeish AS, Harms K, Rey J et al (1979) Re-evaluation of diagnostic criteria for coeliac disease. *Archives of Disease in Childhood* **54:** 783–786.

Mäki M (1992) Use of serological antibody tests in celiac disease. In Branski D, Rozen P & Kagnoff MF (eds) *Gluten Sensitive Enteropathy*, pp 108–129. Basel: Karger.

Mäki M & Holm K (1990) Incidence and prevalence of coeliac disease in Tampere. *Acta Paediatrica Scandinavica* **79:** 980–982.

Mäki M, Hallstrom O, Huupponen T et al (1984) Increased prevalence of coeliac disease in diabetes. *Archives of Disease in Childhood* **59:** 739–742.

Mäki M, Lahdeaho M-L, Hallstrom O et al (1989) Postpubertal gluten challenge in coeliac disease. *Archives of Disease in Childhood* **64:** 1604–1607.

Mäki M, Holm K, Koskimies S et al (1990) Normal small bowel biopsy followed by coeliac disease. *Archives of Disease in Childhood* **65:** 1137–1141.

Mäki M, Aine L. Lipsanen V & Koskimos S (1991) Dental enamel defects in first-degree relatives of coeliac disease patients. *Lancet* **337:** 763–764.

Marks J, Shuster S & Watson AJ (1966) Small bowel changes in dermatitis herpetiformis. *Lancet* **ii:** 1280–1282.

Mayer M, Greco L, Troncone R et al (1989) Early prediction of relapse during gluten challenge in childhood celiac disease. *Journal of Pediatric Gastroenterology and Nutrition* **8:** 474–479.

Mayer M, Greco L, Troncone R et al (1991) Compliance of adolescents with coeliac disease with a gluten free diet. *Gut* **32:** 881–885.

Meeuwisse GW (1970) Round table discussion. Diagnostic criteria in coeliac disease. *Acta Paediatrica Scandinavica* **59:** 461–463.

Mirakian R, Richardson A, Milla PJ et al (1986) Protracted diarrhoea in infancy: evidence in support of an autoimmune variant. *British Medical Journal* **293:** 1132–1136.

Montgomery AMP, Goka AKJ, Kumar PJ et al (1988) Low gluten diet in the treatment of adult coeliac disease: effect on jejunal morphology and serum anti-gluten antibodies. *Gut* **29:** 1564–1568.

Mora S, Weber G, Barera G et al (1993) Effect of gluten free diet on bone mineral content in growing patients with celiac disease. *American Journal of Clinical Nutrition* **57:** 224–228.

Naiman JL, Oski FA, Diamond LK et al (1964) The gastrointestinal effects of iron deficiency anaemia. *Pediatrics* **33:** 83–99.

Nelson R, McNeish AS & Anderson CM (1973) Coeliac disease in children of Asian immigrants. *Lancet* **i:** 348.

Packer SM, Charlton V, Keeling JW et al (1978) Gluten challenge in treated coeliac disease. *Archives of Disease in Childhood* **53:** 449–455.

Paerregaard A, Vilien M, Krasilnikoff PA & Gudmand-Hoyer E (1988) Supposed coeliac disease during childhood and its presentation 14–38 years later. *Scandinavian Journal of Gastroenterology* **23:** 65–70.

Paulley JW (1954) Observations on the aetiology of idiopathic steatorrhoea. *British Medical Journal* **ii:** 1318.

Pelkonen P, Scinala M & Vicopio P (1963) Inherited agammaglobulinaemia with malabsorption and marked alterations in the gastrointestinal mucosa. *Acta Medica Scandinavica* **173:** 549.

Prader A, Schermling DH, Zachmann M & Biro Z (1969) Catch-up growth in coeliac disease. *Acta Paediatrica Scandinavica* **58:** 311.

Rich EJ & Christie DL (1990) Anti-gliadin antibody panel and xylose absorption test in screening for celiac disease. *Journal of Pediatric Gastroenterology and Nutrition* **10:** 174–178.

Rossipal E (1991) The incidence of childhood coeliac disease in Austria: a study covering the period 1969–86. In Kumar PJ & Walker-Smith JA (eds) *Coeliac Disease: One Hundred Years*, pp 299–302. Leeds: Leeds University Press.

Sakula J & Shiner M (1957) Coeliac disease with atrophy of the small intestine mucosa. *Lancet* **ii:** 876.

Sanderson MC, Davis LR & Mowat AP (1975) Failure of laboratory and radiological studies to predict jejunal mucosal atrophy. *Archives of Disease in Childhood* **50:** 526–531.

Sandyk R & Brennan MJW (1983) Isolated ocular myopathy and celiac disease in childhood. *Neurology* **33:** 792.

Saverymuttu SH, Sabbat J, Burke M & Maxwell JD (1991) Impact of endoscopic duodenal biopsy on the detection of small intestinal villous atrophy. *Postgraduate Medical Journal* **67:** 47–49.

Schmitz J, Jos J & Rey J (1978) Transient mucosal atrophy in confirmed coeliac disease. In McNicholl B, McCarthy CF & Fottrell PF (eds) *Perspectives in Coeliac Disease*, pp 259–266. Lancaster, Kluwer Academic Publishers.

Schmitz J, Arnand-Battandier F, Jos J & Rey L (1984) Long-term follow-up of childhood coeliac disease (CD): is there a 'natural recovery'? *Pediatric Research* **18:** 1052.

Scott BB & Losowsky MS (1975) Coeliac disease: a cause of various associated diseases? *Lancet* **ii:** 956–957.

Seah PP, Fry L, Rossiter MA et al (1971) Anti-reticulin antibodies in childhood coeliac disease. *Lancet* **ii:** 681–682.

Shale DJ, Johnston DG, Haeer F & Roberts DF (1982) Coeliac disease in monozygotic twins. *Postgraduate Medical Journal* **58:** 797–798.

Shmerling DH (1977) Questionnaire of the European Society for Paediatric Gastroenterology and Nutrition on coeliac disease. In McNicholl B, McCarthy CF & Fottrell PF (eds) *Perspectives in Coeliac Disease. Proceedings of the Third International Symposium on Coeliac Disease, Galway, September 1977*, pp 245–249. Lancaster: Kluwer Academic Publishers.

Shmerling DH & Franckx J (1986) Childhood celiac disease: a long-term analysis of relapses in 91 patients. *Journal of Pediatric Gastroenterology and Nutrition* **5:** 565–569.

Shmerling DH, Forner JCW & Prader A (1970) Faecal fat and nitrogen in healthy children and in children with malabsorption or maldigestion. *Pediatrics* **46:** 690–695.

Smith SEW & Littlewood JM (1977) The two film barium meal in the exclusion of coeliac disease. *Clinical Radiology* **28:** 629–634.

Stahlberg MR, Savilahti E & Siimes MA (1991) Iron deficiency in coeliac disease is mild and it is detected and corrected by gluten-free diet. *Acta Paediatrica Scandinavica* **80:** 190–193.

Stevens FM, Egan-Mitchell B, Cryan E et al (1987) Decreasing incidence of coeliac disease. *Archives of Disease in Childhood* **62:** 465–468.

Stokes PL, Asquith P, Holmes GKT et al (1972) Histocompatibility antigens associated with adult coeliac disease. *Lancet* **ii:** 162.

Stokes PL, Ferguson R, Holmes GKT & Cooke WT (1976) Familial aspects of coeliac disease. *Quarterly Journal of Medicine* **45:** 567–582.

Tanner JM, Whitehouse RH, Cameron N et al (1983) *Assessment of Skeletal Maturity and Prediction of Adult Height (TW 2 Method)*, 2nd edn. London: Academic Press.

Taylor CJ (1988) Predictive value of intraepithelial lymphocyte counts in childhood coeliac disease. *Journal of Pediatric Gastroenterology and Nutrition* **7:** 532–536.

Tosi R, Visamara D, Tanigaki N et al (1983) Evidence that coeliac disease is associated with a DC locus allelic specificity. *Clinical Immunology and Immunopathology* **28:** 359–404.

Valletta EA & Mastella G (1989) Incidence of coeliac disease in a cystic fibrosis population. *Acta Paediatrica Scandinavica* **78:** 784–785.

Valletta EA, Trevisiol D & Mastella G (1990) IgA antigliadin antibodies in the monitoring of gluten challenge in celiac disease. *Journal of Pediatric Gastroenterology and Nutrition* **10:** 169–173.

Visakorpi JK (1974) Definition of coeliac disease in children. In Hekkens WThJM & Pena AS (eds) *Coeliac Disease. Proceedings of the Second International Coeliac Symposium, Noordwijkerrhout, The Nederlands, 1974*, pp 10–16. Leiden: Stenfert Kroese.

Visakorpi JK & Immonen P (1967) Intolerance to cow's milk and wheat gluten in the primary malabsorption syndrome in infancy. *Acta Paediatrica Scandinavica* **56:** 49–56.

Vitoria JC, Canarero C, Sojo A et al (1982) Enteropathy related to fish, rice and chicken. *Archives of Disease in Childhood* **57:** 44–48.

Walker-Smith JA (1967) Dissecting microscope appearance of small bowel mucosa in children. *Archives of Disease in Childhood* **42:** 626–630.

Walker-Smith JA (1973) Discordance for coeliac disease in monozygotic twins. *Gut* **14:** 374.

Walker-Smith J (1988) *Diseases of the Small Intestine in Childhood*, 3rd edn. London: Butterworths.

Walker-Smith JA (1991) Coeliac disease. In Walker WA, Durie PR, Hamilton JR et al *Paediatric Gastrointestinal Disease*, pp 700–715. Philadelphia: BC Decker.

Walker-Smith JA, Guandalini S, Schmiz J et al (1990) Revised criteria for diagnosis of coeliac disease. *Archives of Disease in Childhood* **65:** 909–911.

Walker-Smith JA, Phillips AD & Richman PI (1991) Intestinal biopsy. In Walker WA, Durie PR, Hamilton JR et al (eds) *Pediatric Gastrointestinal Disease*, vol. 2, pp 1307–1323. Philadelphia: BC Decker.

Wall AJ, Douglas AP, Booth CC & Pearse AGE (1970) Response of the jejunal mucosa in adult coeliac disease to oral prednisolone. *Gut* **2:** 7.

Walters JRF (1994) Bone mineral density in coeliac disease. *Gut* **35:** 150–151.

Walters MP, Kelleher J, Gilbert J & Littlewood JM (1990) Clinical monitoring of steatorrhoea in cystic fibrosis. *Archives of Disease in Childhood* **65:** 99–102.

Weizman Z, Hamilton JR, Kopelman HR et al (1987) Treatment failure in celiac disease due to coexistent exocrine pancreatic insufficiency. *Pediatrics* **80:** 924–926.

Weile B & Krasilnikoff PA (1993) Extremely low incidence of coeliac disease in Denmark. *Journal of Clinical Epidemiology* **46:** 661–664.

Young WF & Pringle EM (1971) 110 Children with coeliac disease. *Archives of Disease in Childhood* **46:** 421–436.

Zubillaga P, Vitoria JC, Arrieta A et al (1993) Down's syndrome and celiac disease. *Journal of Pediatric Gastroenterology and Nutrition* **16:** 168–171.

7

Coeliac disease in adults

GINO R. CORAZZA
GIOVANNI GASBARRINI

Coeliac disease can be defined as a chronic disease in which there is a characteristic, though not specific, mucosal lesion of the small intestine, which impairs nutrient absorption by the involved bowel and which improves on withdrawal of wheat gliadins and barley, rye and oat prolamins from the diet (Trier, 1991). The merit of this definition is that it specifies that the severity of nutrient malabsorption depends largely on the length of small intestine involved. This has important consequences from a clinical standpoint, since it suggests an explanation as to why the clinical presentation of adult coeliac disease can have a protean nature, varying from clinically severe forms to subclinical or silent forms.

This review aims to be practical and is intended to offer appropriate and updated guidelines for the diagnosis and management of adult patients with coeliac disease.

EPIDEMIOLOGICAL ASPECTS

Disease frequency

Particularly in the adult form, owing to the frequent subclinical trend and the consequent difficulty in dating the onset of disease, the frequency of coeliac disease is easier to evaluate in terms of prevalence than of incidence. In Europe, the prevalence rate of adult coeliac disease has been reported as being 1:950 in Sweden (Hallert et al, 1983) and 1:1700 in Scotland (Logan et al, 1986). These figures are based on detected symptomatic cases. However, there is now a wide consensus that the true prevalence of coeliac disease is much greater and that it is close to a rate of 1 in 300 in the general population (Auricchio et al, 1990).

The recent availability of screening tests with adequate sensitivity and specificity has permitted studies on asymptomatic subjects that confirm the figure given above. In Sweden, screening by means of the search for immunoglobulin (Ig)A anti-gliadin antibodies in 1866 blood donors showed that seven completely asymptomatic subjects (1 in 270) had mucosal lesions typical of coeliac disease (Hed et al, 1986). However, if we consider that blood donors are not representative of the general population, that the search for anti-gliadin antibodies is a test with high but not absolute sensitivity, and that not all the donors with positive anti-gliadin antibodies agreed to undergo intestinal biopsy, it can be concluded that the true prevalence of adult coeliac disease in the general population may be even greater.

Using the same screening test in groups of subjects considered at risk for coeliac disease, such as first-degree relatives of coeliac patients who should always be screened for the condition, it was possible to ascertain a prevalence ten times greater than that of the blood donors (Corazza et al, 1992a).

Sex and age frequency

Data from new patients who joined the Coeliac Society of the United Kingdom between 1980 and 1990 show that sex frequency is nearly equal in childhood while in adults the female:male ratio is 2:1 (Howdle and Losowsky, 1992).

The greater frequency of adult disease in females is a well-established finding and is commonly explained by the fact that presentation may be precipitated by pregnancy, that there is a greater likelihood of iron or calcium deficiency in the female during fertile years and that there may be a greater tendency in females to seek medical advice.

In our series of adult patients with coeliac disease diagnosed at the University of Bologna between 1972 and 1989, the female:male ratio progressively decreased in the last few years of the study, parallel to the increase in the number of patients diagnosed with a subclinical form of the disease (Corazza et al, 1993a). Bearing in mind that there is the same prevalence between the sexes in childhood, these results support the suggestion that in adult males coeliac disease is more difficult to diagnose and that undiagnosed adult coeliac patients may be mainly males (Logan et al, 1983).

As far as age is concerned, although adult coeliac disease may be diagnosed at any age, adults present a bimodal peak localized at the fourth or fifth decade for females and at the fifth or sixth decade for males (Howdle and Losowsky, 1992). Females are thus diagnosed a decade earlier than males and, although this may reflect varying patterns of joining the Coeliac Society, it is attributed to the precipitating effect of pregnancy in unmasking a predisposition to coeliac disease (Stewart and Willoughby, 1988).

Clearly, it is one thing to talk of age at diagnosis and another to talk of age at clinical onset (appearance of symptoms) or of true onset (appearance of intestinal lesions). It is believed that symptoms of illness in childhood are present on close investigation in about one-third of adult patients (Barry et al, 1974). This statement agrees with our own experience, but its specificity has obviously not been demonstrated while its sensitivity is certainly low if we admit that coeliac disease can start in a subclinical or even asymptomatic form. On the other hand, there are increasingly detailed and numerous reports that the intestinal lesions can appear, after a phase of latency, in adulthood and not concurrently with the first contact with gluten (Collin et al, 1993).

CLINICAL ASPECTS

Mode of presentation

The classical clinical presenting features of adult coeliac disease were for many years considered to be diarrhoea, steatorrhoea and marked weight loss. These features were reported with surprising precision more than a century ago by Samuel Gee in his admirable article 'On the coeliac affection': '. . . to diarrhoea alba add emaciation and cachexia, and we have a complete picture of the disease . . .' (Gee, 1888). For many years the presence of these symptoms was considered as being a condition *sine qua*

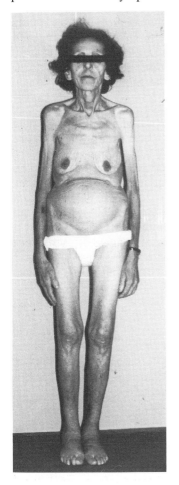 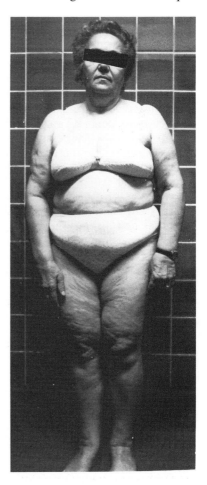

Figure 1. The protean presentation of adult coeliac disease. Left: 60-year-old woman presenting with persistent diarrhoea, steatorrhoea, weight loss, abdominal distension, tetany, bone pain and peripheral oedema. Right: 58-year-old woman, obese, diagnosed in spite of the absence of malabsorption symptoms and haematochemical abnormalities, because of positivity to anti-gliadin antibodies evaluated within a family study.

non for carrying out an intestinal biopsy and, consequently, their prevalence was very high in the earlier series of patients with coeliac disease. That adult disease could present with more subtle and variable clinical expressions, and that gross clinical evidence of malabsorption was no longer an essential criterion for diagnosis, began to be noted in the mid-1960s (Brooks et al, 1966), and since then the lower prevalence of malabsorption has been attributed to the reduced extent of the lesions along the small intestine (MacDonald et al, 1964). It was, however, only some time later that the conviction began to spread that patients with only minimal, transient or extraintestinal symptoms constitute the majority of patients with adult coeliac disease (Mann et al, 1970; Swinson and Levi, 1980; Logan et al, 1983). However, this change in the pattern of clinical presentation is only apparent; adult coeliac disease has not really changed. What has changed in recent years, or rather improved, is the clinician's knowledge of the wide range of possible clinical manifestations. This now makes it possible to diagnose forms of coeliac disease that in the past would never have been diagnosed and were therefore unknown (Figure 1).

We have recently re-examined the presenting features of our series of 226 consecutive patients (Corazza et al, 1993a). As expected, the number of new cases per year has progressively increased over a period of 18 years (Figure 2). The remarkable increase in new cases since 1981—only 36 diagnoses were made in the first half of the study—was partly accounted for by the recognition of patients with a subclinical presentation, i.e. without diarrhoea and/or weight loss, whose number continues to rise. In the last 3 years of the study, cases of subclinical presentation accounted for half of all diagnoses and in 1989 they were double the number of classical presentations. It is also important to note that, if trivial symptoms are duly con-

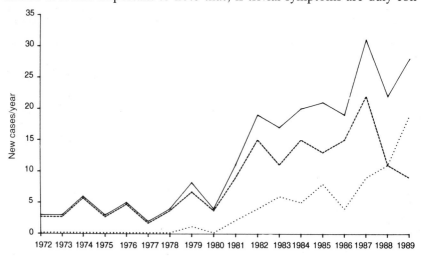

Figure 2. Number of new cases of adult coeliac disease per year, diagnosed at the University of Bologna from 1972 to 1989. All cases (continuous line), classical presentation (dashed line), subclinical presentation (dotted line). Reproduced from Corazza et al (1993a, *Journal of Clinical Gastroenterology* **16:** 16–21) with permission of Raven Press.

sidered, the age of diagnosis can be significantly lowered, thereby confirming the previous suggestion that incomplete knowledge of the full range of presenting symptoms represented the main cause of delay in the diagnosis of adult patients with coeliac disease (Croese et al, 1979).

Specific presenting features

Table 1 shows the frequency of the most important presenting features in seven different series of biopsy-proven adult coeliac patients. Apart from the particularly high prevalence of constipation and aphthous stomatitis in one of these series, the prevalence of the other signs and symptoms is fairly well balanced. Minor variations probably reflect minor differences in the definition of each feature, rather than actual variations in prevalence. Lassitude, diarrhoea and weight loss are the most frequent symptoms, but it should not be forgotten that most of the patients included in these series had been diagnosed before the fact that adult coeliac disease could present with minor, transient or extraintestinal symptoms was common knowledge. In our series weakness, diarrhoea and weight loss had a prevalence of 68, 90 and 90%, respectively, in patients diagnosed between 1972 and 1977, and of 54, 54 and 55%, respectively, in those diagnosed between 1984 and 1989 (Corazza et al, 1993a).

Among the so-called constitutional symptoms, lassitude is very common. Lassitude is an almost impossible symptom to quantify and is often given little consideration by the patient, who has lived with it for a long time. It is often independent of the presence of diarrhoea or anaemia (Cooke and Holmes, 1984), but may at times be accompanied by low blood pressure

Table 1. Frequency (%) of presenting features in seven different series of adult coeliac patients. Reproduced from Corazza et al (1991, *Coeliac Disease: 40 Years Gluten Free*. Dordrecht: Kluwer Academic Publishers) with permission.

	Barry et al (1974) (—)	Dissa-nayake et al (1974) (n = 38)	Stevens (1980) (n = 144)	Cooke and Holmes (1984) (n = 171)	Dawson and Kumar (1985) (n = 168)	Biemond et al (1987) (n = 414)	Corazza et al (1991) (n = 226)
Lassitude	—	—	70	61	79	—	73
Weight loss	50	47	62	41	62	69	70
Diarrhoea	78	53	73	62	70	80	70
Constipation	—	—	33	9	—	—	3
Abdominal distension	24	18	70	40	23	—	54
Abdominal pain	—	26	—	43	42	—	50
Nausea or vomiting	32	18	32	26	18	—	18
Bone pain	2	5	—	13	8	—	27
Cramp or tetany	—	3	50	—	4	—	20
Oedema	16	—	32	5	10	—	27
Menstrual irregularities	—	—	—	30	—	—	23
Aphthous stomatitis	—	—	61	—	28	40	12
Finger clubbing	—	—	—	—	—	—	15
Short stature	—	—	—	19	—	—	6

(Salvesen, 1963). As far as weight loss is concerned, it is important to remember that the suspicion of adult coeliac disease must not be dismissed by the presence of a normal weight or even of obesity (Owen et al, 1980). In a recent study (Corazza et al, 1994) the prevalence of malnutrion, defined as an actual body-weight less than 90% of the ideal, was 67% in adult patients with coeliac disease who presented with the classical symptoms of malabsorption but only 31% in subclinical patients. Thirty-seven per cent of the latter were actually overweight. Although adult coeliac patients have a reputation as a whole for being short, and short stature can constitute an isolated indication of intestinal biopsy in children and adolescents, the height of patients with coeliac disease diagnosed after reaching adulthood does not differ significantly from that of the general population or between adult coeliac patients who have or have not had gastrointestinal symptoms since childhood (Cacciari et al, 1991).

Among the so-called gastrointestinal symptoms, diarrhoea is predominant and can assume greatly differing clinical characteristics. When present, it may be continuous or occur periodically, alternating with phases of normal bowel movements or even of constipation. The latter may even represent the only bowel disorder in untreated coeliac disease. In the early series, the great majority of patients were troubled by nocturnal diarrhoea and some were incontinent (Green and Wollaeger, 1960). The presence of steatorrhoea is suggested by loose, discoloured, greasy and frothy stools, which are fetid and difficult to flush away. At other times the diarrhoea is frankly watery and may be exacerbated by emotional disturbances, leading to a wrong diagnosis of irritable bowel syndrome (Ross and Garabedian, 1970). The latter could also be suggested by concomitant abdominal distention, usually more frequent in the evening and accompanied by abdominal pain.

Because it is a possible source of misdiagnosis, abdominal pain must always be considered with great care and attention. In uncomplicated coeliac disease, pain, when present, is usually mild, but during attacks of diarrhoea it frequently assumes colicky-type characteristics. Severe obstructive-type pain, especially if accompanied by an unexplained relapse of the symptoms, by fever or by lymphadenopathy, must always arouse suspicion of the onset of a complication such as intestinal lymphoma (Cooper and Read, 1987) or ulcerative enteritis (Baer et al, 1980). In the presence of such pain it is advisable to carry out radiological examination and, if this is negative and the condition persists, explorative laparotomy should be considered.

Anorexia is present in about one-third of cases (Cooke and Holmes, 1984) and may be accompanied by nausea and vomiting, which are both less frequent than in childhood coeliac disease. On the contrary, adaptive hyperphagia is sometimes present, although this may not compensate for the weight loss even with an intake of 7000 calories daily (Comfort, 1958).

Since, as we have already said, extraintestinal symptoms often dominate the clinical picture, coeliac patients may seek medical advice in many different hospital departments (Barry et al, 1974). A clear example of this is represented by the bone pain due to metabolic osteopathy. This may be the only sign of adult coeliac disease (Moss et al, 1965) and may be mistaken for rheumatic pain, even though on pressure and percussion bone tenderness is present, representing a simple indicator of metabolic osteopathy. Adult coeliac patients have an increased susceptibility to pathological fractures and pseudofractures, even at a young age. The deficiency of vitamin D that is often present is also responsible for the characteristic myopathy, the symptoms of which are represented by proximal muscle weakness, anserine gait and difficulty in rising from a chair without assistance (Hepner et al, 1978). Our recent results showed that 16 of 17 untreated adult coeliac patients had a bone mineral density in the range of osteoporosis. Bone pain was present in only four of them, and a gluten-free diet, followed for a mean of 52 months improved but did not normalize bone mass. Cramps and tetany are present, particularly in patients in whom profuse diarrhoea has led to severe electrolyte depletion, and it is important to remember that administration of calcium may be ineffective without correcting the potassium and magnesium deficiencies that are often present in such cases (Balint and Hirschowitz, 1961).

In adult coeliac disease, the occurrence of neurological disorders has often been reported (Cooke and Holmes, 1984). The most frequent is mixed peripheral neuropathy, legs being more affected than arms and males more than females. The limbs are weak, numb, trembling and paraesthetic with sensory impairment of glove and stocking type. The response of this neurological syndrome, probably due to electrolyte and metabolic deficiencies, to gluten withdrawal is unpredictable. As far as intellectual ability is concerned, although psychometric examination shows no consistent signs of cognitive impairment in adult coeliac patients (Hallert and Åström, 1983), five patients with brain atrophy and presenile dementia have been recently reported (Collin et al, 1991). All but one were unresponsive to gluten withdrawal and aggressive substitution therapy. As far as psychiatric disorders in adult coeliac disease are concerned, depression is said to be the most frequent and proved to be the commonest reason for granting a disability pension in Swedish adult coeliac patients (Hallert and Derefeldt, 1982).

Reproductive dysfunction is at times present in both sexes. In females there is a tendency to late menarche, amenorrhoea, early menopause and infertility, which respond positively to dietary gluten restriction (Morris et al, 1970). In untreated women, there is also a greater frequency of spontaneous abortion, stillbirth and neonatal death (Ferguson et al, 1982). In males, impotence, decreased sexual activity, infertility, abnormalities of sperm morphology and motility were more frequent than expected (Farthing et al, 1982). The majority of these dysfunctions improved after a gluten-free diet and were accompanied by a pattern of hormonal abnormality indicative of androgen resistance (Farthing et al, 1983).

Although hypoprothrombinaemia is present in many adult patients, overt and severe bleeding has only rarely been reported as the initial presenting feature (Graham et al, 1982).

Physical findings

The variations in height and weight of adult patients with coeliac disease have been discussed above. As far as facial appearance is concerned, classical descriptions report plump faces in females and triangular faces in males (Cooke and Holmes, 1984). Our experience differs in the sense that the triangular appearance, although present in only a certain number of cases, is also fairly common in females. Premature hair greying is frequent and potentially reversible after starting a gluten-free diet. The hair is also fine, the beard scanty and axillary hair is often lost.

Finger clubbing is present in 20% of patients; it is usually mild, decreases after a gluten-free diet and, contrary to common belief, is not more frequent or severe in patients with malignant complications (Cooper et al, 1980). Koilonychia is the expression of iron-deficiency anaemia and disappears after iron replacement.

Skin lesions are frequently found in adult coeliac disease, and the special relationship with dermatitis herpetiformis is discussed in Chapter 9. Dryness is the most frequent skin disorder, perhaps reflecting deficiencies of various nutrients. Pigmentation occurs in a minority of patients but may raise diagnostic doubts. Unlike Whipple's disease, but similar to Addison's disease, with which coeliac disease may have other clinical features in common, the pigmentation may involve the oral mucosa. Unlike Addison's disease it may have pellagroid characteristics (Cooke et al, 1953). Other possible skin lesions include psoriasis, eczema, cutaneous vasculitis, lichen planus and pityriasis rubra pilaris. Our series included two patients with pyoderma gangrenosum and one with hypertrichosis lanuginosa, which had never hitherto been reported in association with adult coeliac disease (Corazza et al, 1991).

Lesions of the oral cavity are of notable diagnostic importance. Recurrent aphthous stomatitis (Ferguson et al, 1975) or dental enamel hypoplasia (Aine et al, 1990) may, in fact, be the only presenting features of adult coeliac disease. The frequency of coeliac disease in aphthous stomatitis was subsequently re-evaluated, and it was recommended that jejunal biopsy be carried out only in those cases where there is evidence of malabsorption (Ferguson et al, 1980). However, since anti-gliadin antibodies seem to be of help in identifying not only patients with coeliac disease but also those with oral ulceration responding to a gluten-free diet even in the absence of jejunal villous atrophy (O'Farrelly et al, 1991), it is suggested that this test may represent the best way to screen patients with aphthous ulcers. This is still an area requiring further clarification. Redness and soreness of the tongue with atrophied papillae, accompanied at times by angular stomatitis and less frequently by cheilosis, are linked to nutritional deficiencies. In cases of iron deficiency, the tongue tends to be smoother and paler. The presence of these symptoms often reflects the general condition of the patient (Cooke and Holmes, 1984).

Peripheral oedema linked to low serum protein levels is considered to be a marker of poor general condition in adult coeliac disease, and, as such, the prevalence of this sign is now less than in the older series. It is probable that it is determined not only by malabsorption but also by protein loss from the damaged mucosa.

Major haematological abnormalities

Low levels of haemoglobin, albumin, calcium, potassium, magnesium and iron are frequently encountered in adult coeliac disease. Although also present in patients with subclinical disease, confirming the occurrence of malabsorption at least from a biochemical standpoint in these patients, they are significantly more common in patients who present with the classical symptoms of malabsorption. Only iron deficiency was equally frequent in both subgroups of patients (Corazza et al, 1993a). This is not surprising since the main site of iron absorption is the duodenum, which is always involved in coeliac patients, even in those with minor symptoms in whom less extensive mucosal damage is present (MacDonald et al, 1964). Anaemia is consequently more often microcytic, but at times a dimorphic picture is present in the blood film owing to the concomitant malabsorption of folate in the upper jejunum (Hoffbrand, 1974). The level of vitamin B_{12} is normal or even high owing to a functional adaptation of the ileum (Mackinnon et al, 1975), and the low serum levels sometimes present are secondary to the severe folate deficiency. It must be kept in mind that anaemia, in particular iron-deficiency anaemia, may be the only indication of adult coeliac disease (Depla et al, 1990) and that the prevalence of unsuspected disease in patients with unexplained anaemia has been reported as being around 5% (Corazza et al, 1995).

Pitted red cells and Howell–Jolly bodies are present in the blood film in about half of adult coeliac patients, and are indicative of dysfunction or atrophy of the spleen. Hyposplenism in coeliac disease is more frequent and severe the later the diagnosis. It does not complicate the childhood form, it regresses at least partially after a gluten-free diet, and it may lead to autoimmunity and fatal infections (Corazza and Gasbarrini, 1983). Adult coeliac disease is the condition most commonly associated with hyposplenism and a diagnosis of asymptomatic coeliac disease should always be considered in patients presenting features of idiopathic hyposplenism (Ferguson et al, 1970). The thrombocytosis that is sometimes present may be due to the impaired splenic function, but has also been related to inflammation of the intestinal mucosa (Nelson et al, 1976).

Hypocholesterolaemia is often present and may be accompanied by hypertriglyceridaemia in some cases of severe malabsorption (Vuoristo et al, 1980).

Associated disorders

Many conditions have been reported in association with coeliac disease. Some of the numerous immunological perturbations (Howdle and Losowsky, 1987), such as the HLA haplotype DR3-DQw2, the anomalous crossing of antigens through the damaged small intestinal mucosa, the deposition in target organs of immune complexes and the reduction in immune surveillance, can explain the association with other conditions that are believed to have an immunological pathogenesis.

The conditions that may be associated with coeliac disease are listed in

Table 2. Coeliac disease and related disorders*.

Insulin-dependent diabetes mellitus	Congenital heart disease
Atopy	Lung cavities
Inflammatory bowel disease	Sjögren's syndrome
Primary biliary cirrhosis	Systemic and cutaneous vasculitis
Primary sclerosing cholangitis	Systemic lupus erythematosus
Epilepsy with cerebral calcification	Polymyositis
IgA mesangial nephropathy	Myasthenia gravis
Thyroid disease	Iridocyclitis or choroiditis
IgA deficiency	Cystic fibrosis
Rheumatoid arthritis	Macroamylasaemia
Sarcoidosis	Addison's disease
Down's syndrome	Autoimmune thrombocytopenic purpura
Bird-fancier's lung	Autoimmune haemolytic anaemia
Recurrent pericarditis	Schizophrenia

* For the disorders listed in column 1 evidence exists of an association that is more than coincidental.

Table 2 (for references see Mulder and Tytgat, 1987; Branski et al, 1992). While the association is real and based on probable causal relationships for some of these conditions, it is likely that for others it is by chance and linked to the relative probability of concurrence with a condition like coeliac disease, which is life-long. The clinical relevance of these associations is two fold: first, adult coeliac disease may present only with the symptoms of the second disease and, second, there is evidence, mostly only anecdotal, that a gluten-free diet may improve the control of the second disease. An active search for coeliac disease, using non-invasive screening tests, has been proposed in insulin-dependent diabetes mellitus (Collin et al, 1989), epilepsy with cerebral calcification (Gobbi et al, 1992), rheumatoid arthritis (O'Farrelly et al, 1988), IgA mesangial nephropathy (Fornasieri et al, 1987) and Down's syndrome (Zubillaga et al, 1993).

The natural course of coeliac disease

When an adult patient is diagnosed, it is difficult to date the start of the symptoms, which have often undergone phases of spontaneous remission and re-occurrence, and practically impossible to date the start of the intestinal lesion. It is equally difficult to predict what would be the spontaneous course of the disease without the institution of a gluten-free diet.

For these reasons the information available on the natural course of untreated adult coeliac disease is extremely limited and derives from early studies on young neglected coeliac patients, i.e. patients diagnosed as having coeliac disease in childhood and subsequently lost to follow-up. In their adult life, the morbidity resulting from non-treatment, in spite of the presence of villous atrophy, was slight in a study dealing with adolescents who had abandoned treatment for just over 10 years (McCrae et al, 1975). In another study dealing with older patients (mean age 30.6 years), complaints varied from moderate to severe during a longer period of exposure to gluten, and five of nine had spent time in hospital (Mortimer et al, 1968). The relative lack of symptoms in patients with neglected coeliac disease is not surprising, since many patients diagnosed for the first time in adult life can be subclinical or even symptomless. However, unlike these latter, in neglected coeliacs it is possible to correlate the symptoms with a precise lifespan of untreated disease.

Although the extent of the risk associated with undiagnosed or untreated disease is not fully known, it is commonly thought that it may be considerable (Holmes, 1992). A retrospective study has shown the mortality rate in those patients diagnosed and treated in childhood to be similar to that in the general population, while it is doubled in those diagnosed in adult life (Logan et al, 1989), suggesting that in this condition exposure to gluten should be as short as possible.

In the elderly, coeliac disease may present with non-specific complaints, particularly unexplained anaemia, although this does not differ greatly from what is currently seen in the adult population. The only differences are represented by a decrease in the female:male ratio and by the greater frequency of small bowel lymphoma, which may be the presenting symptom of coeliac disease (Hankey and Holmes, 1994).

DIAGNOSIS

Intestinal biopsy

Since the definition of coeliac disease is universally given in morphological terms, a duodenal or proximal jejunal biopsy is essential for diagnosis of this condition. In adults too, although less often than in children, there are causes other than coeliac disease for loss of the normal villous architecture of the intestinal mucosa (Katz and Grand, 1979). A second biopsy is therefore necessary to show an improvement of the lesion towards normality after the withdrawal of gluten from the diet. The diagnosis of adult coeliac disease does not require a third biopsy after a period of gluten challenge, although it is mandatory in particularly difficult or borderline cases, or when (and this still occurs too often) the patient has been put on a gluten-free diet without having had a pretreatment biopsy (Howdle and Losowsky, 1992).

It should be pointed out that even lesions milder than subtotal villous atrophy should be classified as coeliac disease if they respond unequivocally to a gluten-free diet. Moreover, since there is evidence that the severity of the lesions may vary in the same patient from one biopsy sample to another taken from an adjacent area, it is recommended that multiple biopsies be carried out (Scott and Losowsky, 1976). Also for this reason, since it is accepted that the diagnostic adequacy of multiple specimens taken by endoscopic forceps is comparable to or even better than that of specimens taken by the classical suction capsules (Mee et al, 1985), more practical wide-channel fibre-optic endoscopes are now routinely used for the diagnosis of this condition.

We recently identified two distinct endoscopic patterns in adult and childhood coeliac disease: the loss or reduction of duodenal folds (Brocchi et

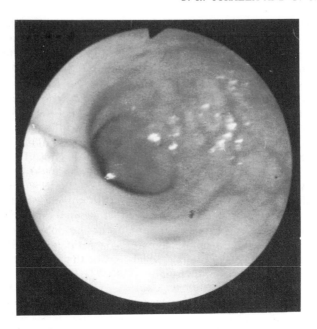

Figure 3. Endoscopic appearance of the descending duodenum of an adult patient with coeliac disease. The disappearance of Kerckring folds is evident at maximal insufflation.

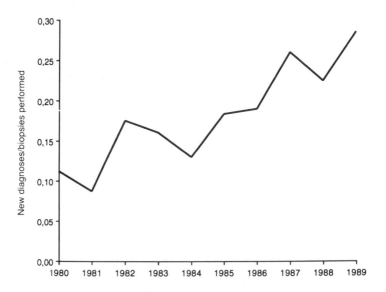

Figure 4. Ratio between the number of new diagnoses of adult coeliac disease and the number of new biopsies per year from 1980 to 1989. Reproduced from Corazza et al (1993a, *Journal of Clinical Gastroenterology* **16:** 16–21) with permission of Raven Press.

al, 1988) and the scalloping of duodenal folds (Corazza et al, 1993b), respectively. In particular, the loss or reduction of folds (Figure 3), whose diagnostic accuracy has been confirmed by other groups (McIntyre et al, 1992; van Bergeijk et al, 1993), permitted us to diagnose some clinically unsuspected adult patients (up to 13 in number) who had undergone upper gastrointestinal endoscopy for completely different reasons (Corazza et al, 1990a).

It has been demonstrated that the diagnostic rate of new adult coeliac patients increases both with the number of biopsies carried out and when the indications for biopsy take into account the full range of presenting symptoms (Swinson and Levi, 1980). Our results confirm these data (Figure 4). From 1980 to 1989, while carrying out the same number of biopsies every year but improving our awareness of the wide clinical spectrum of adult coeliac disease, the ratio between the number of new diagnoses and the number of new biopsies almost tripled (Corazza et al, 1993a).

Radiology

Radiology has practically no role in the diagnosis of uncomplicated untreated coeliac disease unless intestinal malignancy, strictures or ulceration are suspected. However, the reduction in the number of jejunal folds and the increase in the number of ileal folds evident with small bowel enema are considered specific features of coeliac disease (Herlinger and Maglinte, 1986). This reversal pattern is particularly evident in patients with long-standing or non-responsive disease (Mike et al, 1990).

Screening tests

In the past few years, the wide recognition of the concept of subclinical or silent coeliac disease has made necessary a significant change in diagnostic policy. The availability of new screening tests has contributed towards this change and also to a better knowledge of the increasingly wide spectrum of possible clinical presentations of the disease.

The determination of serum levels of IgG and IgA anti-gliadin antibodies is commonly considered to be a valuable screening assay in terms of sensitivity, specificity, convenience and expense (see Chapter 3). Their diagnostic predictability has proved greater than that of five other non-invasive tests for the screening of adult coeliac disease, including the D-xylose test and reticulin antibodies (Corazza et al, 1990b). Authorities now agree that tests which explore small bowel malabsorption, such as the D-xylose test or the 3-day quantitative test for faecal fat, are no longer valid in coeliac disease screening, particularly in patients with more subtle clinical manifestations who are in most need of a good screening test (Shanahan and Weinstein, 1988). Tests that quantify the increased intestinal permeability in coeliac disease also have a high degree of sensitivity (Juby et al, 1989) but, since they give abnormal results in many other conditions, their clinical use should be considered as complementary to that of anti-gliadin antibody estimation.

IgA anti-endomysium antibodies, directed at the lining of smooth muscle bundles of primates, seem to be closely related to previous reticulin antibodies (Chorzelsky et al, 1983). Their diagnostic predictability is greater than that of anti-gliadin antibodies (Ferreira et al, 1992; Corrao et al, 1994), some authors report high predictability also with the similar IgA reticulin antibodies (Mäki et al, 1984) (see Chapter 3). One recent study showed that serological screening increased the overall incidence of adult coeliac disease in the UK by up to 12% (Unsworth and Brown, 1994).

In clinical practice there are no precise guidelines with respect to the best screening procedure for coeliac disease in various clinical settings. Our recent results (Corrao et al, 1994) suggest that in patients referred for suspected coeliac disease intestinal biopsy should be performed directly, without any serological screening. On the contrary, in settings in which the expected prevalence of the disease is lower, a two-step procedure, measuring IgA anti-gliadin antibodies as the first step and performing anti-endomysium antibody testing as a confirmatory test only in subjects positive for anti-gliadin antibodies, was recommended particularly in view of the high costs involved in anti-endomysium measurement. Risk groups to be screened include patients with traditional symptoms in a monosymptomatic, mild or transient form, first-degree relatives of known coeliac patients, and those with certain associated diseases (Visakorpi, 1992).

TREATMENT

The gluten-free diet

Ever since Dicke published his thesis on the effect of gluten on coeliac children, a gluten-free diet has become the standard treatment for coeliac disease (van Berge-Henegouwen and Mulder, 1993). Diet may be the only therapy necessary in more than 70% of adult coeliac patients. Only some will also need symptomatic therapy, while very few patients will not respond either clinically or histologically to withdrawal of gluten from the diet.

There is also sufficient evidence to show that not only wheat gluten but also rye, barley and oat prolamins, which have close taxonomic relationships with wheat, should also be withdrawn from the diet of coeliac patients (Anand et al, 1978). It has, for example, been shown that a pint of beer contains a significant quantity of hordein, the prolamin contained in barley, and this drink must therefore be considered unsuitable for coeliac patients (Ellis et al, 1990). On the contrary, foods containing other cereals less closely related on a taxonomic level to wheat, such as rice, maize, buckwheat, millet and sorghum, are not toxic to the mucosa of coeliac patients and do not have to be eliminated from the diet (Campbell, 1982).

Sensitivity to gluten varies among patients and may also vary in the same patient at different times of life. As far as the first point is concerned, some adult patients can tolerate up to 5 g gluten daily, even for prolonged periods, without developing symptoms or gross morphological changes (Montgomery et al, 1988), while in others a single Communion wafer taken once a week can produce partial villous atrophy and reversible growth retardation

(Scotta et al, 1982). As far as the second point is concerned, as has already been stated regarding so-called neglected coeliac disease, the reintroduction of gluten in treated adult patients is not always accompanied by a recurrence of symptoms. Moreover, at least one adult case of non-histological relapse after 2 years of a gluten-containing diet has been reported (Kumar et al, 1979). Such a relapse may occur, however, after longer periods of gluten tolerance, and since the evidence in favour of temporary gluten tolerance is stronger than that of temporary intolerance, our conclusion is that a gluten-free diet should constitute a life-time commitment in all patients.

We are convinced that the gluten-free diet must be as strict as possible at all ages. In teenagers, the strong need for peer identification means that compliance with the diet is particularly poor. Even if their biochemical parameters are within the normal range (Kumar et al, 1988), poor compliance results in a suboptimal state of health and persistence of active enteropathy (Colaco et al, 1987). Moreover, it has been shown that, in teenagers, continuing ingestion of small amounts of gluten maintains local intestinal immunity in a state of continuous activation and this can, in the long term, theoretically predispose to T-cell lymphoma (Mayer et al, 1991).

Having said this, it should be added that a strict gluten-free diet is easy to prescribe but difficult to follow. Wheat gluten is contained in many pharmaceutical products (Patel et al, 1985), in nominally gluten-free products (Ciclitira et al, 1984) and in numerous canned, frozen and convenience-type processed foods that are commonly part of a Western diet. Several immunological methods for measuring gluten content in foods have been developed, but none seems to be particularly practical, easy or cheap enough to be used in normal everyday life (Howdle and Losowsky, 1990). The key to good compliance with a gluten-free diet is education; it is therefore essential to maintain a good patient–physician relationship, and we agree that coeliac patients should receive life-long follow-up (Howdle and Losowsky, 1992). Physicians and dietitians must therefore assist the patient in avoiding intentional and unintentional lapses, and non-invasive tests to verify adherence to a gluten-free diet would thus be very useful. Although serological and permeability tests are used for this purpose, we believe that asking the patient to keep a diary of everything eaten over a 2-week period, which is then analysed by an expert dietician, is still perhaps the best method for ascertaining the suitability of the diet. In our experience, compliance is much better if the patient has joined a branch of the Coeliac Society, which also publishes handbooks and up-to-date lists of gluten-free products and recipes (PO Box 220, High Wycombe, Bucks, UK).

It must be stressed that the need for treatment concerns not only symptomatic patients but also those with subclinical and silent disease. Apart from the fact that without treatment the latter may well worsen clinically and are more likely to develop associated disorders, patients often recognize the precariousness of their previous state of health only after having experienced the benefits consequent upon gluten withdrawal from the diet. Furthermore, it has now been shown that a strict gluten-free diet can prevent malignancy (Holmes et al, 1989) and that malignancy may also occur in patients with a silent (Freeman et al, 1977) or even latent form of the disease (Freeman and Chiu, 1986). Diagnosis and treatment should also be as prompt as possible since life-threatening complications such as malignancy (Cooper et al, 1982), poor response to gluten withdrawal (Nielsen et al, 1985) and splenic atrophy (Corazza and Gasbarrini, 1983) are particularly likely to arise in coeliac patients diagnosed late in life.

Unresponsiveness to a gluten-free diet

Failure to respond to the diet may occur from the outset or after many years of treatment. In the first instance the diagnosis of coeliac disease must, by definition, be questioned since the patient could be affected by other disorders causing a flat mucosa (Katz and Grand, 1979). In these patients the positivity of anti-gliadin or anti-endomysium antibodies, a blood film indicative of hyposplenism or a typical HLA phenotype are strong indications of coeliac disease already complicated by dietary unresponsiveness before diagnosis. In the second instance, it must always be ascertained whether failure to respond, is merely apparent, as in the large majority of cases, and is due to non-compliance to the gluten-free diet (Howdle, 1991). If compliance is considered to be good, the state of true non-responsiveness may be caused by associated conditions such as exocrine pancreatic insufficiency (Regan and Di Magno, 1980) or by intolerance to other foods such as milk (Cooke and Holmes, 1984), soya (Haeney et al, 1982), egg, chicken and tuna (Baker and Rosenberg, 1978). Once these conditions have been excluded, the possible presence of specific complications as more serious causes of unresponsiveness to a gluten-free diet must be carefully evaluated. Treatment of malignancy and ulcerative enteritis is dealt with in Chapter 8.

There are cases in which a dramatic worsening of the clinical condition is not linked to the presence of specific complications. Some of these patients respond to the administration of steroids or azathioprine (Hamilton et al, 1976), even in the presence of extensive subepithelial collagen deposition (Holdstock and Oleesky, 1973). More recently the safer drug, cyclosporin has been used, leading to remission in an adult patient, which persisted even after suspension of the drug (Longstreth, 1993). Other cases reported in the literature failed to respond to all measures, probably because the jejunal mucosal abnormalities had become irreversible. Total parenteral nutrition is the only treatment available for such cases (Howdle, 1991).

Nutritional supplementation

The use of supplementary therapy in coeliac disease is generally needed only in the initial stage of a gluten-free diet, i.e. when the still-damaged mucosa does not yet permit adequate nutrient absorption. We believe that this should be limited as far as possible and aimed not so much at the correction of specific laboratory parameters as at control of the symptoms linked to such deficits. If necessary, however, fluids, albumin, vitamins, iron, folic acid, calcium, potassium and magnesium must be administered, but both the physician and the patient must be fully aware that the state of health can be achieved and maintained only with a strict diet. It has been reported that untreated adult patients had prolongation of the QT interval on electrocardiography (Corazza et al, 1992b). Since this alteration predisposes to ventricular tachyarrhythmias and sudden death, the QT interval should be evaluated in untreated patients and any electrolyte deficiency should be promptly corrected. Finally, in patients with a blood film indicative of hyposplenism, immunization with polyvalent pneumococcal vaccine is recommended, and infections should be treated promptly (Corazza and Gasbarrini, 1983).

CONCLUSIONS

Few diseases have changed so much and so quickly in terms of their clinical pattern as the adult form of coeliac disease. The increasing practice by specialists of diagnosing subclinical and even silent forms is also changing the epidemiology of this condition, which is no longer considered a rare disease. It is the opinion of many physicians involved in this field that some clinical aspects of this protean disease have still to be discovered. The fact that coeliac disease is less underdiagnosed than in the past has obvious positive repercussions, since the prompt institution of a strict gluten-free diet prevents its feared complications. The availability of non-invasive and increasingly more sensitive screening tests now makes population surveys possible among healthy individuals, which should explain many aspects of this condition that are not yet clear.

SUMMARY

Coeliac disease is a chronic disease characterized by small bowel villous atrophy which impairs nutrient absorption and improves on withdrawal of wheat gliadins and barley, rye and oat prolamins from the diet. Knowledge of the adult form of coeliac disease has greatly improved in recent years. Although this knowledge is not yet sufficiently widespread among referring clinicians, it has, over the past few years, allowed an increasing number of patients to be diagnosed with subclinical forms characterized by minor, transient or apparently unrelated symptoms. As a consequence, our views on the clinical and epidemiological aspects of this condition, the prevalance of which in the general population is believed to be close to 1 in 300, have changed and are still changing. Since it has been demonstrated that a strict gluten-free diet is protective against the complications of adult coeliac disease, it is important that even subclinical and silent forms are diagnosed and treated as early as possible. Non-invasive screening tests, such as anti-gliadin and anti-endomysium antibody estimation, should therefore be used systematically in groups considered to be at risk of coeliac disease. These include first-degree relatives of coeliac patients and patients with insulin-dependent diabetes mellitus, iron-deficiency anaemia, epilepsy with cerebral calcification, recurrent aphthous stomatitis and dental enamel hypoplasia. Other conditions will probably be identified in the near future.

Acknowledgements

The authors thank Ms Susan West for translation assistance and Drs Federico Biagi and Giovanna Brusco for help in preparing the manuscript.

REFERENCES

Aine L, Mäki M, Collin P & Keyriläinen O (1990) Dental enamel defects in celiac disease. *Journal of Oral Pathology and Medicine* **19:** 241–245.
Anand BS, Piris J & Truelove SC (1978) The role of various cereals in coeliac disease. *Quarterly Journal of Medicine* **47:** 101–110.
Auricchio S, Greco L & Troncone R (1990) What is the true prevalence of coeliac disease? *Gastroenterology International* **3:** 140–142.
Baer AN, Bayless TM & Yardley JH (1980) Intestinal ulceration and malabsorption syndromes. *Gastroenterology* **79:** 754–765.
Baker AL & Rosenberg IH (1978) Refractory sprue: recovery after removal of nongluten dietary proteins. *Annals of Internal Medicine* **89:** 505–508.
Balint JA & Hirschowitz BJ (1961) Hypomagnesemia with tetany in non-tropical sprue. *New England Journal of Medicine* **265:** 631–633.
Barry RE, Baker P & Read AE (1974) Coeliac disease. The clinical presentation. *Clinics in Gastroenterology* **3:** 55–69.
Biemond I, Peña AS, Groenland F et al (1987) Coeliac disease in the Netherlands: demographic data of a patient survey among the members of the Dutch Coeliac Society. *Netherland Journal of Medicine* **31:** 263–268.
Branski D, Ashkenazi A, Freier S et al (1992) Extraintestinal manifestations and associated disorders of celiac disease. In Branski D, Rozen P & Kagnoff MF (eds) *Gluten-Sensitive Enteropathy*, pp 164–175. Basel: Karger.
Brocchi E, Corazza GR, Caletti G et al (1988) Endoscopic demonstration of loss of duodenal folds in the diagnosis of celiac disease. *New England Journal of Medicine* **319:** 741–744.
Brooks FP, Powell KC & Cerda JJ (1966) Variable clinical course of adult celiac disease. *Archives of Internal Medicine* **117:** 789–794.
Cacciari E, Corazza GR, Salardi S et al (1991) What will be the adult height of coeliac patients? *European Journal of Pediatrics* **150:** 407–409.
Campbell JA (1982) Foods for patients with celiac disease. *Canadian Medical Association Journal* **127:** 963–965.
Chorzelsky TP, Sulej J & Tchorzewska H (1983) IgA class endomysium antibodies in dermatitis herpetiformis and coeliac disease. *Annals of the New York Academy of Sciences* **420:** 325–334.
Ciclitira PJ, Ellis HJ & Fagg NLK (1984) Evaluation of a gluten free product containing wheat gliadin in patients with coeliac disease. *British Medical Journal* **289:** 83.
Colaco J, Egan-Mitchell B, Stevens FM et al (1987) Compliance with gluten free diet in coeliac disease. *Archives of Disease in Childhood* **62:** 706–708.
Collin P, Salmi J, Hällström O et al (1989) High frequency of coeliac disease in adult patients with type-I diabetes. *Scandinavian Journal of Gastroenterology* **24:** 81–84.
Collin P, Pirttilä T, Nurmikko T et al (1991) Celiac disease, brain atrophy, and dementia. *Neurology* **41:** 372–375.
Collin P, Helin H, Mäki M et al (1993) Follow-up of patients positive in reticulin and gliadin antibody tests with normal small-bowel biopsy findings. *Scandinavian Journal of Gastroenterology* **28:** 595–598.
Comfort MW (1958) Non-tropical sprue: diagnosis and therapy. *Gastroenterology* **34:** 476–483.
Cooke WT & Holmes GKT (1984) *Coeliac Disease.* Edinburgh: Churchill Livingstone.
Cooke WT, Peeney ALP & Hawkins CF (1953) Symptoms, signs and diagnostic features of idiopathic steatorrhoea. *Quarterly Journal of Medicine* **22:** 59–77.
Cooper BT & Read AE (1987) Coeliac disease and lymphoma. *Quarterly Journal of Medicine* **240:** 269–274.
Cooper BT, Holmes GKT, Ferguson R & Cooke WT (1980) Coeliac disease and malignancy. *Medicine* **59:** 249–261.

Cooper BT, Holmes GKT & Cooke WT (1982) Lymphoma risk in coeliac disease of later life. *Digestion* **23:** 89–92.

Corazza GR & Gasbarrini G (1983) Defective splenic function and its relation to bowel disease. *Clinics in Gatroenterology* **12:** 651–669.

Corazza GR, Brocchi E, Caletti G & Gasbarrini G (1990a) Loss of duodenal folds allows diagnosis of unsuspected coeliac disease. *Gut* **31:** 1080–1081.

Corazza GR, Volta U, Frisoni M et al (1990b) Comparison of six non-invasive tests for the screening of adult coeliac disease. In Kumar PJ & Walker-Smith JA (eds) *Coeliac Disease: 100 Years*, pp 269–272. Leeds: University Printing Press.

Corazza GR, Frisoni M, Treggiari EA et al (1991) Clinical features of adult coeliac disease in Italy. In Mearin ML & Mulder CJJ (eds) *Coeliac Disease: 40 Years Gluten Free*, pp 117–121. Dordrecht: Kluwer Academic Publishers.

Corazza GR, Valentini RA, Frisoni M et al (1992a) Gliadin immune reactivity is associated with overt and latent enteropathy in relatives of celiac patients. *Gastroenterology* **103:** 1517–1522.

Corazza GR, Frisoni M, Filipponi C et al (1992b) Investigation of QT interval in adult coeliac disease. *British Medical Journal* **304:** 1285.

Corazza GR, Frisoni M, Treggiari EA et al (1993a) Subclinical celiac sprue: increasing occurrence and clues to its diagnosis. *Journal of Clinical Gastroenterology* **16:** 16–21.

Corazza GR, Caletti GC, Lazzari R et al (1993b) Scalloped duodenal folds in childhood celiac disease. *Gastrointestinal Endoscopy* **39:** 543–545.

Corazza GR, Di Sario A, Sacco G et al (1994) Subclinical coeliac disease: an anthropometric assessment. *Journal of Internal Medicine* **236:** 183–187.

Corrao G, Corazza GR, Andreani ML et al (1994) Serological screening of coeliac disease: choosing the optimal procedure according to various prevalence levels. *Gut* **35:** 771–775.

Corazza GR, Valentini RA, Andreani ML et al (1995) Subclinical coeliac disease is a frequent cause of iron-deficiency anaemia. *Scandinavian Journal of Gastroenterology* (in press).

Croese J, Harris O & Bain B (1979) Coeliac disease. Haematological features and delay in diagnosis. *Medical Journal of Australia* **2:** 335–338.

Dawson AM & Kumar PJ (1985) Coeliac disease. In Booth CC & Neale G (eds) *Disorders of the Small Intestine*, pp 153–178. Oxford: Blackwell.

Depla ACTM, Bartelsman JFWM, Mulder CJJ & Tytgat GNJ (1990) Anemia: monosympto-matic coeliac disease. *Hepato-gastroenterology* **37:** 90–91.

Dissanayake AS, Truelove SC & Whitehead R (1974) Jejunal mucosal recovery in coeliac disease in relation to the degree of adherence to a gluten free diet. *Quarterly Journal of Medicine* **43:** 161–185.

Ellis HJ, Freedman AR & Ciclitira PJ (1990) Detection and estimation of the barley prolamin content of beer and malt to assess their suitability for patients with coeliac disease. *Clinica Chimica Acta* **189:** 123–130.

Farthing MJG, Edwards CRW, Rees LH & Dawson AM (1982) Male gonadal function in coeliac disease: 1. Sexual dysfunction, infertility, and semen quality. *Gut* **23:** 608–614.

Farthing MJG, Rees LH, Edwards CRW & Dawson AM (1983) Male gonadal function in coeliac disease: 2. Sex hormones. *Gut* **24:** 127–135.

Ferguson A, Hutton MM, Maxwell JD & Murray D (1970) Adult coeliac disease in hyposplenic patients. *Lancet* **i:** 163–164.

Ferguson MM, Wray D, Carmichael HA et al (1980) Coeliac disease associated with recurrent aphthae. *Gut* **21:** 223–226.

Ferguson R, Basu MK, Asquith P & Cooke WT (1975) Jejunal mucosal abnormalities in patients with recurrent aphthous ulceration. *British Medical Journal* **i:** 11–13.

Ferguson R, Holmes GKT & Cooke WT (1982) Coeliac disease, fertility, and pregnancy. *Scandinavian Journal of Gastroenterology* **17:** 65–68.

Ferreira N, Lloyd Davies S, Butler M et al (1992) Endomysial antibody: is it the best screening test for coeliac disease? *Gut* **33:** 1633–1637.

Fornasieri A, Sinico SA, Maldifassi P et al (1987) IgA-antigliadin antibodies in IgA mesangial nephropathy (Berger's disease). *British Medical Journal* **295:** 78–80.

Freeman HJ & Chiu BK (1986) Multifocal small bowel lymphoma and latent celiac sprue. *Gastroenterology* **90:** 1992–1997.

Freeman HJ, Weinstein WM, Shnitka TK et al (1977) Primary abdominal lymphoma.

Presenting manifestation of celiac sprue or complicating dermatits herpetiformis. *American Journal of Medicine* **63**: 585–594.

Gee S (1888) On the coeliac affection. *Saint Bartholomew's Hospital Reports* **24**: 17–20.

Gobbi G, Bouquet F, Greco L et al (1992) Coeliac disease, epilepsy, and cerebral calcifications. *Lancet* **340**: 439–443.

Graham DR, Bellingham AJ, Alstead E et al (1982) Coeliac disease presenting as acute bleeding disorders. *Postgraduate Medical Journal* **58**: 178–179.

Green PA & Wollaeger EE (1960) The clinical behaviour of sprue in the United States. *Gastroenterology* **38**: 399–418.

Haeney MR, Goodwin BJF, Barratt MEJ et al (1982) Soya protein antibodies in man: their occurrence and possible relevance in coeliac disease. *Journal of Clinical Pathology* **35**: 319–322.

Hallert C & Åström J (1983) Intellectual ability after lifelong intestinal malabsorption due to coeliac disease. *Journal of Neurology, Neurosurgery and Psychiatry* **46**: 87–89.

Hallert C & Derefeldt T (1982) Psychic disturbances in adult coeliac disease. I. Clinical observations. *Scandinavian Journal of Gastroenterology* **17**: 17–19.

Hallert C, Gotthard R, Jansson G et al (1983) Similar prevalence of coeliac disease in children and middle-aged adults in a district of Sweden. *Gut* **24**: 389–391.

Hamilton JD, Chambers RA & Wynn-Williams A (1976) Role of gluten, prednisone, and azathioprine in non-responsive coeliac disease. *Lancet* **i**: 1213–1216.

Hankey GL & Holmes GKT (1994) Coeliac disease in the elderly. *Gut* **35**: 65–67.

Hed J, Lieden G, Ottosson E et al (1986) IgA anti-gliadin antibodies and jejunal mucosal lesions in healthy blood donors. *Lancet* **ii**: 215.

Hepner GW, Jowsey J, Arnaud C et al (1978) Osteomalacia and celiac disease. Response to 25-hydroxyvitamin D. *American Journal of Medicine* **65**: 1015–1020.

Herlinger H & Maglinte DDT (1986) Jejunal fold separation in adult celiac disease: relevance of enteroclysis. *Radiology* **158**: 605–611.

Hoffbrand AV (1974) Anaemia in adult coeliac disease. *Clinics in Gastroenterology* **3**: 71–89.

Holdstock DJ & Oleesky S (1973) Successful treatment of collagenous sprue with combination of prednisolone and gluten-free diet. *Postgraduate Medical Journal* **49**: 664–667.

Holmes GKT (1992) Long-term health risks for unrecognized coeliac patients. In Auricchio S & Visakorpi JK (eds) *Common Food Intolerances 1: Epidemiology of Coeliac Disease*, pp 105–118. Basel: Karger.

Holmes GKT, Prior P, Lane MR et al (1989) Malignancy in coeliac disease—effect of a gluten free diet. *Gut* **30**: 333–338.

Howdle PD (1991) Coeliac disease: therapeutic choices in non-responders to conventional therapy. In Dobrilla G, Bardhan KD & Steele A (eds) *Non-Responders in Gastroenterology*, pp 129–139. Verona: Cortina International.

Howdle PD & Losowsky MS (1987) The immunology of coeliac disease. *Baillière's Clinical Gastroenterology* **1**: 507–529.

Howdle PD & Losowsky MS (1990) Review of methods for measuring gliadins in food. *Gut* **31**: 712–713.

Howdle PD & Losowsky MS (1992) Coeliac disease in adults. In Marsh MN (ed.) *Coeliac Disease*, pp 49–80. Oxford: Blackwell.

Juby LD, Rothwell J & Axon ATR (1989) Cellobiose/mannitol sugar test—a sensitive tubeless test for coeliac disease: results on 1010 unselected patients. *Gut* **30**: 476–480.

Katz AJ & Grand RJ (1979) All that flattens is not 'sprue'. *Gastroenterology* **76**: 375–377.

Kumar PJ, O'Donoghue DP, Stenson K & Dawson AM (1979) Reintroduction of gluten in adults and children with treated coeliac disease. *Gut* **20**: 743–749.

Kumar PJ, Walker-Smith J, Milla P et al (1988) The teenage coeliac: follow up study of 102 patients. *Archives of Diseases in Childhood* **63**: 916–920.

Logan RFA, Tucker G, Rifkind EA et al (1983) Changes in clinical features of coeliac disease in adults in Edinburgh and the Lothians 1960–79. *British Medical Journal* **286**: 95–97.

Logan RFA, Rifkind EA, Busuttil A et al (1986) Prevalence and 'incidence' of celiac disease in Edinburgh and the Lothian region of Scotland. *Gastroenterology* **90**: 334–342.

Logan RFA, Rifkind EA, Turner IA & Ferguson A (1989) Mortality in celiac disease. *Gastroenterology* **97**: 265–271.

Longstreth GF (1993) Successful treatment of refractory sprue with cyclosporine. *Annals of Internal Medicine* **119**: 1014–1016.

McCrae WM, Eastwood MA, Martin MR & Sircus W (1975) Neglected coeliac disease. *Lancet* **i:** 187–190.

MacDonald WC, Brandborg LL, Flick AL et al (1964) Studies of celiac sprue. IV. The response of the whole length of the small bowel to a gluten-free diet. *Gastroenterology* **47:** 573–589.

McIntyre AS, Ng DPK, Smith JA et al (1992) The endoscopic appearance of duodenal folds is predictive of untreated adult celiac disease. *Gastrointestinal Endoscopy* **38:** 148–151.

Mackinnon AM, Short MD, Elis E & Dowling RH (1975) Adaptive changes in vitamin B_{12} absorption in celiac disease and after small-bowel resection in man. *Digestive Diseases* **20:** 835–840.

Mäki M, Hällström O, Vesikari T & Visakorpi JK (1984) Evaluation of a serum IgA-class reticulin antibody test for the detection of childhood celiac disease. *Journal of Pediatrics* **105:** 901–905.

Mann JG, Brown WR & Kern F Jr (1970) The subtle and variable clinical expressions of gluten induced enteropathy. *American Journal of Medicine* **48:** 357–366.

Mayer M, Greco L, Troncone R et al (1991) Compliance of adolescents with coeliac disease with a gluten free diet. *Gut* **32:** 881–885.

Mee AS, Burke M, Vallon AG et al (1985) Small bowel biopsy for malabsorption: comparison of the diagnostic adequacy of endoscopic forceps and capsule biopsy specimens. *British Medical Journal* **291:** 769–772.

Mike N, Udeshi U, Asquith P & Ferrando J (1990) Small bowel enema in non-responsive coeliac disease. *Gut* **31:** 883–885.

Montgomery AMP, Goka AKJ, Kumar PJ et al (1988) Low gluten diet in the treatment of adult coeliac disease: effect on jejunal morphology and serum anti-gluten antibodies. *Gut* **29:** 1564–1568.

Morris JS, Adjukiewicz AB & Read AE (1970) Coeliac infertility: an indication for dietary gluten restriction? *Lancet* **i:** 213–214.

Mortimer PE, Stewart JS, Norman AP & Booth CC (1968) Follow-up study of coeliac disease. *British Medical Journal* **2:** 7–9.

Moss AJ, Waterhouse C & Terry R (1965) Gluten-sensitive enteropathy with osteomalacia but without steatorrhea. *New England Journal of Medicine* **272:** 825–830.

Mulder CJJ & Tytgat GNJ (1987) Coeliac disease and related disorders. *Netherland Journal of Medicine* **31:** 286–299.

Nelson EW, Ertan A, Brooks FP & Cerda JJ (1976) Thrombocytosis in patients with coeliac sprue. *Gastroenterology* **70:** 1042–1044.

Nielsen HO, Jacobsen O, Rask Pedersen E et al (1985) Nontropical sprue. Malignant disease and mortality rate. *Scandinavian Journal of Gastroenterology* **20:** 13–18.

O'Farrelly C, Marten D, Melcher D et al (1988) Association between villous atrophy in rheumatoid arthritis and a rheumatoid factor and gliadin-specific IgG. *Lancet* **ii:** 819–822.

O'Farrelly C, O'Mahony C, Graeme-Cook F et al (1991) Gliadin antibodies identify gluten-sensitive oral ulceration in the absence of villous atrophy. *Journal of Oral Pathology and Medicine* **20:** 476–478.

Owen DA, Thorlakson TK & Walli JE (1980) Coeliac disease in a patient with morbid obesity. *Annals of Internal Medicine* **140:** 1380–1383.

Patel DG, Krogh CME & Thompson WG (1985) Gluten in pills: a hazard for patients with celiac disease. *Canadian Medical Association Journal* **133:** 114–115.

Regan PT & Di Magno EP (1980) Exocrine pancreatic insufficiency in celiac sprue: a cause of treatment failure. *Gastroenterology* **78:** 484–487.

Ross JR & Garabedian M (1970) Systemic manifestations of gluten enteropathies in some other diseases. In Glass GBJ (ed.) *Progress in Gastroenterology*, vol. 2, pp 430–449. New York: Grune & Sratton.

Salvesen HA (1963) The blood pressure in idiopathic and symptomatic steatorrhoea. *Acta Medica Scandinavica* **144:** 303–312.

Scott BB & Losowsky MS (1976) Patchiness and duodeno-jejunal variation of the mucosal abnormality in coeliac disease and dermatitis herpetiformis. *Gut* **17:** 984–992.

Scotta MS, De Giacomo C, Maggiore G et al (1982) Eucharistic problems for coeliac patients. *New England Journal of Medicine* **307:** 898.

Shanahan F & Weinstein WM (1988) Extending the scope in celiac disease. *New England Journal of Medicine* **319:** 782–783.

Stevens FM (1980) Celiac disease: clinical manifestation. *Practical Gastroenterology* **4:** 10–15.

Stewart K & Willoughby JMT (1988) Postnatal presentation of coeliac disease. *British Medical Journal* **297:** 1245.

Swinson CM & Levi AJ (1980) Is coeliac disease underdiagnosed? *British Medical Journal* **281:** 1258–1260.

Trier JS (1991) Celiac sprue. *New England Journal of Medicine* **325:** 1709–1719.

Unsworth DJ & Brown DL (1994) Serological screening suggests that adult coeliac disease is underdiagnosed in the UK and increases the incidence by up to 12%. *Gut* **35:** 61–64.

van Berge-Henegouwen GP & Mulder CJJ (1993) Pioneer in the gluten free diet: Willem-Karel Dicke 1905–1962, over 50 years of gluten free diet. *Gut* **34:** 1473–1475.

van Bergeijk JD, Meijer JWR & Mulder CJJ (1993) Endoscopic abnormalities in patients screened for coeliac disease. *Journal of Clinical Nutrition and Gastroenterology* **8:** 136–139.

Visakorpi JK (1992) Silent coeliac disease: the risk groups to be screened. In Auricchio S & Visakorpi JS (eds) *Common Food Intolerances 1: Epidemiology of Coeliac Disease*, pp 84–92. Basel: Karger.

Vuoristo M, Tarpila S & Miettinen TA (1980) Serum lipids and fecal steroids in patients with celiac disease: effects of gluten-free diet and cholestyramine. *Gastroenterology* **78:** 1518–1525.

Zubillaga P, Vitoria JC, Arrieta A et al (1993) Down's syndrome and coeliac disease. *Journal of Pediatric Gastroenterology and Nutrition* **16:** 168–171.

8

The major complications of coeliac disease

D. H. WRIGHT

Nutritional, haematological (Hoffbrand, 1974) and osteopenic compli-cations dominate the clinical progression of untreated coeliac disease and were a major cause of death before the recognition of the role of gluten in this disease. It is claimed that adherence to a gluten-free diet returns patients with coeliac disease to a normal life expectancy and that they ultimately die from unrelated causes (Trier, 1991). While this may be true for the indi-vidual patient, the mortality rate for all patients with coeliac disease is increased above that of the general population (Neilsen et al, 1985; Logan et al, 1989). This increased mortality rate is due largely to an increased preva-lence of malignant disease, particularly malignant lymphoma. The excess mortality could result from non-compliance with a strict gluten-free diet in patients with established disease. The major reason, however, almost cer-tainly relates to the fact that a large number of patients have subclinical or latent coeliac disease, and present in adult life, often synchronously, with one of the major complications of the disease. This interpretation is sup-ported by the observation that the increased mortality rate is greatest within 1 year of diagnosis and steadily declines with time, and that the rate of those diagnosed in childhood as having coeliac disease is similar to that of the general population (Logan et al, 1989). It is not, however, entirely in keeping with the report of Harris et al (1967), who observed 14 lymphomas and 13 gastrointestinal tract carcinomas in a series of 202 adult patients with coeliac disease. The mean duration of disease in this series was 21.2 years before the diagnosis of lymphoma and 38.5 years before that of gastro-intestinal carcinoma.

The major complications of coeliac disease have been identified from studies of mortality in cohorts of patients with the disease (Logan et al, 1989), from autopsy reports of patients (Thompson, 1974; Pollock, 1977) and from individual case studies. In such studies, the criteria used to identify patients with coeliac disease are important. It is likely, however, that these data give an incomplete evaluation of the extent of complications, in view of the prevalence of undiagnosed, subclinical or latent coeliac disease in the general population (Catassi et al, 1994). The use of antibody screening tests and HLA genotyping, together with intestinal biopsy to establish the preva-lence of the disease in different communities, will eventually lead to a more complete assessment of the complications.

Baillière's Clinical Gastroenterology—
Vol. 9, No. 2, June 1995
ISBN 0–7020–1953–4

MALIGNANT LYMPHOMA

The recognition of the association of sprue and malignant lymphoma is attributed to Fairley and Mackie (1937), who proposed that lymphatic obstruction was the cause of malabsorption. Gough et al (1962) reported three patients with lymphoma and steatorrhoea, and noted that 29 such patients had been reported since the publication of Fairley and Mackie (1937). They observed that malabsorption frequently predated the diagnosis of lymphoma by as much as 20–25 years and proposed that the lymphoma was a complication of idiopathic steatorrhoea, rather than being the cause. Subsequent studies have supported this view (Thompson, 1974; Swinson et

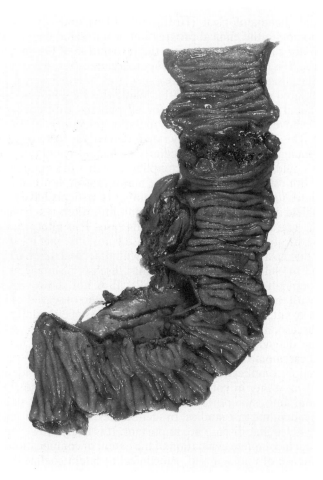

Figure 1. Resected length of small intestine showing a typical circumferential ulcer of enteropathy-associated T-cell lymphoma. Smaller, linear ulcers are often hidden in the oedematous folds of small intestinal mucosa.

al, 1983b). However, whereas some patients have a long history of malabsorption before the diagnosis of lymphoma (Harris et al, 1967), in many the duration of coeliac disease is short and is often diagnosed in the same clinical episode as the lymphoma. Isaacson and Wright (1978a) reported 18 patients with small intestinal lymphoma, showing villous atrophy and crypt hyperplasia in the adjacent, uninvolved, small bowel mucosa. Five of these patients had a preceding history of adult-onset coeliac disease. They proposed that the lymphoma was of a single histological type, which they designated as malignant histiocytosis of the intestine, based on morphology and the limited immunohistochemical markers available at that time. Subsequent studies based on clonal rearrangements of T-cell receptor (TCR) genes and immunohistochemical markers, have shown that the tumour cells

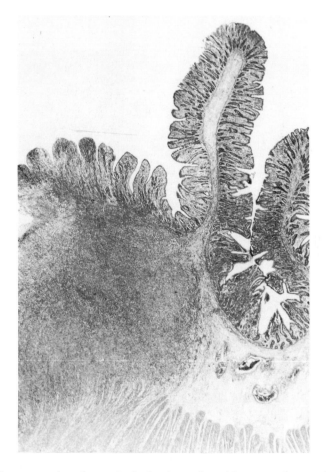

Figure 2. Low-power view of a neoplastic ulcer in a patient with enteropathy-associated T-cell lymphoma. The mixed infiltrate of tumour cells and inflammatory cells can be seen extending deep to the ulcer into the muscularis. The adjacent small bowel mucosa shows villous atrophy. Haematoxylin and eosin stain, original magnification × 12.

are, in fact, of the T-cell lineage (Isaacson et al, 1985; Salter et al, 1986; Stein et al, 1988). In addition to the expression of T-cell lineage markers, these tumours also express the activation marker, CD30, and the intraepithelial T-cell marker, HML-1. The tumour has now been designated as enteropathy-associated T-cell lymphoma (EATCL).

EATCL typically occurs in the fifth to seventh decades of life. Most patients present with acute intestinal obstruction or perforation, preceded by abdominal pain and weight loss. Patients with diagnosed coeliac disease usually become unresponsive to a gluten-free diet and have diarrhoea and steatorrhoea. Other recorded features include pyrexia, finger clubbing and an ichthyotic skin rash (Hodges et al, 1979). Abdominal pain, intestinal obstruction, haemorrhage and perforation usually lead to laparotomy and small bowel resection. The resected bowel is often oedematous, proximally dilated and shows multiple circumferential ulcers (Figures 1 and 2). Tumour

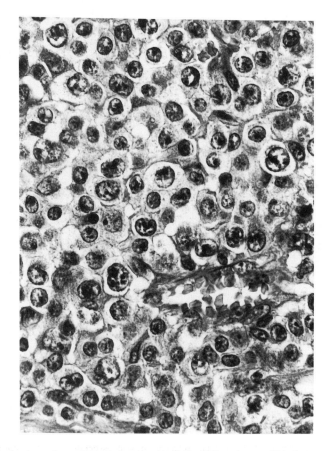

Figure 3. Section of an enteropathy-associated T-cell lymphoma. This is a monomorphic tumour. Greater degrees of pleomorphism may be seen. Haematoxylin and eosin stain, original magnification × 480.

masses are less common. Mesenteric lymphadenopathy may be due to reactive hyperplasia or tumour involvement. The lesions are most common in the jejunum, but may be found throughout the small intestine and rarely in the stomach and colon. The tumours are high-grade blastic lymphomas with variable morphology, usually regular (Figure 3) but sometimes extremely pleomorphic. The adjacent small intestine shows villous atrophy, plasma cell infiltration of the lamina propria, and intraepithelial lymphocytosis (Figure 4). If the resection is from the distal small bowel or the patient is on a gluten-free diet, the adjacent mucosa may appear histologically normal. The phenotype of the intraepithelial lymphocytes is similar to that found in coeliac disease (Spencer et al, 1989).

Not all authors have accepted the view that EATCL is the consequence, rather than the cause, of malabsorption, nor yet that the enteropathy associated with this tumour is coeliac disease. Eakins et al (1964) noted that very few patients had been reported who had a long history of coeliac disease. They suggested that in at least some cases the malabsorption might be a consequence of the tumour. Hourihane and Weir (1970) also supported the view that the lymphomatous process caused the whole clinicopathological syndrome. They suggested an analogy with mycosis fungoides in which a 'pre-lymphomatous' infiltrate (low-grade lymphoma) was the cause of the enteropathy and from which a high-grade lymphoma evolved. Wright

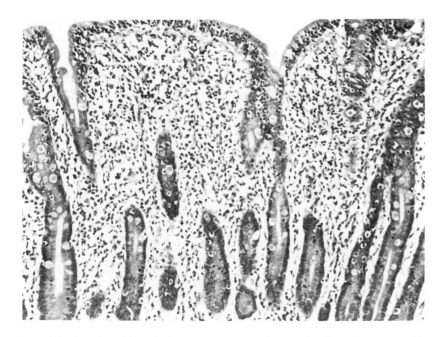

Figure 4. Section of small bowel adjacent to an enteropathy-associated T-cell lymphoma. Note villous atrophy and crypt hyperplasia. There is a marked infiltration of lymphocytes and plasma cells in the lamina propria. Intraepithelial lymphocytosis is apparent, particularly in the surface epithelium. Haematoxylin and eosin stain, original magnification × 120.

et al (1991) reported a patient with widespread small intestinal lymphocytosis in whom the lymphocytes were found to be clonal by gene rearrangement studies and to have clonal cytogenetic abnormalities. They suggested that this case might support the analogy between EATCL and mycosis fungoides. This patient has, however, not gone on to develop a high-grade lymphoma and possibly represents a rare epitheliotropic T-cell lymphoma, distinct from EATCL (Foucar et al, 1984).

O'Farrelly et al (1986) compared 76 patients with coeliac disease (CD) with 16 with EATCL. They noted that 93% of the coeliac patients had raised levels of α-gliadin antibody and responded to a gluten-free diet, whereas none of those with EATCL had raised α-gliadin antibodies and the majority showed no response or only a partial response to gluten withdrawal. The ratio of women to men in the group with CD was 2.2 : 1, whereas in the group with EATCL it was 1 : 1.6. They suggested the presence of two forms of enteropathy, one benign and sensitive to wheat protein and the other running a malignant course, perhaps analogous to mycosis fungoides. However, the specificity of raised antibody levels to α-gliadin for the diagnosis of coeliac disease is not absolute (Levenson et al, 1985; Loft and Marsh, 1986; Trier, 1991) and the poor response to gluten withdrawal might be related to the presence of tumour. The sex difference between EATCL and uncomplicated coeliac disease remains a distinguishing feature, although, in other series, the ratio of women to men with EATCL is nearer unity.

To investigate the relationship of coeliac patients with lymphoma and other malignancy to those with uncomplicated coeliac disease, O'Driscoll et al (1982) undertook HLA serotyping in both groups. They found that, of the patients with malignancy, 69% expressed HLA-B8 and 71% DR3. The coresponding values for patients with uncomplicated disease were 76% and 84%, respectively, with 43% and 44% in the local non-coeliac population. Similarly, Swinson et al (1983a), in a study of 44 patients with coeliac disease and malignancy and of 57 with uncomplicated disease, found 93% positive for DR3 and 38% positive for DR7, with no difference between the groups. In contrast, O'Farrelly et al (1986) found the DR3 antigen in 90% of patients with uncomplicated coeliac disease, but in only two of five patients with EATCL (the small number of cases in the latter category limits the significance of this finding).

In recent years, serology has given way to the detection of HLA polymorphisms at the DNA level using polymerase chain reaction (PCR) amplification, followed by oligonucleotide probing or DNA sequencing. Susceptibility to coeliac disease appears to be conferred by a particular HLA-DQ heterodimer encoded by the DQA1∗0501 and DQB1∗0201 genes in cis- or trans-configuration (Kagnoff, 1990; Sollid and Thorbsy, 1993). We have recently conducted a study of the genetic relationship between coeliac disease and EATCL using PCR-SSOP typing on biopsy tissue from 17 patients with coeliac disease and 47 with EATCL in comparison with 151 unrelated controls (Howell et al, in press). The DQA1∗0501, DQB1∗0201 phenotype was expressed by 88% of coeliac patients, by 93% of those with EATCL but by only 23% of controls. DRB1∗03 frequencies were also raised in both patient groups (CD, 71%; EATCL, 95%), compared with controls

(21%). These results confirm the previously published HLA associations in coeliac disease and show that EATCL arises in individuals with the DQA1*0501, DQB1*0201, coeliac disease-predisposing phenotype. However, differences also emerge between patients with uncomplicated coeliac disease and those with EATCL. The patients with EATCL expressed an increased frequency of DQB1*0301/0302 and of DRB1*0304 heterozygotes, in comparison with the coeliac disease and control groups. These findings suggest that, while EATCL arises in patients with the DQA1*0501, DQB1*0201, coeliac disease-associated phenotype, additional HLA-DR/DQ alleles may represent risk factors for EATCL.

Alfsen et al (1989) reported a patient with coeliac disease and EATCL who showed marked lymphocytosis in the adjacent enteropathic bowel. The small intraepithelial lymphocytes were CD3 and CD7 positive, but CD1, 2, 4, 5 and 8 negative. Southern blot analysis showed a clonal rearrangement of the TCR-β gene in DNA extracted from this enteropathic bowel. The authors suggested that the EATCL had arisen as a result of transformation of this low-grade T-cell lymphoma, giving some support for the analogy with mycosis fungoides, originally suggested by Hourihane and Weir (1970). We have recently conducted an immunohistochemical and molecular biological analysis of specimens from 23 patients with EATCL (Murray et al, in press). Specimens from 14 of these patients were investigated for the presence of clonal T-cell gene rearrangements in both the tumour and adjacent entero-pathic intestine, using PCR. Primers for TCR-β and TCR-γ genes were used in a combination that permits the identification of approximately 90% of TCR rearrangements. Clonal rearrangements of the TCR were found in 13 of the 14 tumours studied. Specimens of enteropathic bowel resected with the tumour, but showing no morphological or immunohistochemical evidence of tumour involvement, showed clonal TCR gene rearrangements in 11 cases. In ten of these, the amplified DNA was of the same molecular weight in the enteropathic bowel as in the corresponding tumour. In two cases, sequencing the PCR product showed identical TCR gene rearrangements in the tumour and adjacent intestine.

One patient in our series was of particular interest. This man was diag-nosed in childhood as having coeliac disease and was treated with a gluten-free diet until the age of 12 years, when he resumed a normal diet. Thirty-five years later, he presented with abdominal pain, weight loss and melaena. A small bowel resection showed an EATCL. After operation, he was given chemotherapy and was re-started on a gluten-free diet. Nine years later he re-presented with obstruction and a further small bowel resection was performed which showed EATCL causing a stricture. He was given a further course of chemotherapy and remains alive and well 16 years after the first tumour was resected. Most patients with EATCL die within a few months of diagnosis (Mead et al, 1987), so this history alone is remarkable. Analysis of both tumours showed identical rearrangements of the TCR-β gene. The same clone was not identified in the adjacent enteropathic bowel but identi-cal rearrangements of the TCR-γ gene were found in both resection specimens in the enteropathic bowel. It seems improbable that the recur-rence, 9 years after the first resection, was due to regrowth of the high-grade tumour, since these tumours show a high proliferation index. One possible explanation is that a persistent low-grade clone in the enteropathic bowel eventually transformed into a high-grade tumour. Gluten withdrawal, instituted after the first resection, may possibly have contributed to the latency of this clone.

Uniform staining of tumour cell nuclei for p53 (Figure 5) was seen in 22 of the 23 tumours, and in 9 of 19 cases studied, collections of small lymphocytes in the lamina propria and within the epithelium of the enteropathic bowel expressed p53 (Figure 6). In all but one of these specimens a clonal rearrangement of the TCR genes was identified. We do not know whether the p53 expression is due to mutation or stabilization. However, it does appear to be a marker of a neoplastic clone and, as such, may be a valuable means of identifying malignancy in biopsies from patients with coeliac disease.

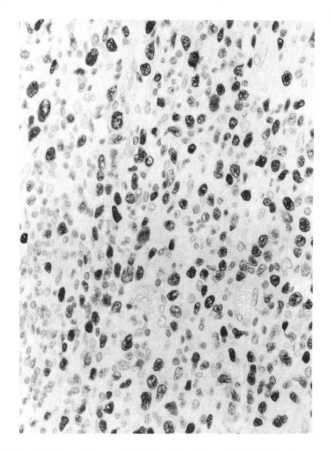

Figure 5. Section of enteropathy-associated T-cell lymphoma stained by the immunoperoxidase technique to show p53. Nuclear staining can be seen in a high proportion of the tumour cells. The intervening unstained nuclei represent stromal and inflammatory cells, including large numbers of histiocytes. Immunoperoxidase stain, original magnification × 300.

In summary, our findings in recent years indicate that EATCL arises in patients with the HLA genotype associated with coeliac disease. The detection of clonal T cells in the enteropathic bowel, adjacent to the high-grade tumours, could be due to intramucosal spread of the tumour. This, however, appears unlikely, since tumour cells cannot be identified either by morphological means or by immunohistochemistry and, in a number of cases, clonal rearrangements were found in blocks taken distant from the tumour, with intervening blocks showing no clonality. The findings might be interpreted as favouring the 'mycosis fungoides' hypothesis proposed by Hourihane and Weir (1970), namely, that the enteropathy itself is due to a low-grade lymphomatous infiltrate. Against this hypothesis, however, is the observation that, when multiple blocks of enteropathic bowel were analysed, clonal T cells were identified only in occasional blocks. The hypothesis that best fits our observations is that EATCL arises in patients

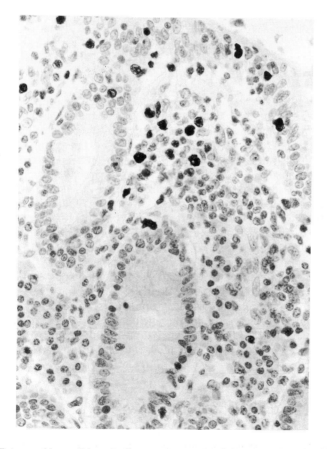

Figure 6. Enteropathic small bowel adjacent to an enteropathy-associated T-cell lymphoma stained for p53. Staining of lamina propria and intraepithelial lymphocyte nuclei. Immuno-peroxidase stain, original magnification × 300.

with coeliac disease and that clonal T-cell populations emerge from the inflammatory T-cell infiltrate, with one of these clones eventually transforming into a high-grade EATCL.

The majority of patients with EATCL do not give a clear history of coeliac disease from childhood. Most present with adult-onset disease or have no previous history of gluten-sensitive enteropathy prior to presentation with EATCL. This is one of the reasons why the relationship between EATCL and coeliac disease has been disputed. The probable explanation for this apparant paradox lies in the fact that coeliac disease may be latent, for example in patients with dermatitis herpetiformis, in relatives of patients with coeliac disease and in the general population (Trier, 1991; Catassi et al, 1994). Patients diagnosed with coeliac disease in childhood will be treated by gluten withdrawal. There is evidence that those who adhere to a gluten-free diet remain well indefinitely and that this diet protects against malignancy (Holmes et al, 1989). Patients with latent coeliac disease, taking a normal diet, will not be so protected and may therefore be the population at greatest risk of developing EATCL.

OTHER MALIGNANCIES

In their study of 259 malignancies occurring in 235 patients with coeliac disease, Swinson et al (1983b) identified 133 malignant lymphomas and 116 invasive non-lymphomatous malignancies. A comparison of observed over expected malignancies at different sites showed twice the expected frequency of gastrointestinal tumours, owing to an increased incidence of adenocarcinoma of the small intestine and of squamous cell carinoma of the pharynx and oesophagus. Nineteen carcinomas of the small intestine were observed, against 0.23 expected. The cause of this increased incidence of adenocarcinoma is unknown, but may be related to the crypt hyperplasia that occurs in coeliac disease. From a practical point of view, it indicates the need to exclude a diagnosis of coeliac disease in any patient presenting with small intestinal adenocarcinoma. Squamous carcinoma of the upper gastrointestinal tract may be related to vitamin A deficiency, which has been implicated as a possible reason for the wide geographical variation seen in the incidence of carcinoma of the oesophagus. Swinson et al (1983b) also found a significant increase in the incidence of testicular neoplasm in patients with coeliac disease. The implications of this observation, at a time when the incidence of testicular germ-cell tumours is increasing, is not apparent.

CHRONIC ULCERATIVE ENTERITIS

The association of malabsorption with small intestinal ulceration was first described by Nyman (1949) and has been variously named (Mills et al, 1980). It is a rare condition. In 1980, Mills et al reported five cases and found only 27 others in the English literature. The clinical features of chronic ulcerative enteritis are similar to those of EATCL. Thus, of 32 patients reviewed by Mills and co-workers, 8 developed melaena, 12 intestinal obstruction and 9 intestinal perforation. The abdominal catastrophe resulted in laparotomy and small bowel resection in 30 of the 32 patients. At operation, the bowel was found to be oedematous and proximally dilated, and showed stricture formation with circumferential mucosal ulcers. Mesenteric lymphadenopathy was noted in many cases. The survival rate was almost as low as that for EATCL, with 62.5% of patients dead within 5–120 months (mean 37 months).

Many patients display features of coeliac disease. Thus, of the 32 patients reviewed by Mills et al, 8 of 18, in whom serum immunoglobulins had been recorded, showed abnormal levels of IgA. Asquith et al (1969) had previously shown that IgA levels in adult patients with untreated coeliac disease are high compared with those in patients on a gluten-free diet or in normal controls. Twenty of 25 patients subjected to small bowel biopsy showed villous atrophy, although ulceration was seen in only one of these. Twelve of 26 patients showed clinical improvement on gluten withdrawal, but histological improvement on small bowel re-biopsy was recorded in only three of these. Using the criteria of Booth (1974), Mills et al accepted only these three cases as having established coeliac disease. Fourteen had villous atrophy unaffected by gluten withdrawal, ten had normal intestinal mucosa, and in five the state of the intervening mucosa was unknown. Three of the five patients reported by Mills and colleagues (1980) had splenic atrophy and features of hyposplenism.

Bayless et al (1967) listed 12 possible causes of small intestinal ulceration, many of which, such as typhoid and syphilis, would not realistically come into the differential diagnosis of chronic ulcerative enteritis. Hourihane and Weir (1970) reported two patients with long-standing malabsorption and intestinal ulceration. They noted that the ulcers were associated with microscopic aggregates of neoplastic cells that did not form gross tumours. They proposed that prelymphoma cells were responsible for the enteropathy and ulceration. The lack of response to gluten withdrawal led them to conclude that their patients did not have coeliac disease. The close association of ulcerative enteritis and lymphoma is illustrated by Freeman et al (1977), who reported seven patients with coeliac-associated lymphoma of whom four were originally diagnosed as benign ulcerative enteritis. Isaacson and Wright (1978b) went further in proposing that ulcerative jejunitis and EATCL are essentially the same condition. They based this opinion on the study of seven cases of EATCL, four of which were originally diagnosed as benign ulcerative enteropathy. In these cases, the neoplastic cells were often present in small numbers and mixed with a prominent infiltrate of small lymphocytes and other inflammatory cells (Figure 7). After this study, Mills et al (1980) examined five cases of chronic ulcerative enteritis but were unable to identify neoplastic cells in any of these. The subsequent development of lymphoma in such patients has been reported (Whitehead, 1968; Baer et al, 1980), although in many with chronic ulcerative enteritis rapid death precludes follow-up.

The current situation is that chronic ulcerative enteritis is recognized as a

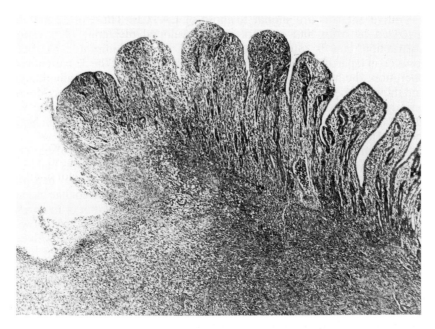

Figure 7. Section of small bowel from a patient with enteropathy-associated T-cell lymphoma showing an apparently inflammatory, non-neoplastic ulcer. In such cases a careful search may be needed to identify occasional clusters of neoplastic cells. Haematoxylin and eosin stain, original magnification × 30.

rare complication of coeliac disease, although its relationship to both coeliac disease and lymphoma is disputed. With advances in our understanding of EATCL we are now in a position to explain the nature of chronic ulcerative enteritis and to diagnose such cases in the future. If EATCL evolves in the setting of coeliac disease from reactive lymphocytes to low-grade lymphoma which then transforms to high-grade lymphoma, the appearance of the associated ulcers will vary with the stage of evolution. Thus, ulcers that arise when the neoplastic cells are of low grade (lymphocytic) will appear inflammatory and will not be recognized as neoplasms. At this stage the neoplastic lymphocytes may not be influenced by gluten, making it unrealistic in such patients to base the diagnosis of coeliac disease on a histological response to gluten withdrawal, as proposed by Booth (1974).

Mills et al (1980) expressed puzzlement at the fact that one of their own cases, and three of ulcerative enteritis reported in the literature, showed a combination of colonic and small bowel ulceration with generalized villous atrophy. They noted that none of these patients had evidence of inflammatory bowel disease. Wolber et al (1990) examined colonic biopsies from 39 patients with coeliac disease and found striking lymphocytic infiltration of the superficial colonic epithelium in 12. Two of four patients with coeliac disease and colonic lymphocytosis, who had gastric biopsies, also showed gastric lymphocytosis. These observations would account for the rare finding of gastric and colonic tumours in patients with EATCL and also for the colonic ulceration observed by Mills et al (1980) in patients with chronic ulcerative enteritis.

In the future, cases of chronic ulcerative enteritis need to be investigated using conventional criteria for the diagnosis of coeliac disease, including HLA genotyping. High-grade tumour cells in the ulcers will be highlighted by immunohistochemical staining for CD30 (Isaacson, 1992) and high- and low-grade tumour cells may be identified by anomalous p53 expression. Clonality of the T cells in the infiltrate can be established using Southern blot analysis techniques or PCR. With the exception of Southern blot analysis, all of these techniques can be applied to archival cases.

LIVER DISEASE

Pollock (1977) studied the liver sections of 19 cases of malabsorption coming to post-mortem at the London Hospital since 1930. Five of these had proven coeliac disease. The other 14 were presumed to have the condition since other causes of malabsorption were excluded and several exhibited other features of coeliac disease, such as splenic atrophy. One patient had cirrhosis and hepatoma and three showed chronic hepatitis with piecemeal necrosis and fibrosis. The coeliac group, as a whole, showed increased portal fibrosis and inflammatory infiltrates, compared with age- and sex-matched controls. Hagander et al (1977) reported 13 liver biopsies from 74 coeliac patients. Seven of these showed cirrhosis and/or chronic active hepatitis, one having cirrhosis and hepatocellular carcinoma. Five further patients had reactive hepatitis, giving a 16% incidence of histological abnormalities in the whole group. Twenty-nine of 53 patients had abnormal liver function tests which responded to gluten withdrawal. Looked at in reverse, Lindberg et al (1979) found total or subtotal villous atrophy in 3 of 16 patients with chronic active hepatitis. Only one of these patients had malabsorption, and response to gluten withdrawal was not recorded. The authors suggested that there might be genetic linkage between these two diseases, both of which are associated with HLA-B8. Logan et al (1978) reported four patients with primary biliary cirrhosis and adult coeliac disease, and suggested that this association is more than a chance occurrence, although the total population from which these cases were drawn was not identified. More recently, Behr and Barnert (1986) reported a woman of 45 years with coeliac disease and primary biliary cirrhosis, drawing attention to the fact that malabsorption, weight loss, bone disease and raised alkaline phosphatase activity are features common to both diseases. Hay et al (1988) reported three patients with coeliac disease and primary sclerosing cholangitis. The significance of this association is, however, questionable, as two of the patients also had chronic ulcerative colitis, a condition known to be associated with sclerosing cholangitis.

It does appear, from the literature, that there is an increased risk of chronic hepatitis of various types in adult coeliac disease. The cause of this association is unclear. Suggestions include absorption of antigens from the gut, immune complex formation, aberrant T-cell function, dietary factors and HLA associations. The possible association of coeliac disease with chronic liver disease should be borne in mind in the investigation and management of coeliac patients.

LUNG DISEASE

There are many reports in the literature of an increased prevalence of lung disease in patients with coeliac disease. These include an association with sarcoidosis (Douglas et al, 1984), idiopathic pulmonary haemosiderosis (Wright et al, 1981) and bird-fancier's lung (Hood and Mason, 1970; Berrill et al, 1975; Eade and Berrill, 1978; Konig et al, 1982). Other workers have disputed the association with bird-fancier's lung. Hendrick and colleagues (1978) performed small bowel biopsy on 12 patients with bird-fancier's lung and found no evidence of coeliac disease. Conversely, they found three possible cases of bird-fancier's lung among 61 patients with coeliac disease, but only one of these responded to a provocation test. In a national survey of 143 patients with bird-fancier's lung, symptoms of malabsorption were displayed by 25. Fourteen of these patients agreed to undergo small bowel biopsy; five of these showed villous atrophy. A further two showed increased lymphocytosis (British Thoracic Society, 1984). The confusion concerning the relationship of coeliac disease and bird-fancier's lung appears to be due, at least in part, to the fact that patients with coeliac disease develop precipitins to hen's egg yolk, possibly because of abnormal absorption of protein by damaged intestinal mucosa (Faux et al, 1978). These precipitins differ from those seen in patients with bird-fancier's lung. Edwards et al (1985) observed that many of the foregoing studies lacked histological confirmation. They reported the necropsy findings in a patient with coeliac disease and lung fibrosis, and the biopsy findings in 13 of 73 patients with coeliac disease who had respiratory problems of sufficient severity to justify transbronchial biopsy. The histological appearances ranged from normal to generally mild degrees of interstitial peribronchial and perivascular fibrosis. The reasons for the association of lung disorders with coeliac disease and the pathogenesis of these disorders are obscure. HLA linkage, dietary and immunological factors have been proposed.

Stevens et al (1990) reported seven patients with coeliac disease who developed lung abscesses or cavities, observed over a period of 20 years, when approximately 600 coeliac patients were seen and 50 died. Six of the patients in this study died. In four the cavities were due to staphylococcal infection, *Klebsiella* pneumonia, tuberculosis and bronchial carcinoma. In three no definite cause could be identified. The group was characterized by malnutrition and hyposplenism. The authors noted that, in their population, lung abscess was second only to malignancy as a cause of death in patients with coeliac disease.

NEUROLOGICAL DISORDERS

The association of adult coeliac disease and neurological disorders was recorded by Cook and Smith in 1966. Spinocerebellar degeneration, often rapidly progressive, has been recorded in patients with diagnosed and occult coeliac disease (Hermaszewski et al, 1991). The pathogenesis of this disease is unknown, but speculation has included the role of vitamin E deficiency resulting from malabsorption. However, patients with established disease appear not to respond to vitamin supplements, nor to gluten withdrawal.

Chapman et al (1978) identified nine patients with epilepsy amongst 185 aged 17–63 years with coeliac disease, giving a prevalence of 5.5%, compared with a national average of 0.5%. Seven of these patients had temporal lobe epilepsy. Correction of calcium, magnesium or folate deficiencies did not control the epilepsy. In three patients gluten withdrawal improved epileptic control. Recently, a syndrome of bilateral occipital calcification, epilepsy and coeliac disease has been described, with most patients reported from Italy (Fois et al, 1992; Gobbi et al, 1992; Bye et al, 1993; Maguadda et al, 1993). In the largest study by the Italian Working Group on Coeliac Disease and Epilepsy (Gobbi et al, 1992), 24 of 31 patients with cerebral calcification and epilepsy of unexplained origin were found to have coeliac disease, and 5 of 12 patients with coeliac disease and epilepsy were found to have cerebral calcification on computed tomography. The patients ranged in age from 4.6 to 30.7 years. Gluten withdrawal had a beneficial effect on the course of the epilepsy, only when initiated soon after the onset of epilepsy. The pathogenesis of this syndrome is unknown, with little evidence to support a role for vitamin or mineral deficiency, nor a direct toxic effect of gliadin. The clinical importance of these observations is that coeliac disease should be suspected in patients with unexplained epilepsy and cerebral cortical calcification, and that cerebral calcification should be sought in patients with coeliac disease and epilepsy. Early gluten withdrawal is indicated if serious, long-lasting epilepsy and intellectual deterioration are to be avoided.

HYPOSPLENISM

The haematological manifestations of hyposplenism include pitting and poikilocytosis of red blood cells and the presence of Howell–Jolly bodies, and are found in the blood films of 10–15% of patients with adult coeliac disease (Hoffbrand, 1974). The reported incidence of hyposplenism in coeliac disease varies from 16% to 77%. This wide variation is undoubtedly due, at least in part, to the small number of patients in some studies and the variations in the methods used to measure splenic function (Corazza et al, 1981). O'Grady et al (1984) assessed splenic function using pitted erythrocyte counts in 177 patients with gluten-sensitive enteropathy, compared with those in 118 healthy volunteers and 77 splenectomized subjects. Hyposplenism was present in 76% of adult patients with untreated coeliac disease, and splenic function improved after gluten withdrawal. Hyposplenism was found in 69–79% of patients with abnormal mucosal biopsies, compared with 8.6% of those with normal, or near normal, mucosa. As measured by pitted erythrocyte count, hyposplenism became more marked with age, presumably as a result of age-related splenic atrophy. The cause of the hyposplenism is not known but most speculation relates to the absorption of antigens through damaged bowel mucosa and the formation of circulating antigen–antibody complexes, an explanation that could also be invoked to explain the hyposplenism associated with inflammatory bowel disease (Corazza and Gasbarrini, 1983).

The marginal zone lymphocytes of the spleen appear to be the main source of immunoglobulin M antibodies to polysaccharides. Thus, loss of splenic function, particularly in early life, leads to a susceptibility to infection with capsulated bacteria, primarily the pneumococcus, but including *Haemophilus influenzae* and meningococcus. Infections with these organisms can be overwhelming in patients with hyposplenism. In practice, this does not appear to be a common complication of coeliac disease, perhaps because splenic function is not lost early in life. Thus, in a study of mortality in 653 patients with coeliac disease, Logan et al (1989) attributed death to possible hyposplenism in only two patients. One of these patients died from pneumococcal meningitis 3 years after a routine blood film had shown evidence of hyposplenism; the other had salmonella septicaemia.

Splenic atrophy may be only part of a more generalized reticuloendothelial abnormality in coeliac disease. Lymph node enlargement (Paulley, 1954; Simmonds and Rosenthal, 1981) or atrophy (McCarthy et al, 1966) has been described and there are reports of central caseation in abdominal lymph nodes (Matuchansky et al, 1984), which also ocurs in association with lymphoma and coeliac disease (Freeman and Chin, 1986).

SUMMARY

Neoplasms constitute the major complication of coeliac disease, and high-grade T-cell lymphoma of the small intestine (enteropathy-associated T-cell lymphoma) is the most common neoplasm in this category. HLA genotyping indicates that in patients with enteropathy-associated T-cell lymphoma have the coeliac disease associated DQA1*0501, DQB1*0201 phenotype, although additional HLA-DR/DQ alleles may represent risk factors for lymphoma development. Molecular biological and immunohistochemical studies have shown that the intestinal mucosa distant from the tumour contains clonal populations of small T cells, often of the same clone as the high-grade T-cell lymphoma. These findings suggest that enteropathy-associated T-cell lymphoma arises in the setting of coeliac disease and evolves from reactive intraepithelial lymphocytes through a low-grade lymphocytic neoplasm to a high-grade tumour, which is usually the cause of the presenting symptoms. Most cases of chronic ulcerative enteropathy (ulcerative jejunitis) are probably part of the same disease process. If the ulceration occurs at a time when the neoplastic T-cells are of a low grade, morphological recognition of tumour cells in the ulcers may be impossible.

Carcinoma of the pharynx and oesophagus, and adenocarcinoma of the small intestine, are increased in frequency in patients with coeliac disease. The increased risk of carcinoma of the oesophagus may be related to vitamin A deficiency.

A number of reports have indicated an increased prevalence of various types of chronic hepatitis in patients with coeliac disease, but no coherent view of the cause of this association has emerged. Similarly, patients with coeliac disease have been reported to have various forms of fibrosing lung disease of uncertain causation. In recent years, there have been several reports, mainly from Italy, of a syndrome of epilepsy and bilateral brain calcification occurring in coeliac patients. The pathogenesis of this condition is not known and its prevalence in other communities is uncertain.

Splenic atrophy occurs frequently in patients with coeliac disease and is related to the severity of the disease and degree of dietary control. Splenic atrophy predisposes to infection with capsulated bacteria, although mortality studies indicate that infection with these organisms is not a major cause of death in patients with coeliac disease.

REFERENCES

Alfsen GC, Beiske K, Bell H & Marton PF (1989) Low-grade intestinal lymphoma of intra-epithelial T-lymphocytes with concomitant enteropathy-associated T-cell lymphoma: case report suggesting a possible histogenetic relataionship. *Human Pathology* **20:** 909–913.

Asquith P, Thompson RA & Cooke WT (1969) Serum-immunoglobulins in adult coeliac disease. *Lancet* **ii:** 129–131.

Baer AN, Bayless TM & Yardley JH (1980) Intestinal ulceration and malabsorption syndromes. *Gastroenterology* **79:** 754–765.

Bayless TM, Kapelowitz RF, Shelley WM et al (1967) Intestinal ulceration—a complication of celiac disease. *New England Journal of Medicine* **276:** 996–1000.

Behr W & Barnert J (1986) Adult onset celiac disease and primary biliary cirrhosis. *American Journal of Gastroenterology* **81:** 796–799.

Berrill WJ, Eade OE, Fitzpatrick TF et al (1975) Bird fancier's lung and jejunal villous atrophy. *Lancet* **ii:** 1006–1008.

Booth CC (1974) Definition of adult coeliac disease. In Hekken WThJM & Pena AS (eds) *Coeliac Disease*, pp 17–21. Leiden: Sternfert Kroese.

British Thoracic Society (1984) A national survey of bird fancier's lung: including its possible association with jejunal villous atrophy. *British Journal of Diseases of the Chest* **78:** 75–87.

Bye AME, Andermann F, Robitaille Y et al (1993) Cortical vascular abnormalities in the syndrome of celiac disease, epilepsy, bilateral occipital calcifications and folate deficiency. *Annals of Neurobiology* **34:** 399–403.

Catassi C, Rätsch I-M, Fabiani E et al (1994) Coeliac disease in the year 2000; exploring the iceberg. *Lancet* **343:** 200–203.

Chapman RWG, Laidlow SM & Colin-Jones D (1978) Increased prevalence of epilepsy in coeliac disease. *British Medical Journal* **2:** 250–251.

Cook WT & Smith WT (1966) Neurological disorders associated with adult coeliac disease. *Brain* **89:** 683–722.

Corazza GR & Gasbarrini G (1983) Defective splenic function and its relation to bowel disease. *Clinics in Gastroenterology* **12:** 651–669.

Corazza GR, Bullen AW, Hall R et al (1981) Simple method of assessing splenic function in coeliac disease. *Clinical Science* **60:** 109–113.

Douglas JG, Gillon J, Logan RFA et al (1984) Sarcoidosis and coeliac disease: an association: *Lancet* **ii:** 13–15.

Eade OE & Berrill WJ (1978) Coeliac lung disease. *Lancet* **i:** 1262–1263.

Eakins D, Fulton T & Hadden DR (1964) Reticulum cell sarcoma of the small bowel and steatorrhoea. *Gut* **5**: 315–323.

Edwards C, Williams A & Asquith P (1985) Bronchopulmonary disease in coeliac patients. *Journal of Clinical Pathology* **38**: 361–367.

Fairley NH & Mackie FP (1937) The clinical and biochemical syndrome in lymphadenoma and allied diseases involving the mesenteric lymph glands. *British Medical Journal* **i**: 375–380.

Faux JA, Hendrick DJ & Anand BS (1978) Precipitins to different avian serum antigens in bird fancier's lung and coeliac disease. *Clinical Allergy* **8**: 101–108.

Fois A, Balestri P, Vascotto M et al (1992) Epilepsy, progressive cerebral calcifications and coeliac disease. *Lancet* **340**: 1095.

Foucar K, Foucar E, Mitros F et al (1984) Epitheliotropic lymphoma of the small bowel. Report of a fatal case with cytotoxic/suppressor T-cell immunophenotype. *Cancer* **54**: 54–60.

Freeman HJ & Chin BK (1986) Small bowel malignant lymphoma complicating celiac sprue and the mesenteric lymph node cavitation syndrome. *Gastroenterology* **90**: 2008–2012.

Freeman HJ, Weinstein WM, Shnitta TK et al (1977) Primary abdominal lymphoma. Presenting manifestation of celiac sprue or complicating dermatitis herpetiformis? *American Journal of Medicine* **63**: 585–594.

Gobbi G, Bouquet F, Greco L et al (1992) Coeliac disease, epilepsy and cerebral calcifications. *Lancet* **340**: 439–443.

Gough KR, Read AE & Naish JM (1962) Intestinal reticulosis as a complication of idiopathic steatorrhoea. *Gut* **3**: 232–239.

Hagander B, Berg NO, Brandt L et al (1977) Hepatic injury in adult coeliac disease. *Lancet* **ii**: 270–272.

Harris OD, Cooke WT, Thompson H & Waterhouse JAH (1967) Malignancy in adult celiac disease and idiopathic steatorrhoea. *American Journal of Medicine* **42**: 899–912.

Hay JE, Wiesner RH, Shorter RG et al (1988) Primary sclerosing cholangitis and celiac disease. A novel association. *Annals of Internal Medicine* **109**: 713–717.

Hendrick DJ, Faux JA, Anand B et al (1978) Is bird fancier's lung associated with coeliac disease? *Thorax* **33**: 425–428.

Hermaszewski RA, Rigby S & Dalgleish AG (1991) Coeliac disease presenting with cerebellar degeneration. *Postgraduate Medical Journal* **67**: 1023–1024.

Hodges JR, Isaacson P, Smith CL & Sworn MJ (1979) Malignant histiocytosis of the intestine. *Digestive Diseases and Sciences* **24**: 631–638.

Hoffbrand AV (1974) Anaemia in adult coeliac disease. *Clinics in Gastroenterology* **3**: 71–89.

Holmes GKT, Prior P, Lane MR et al (1989) Malignancy in coeliac disease—effect of a gluten-free diet. *Gut* **30**: 333–338.

Hood J & Mason AMS (1970) Diffuse pulmonary disease with transfer defect occurring with coeliac disease. *Lancet* **i**: 445–448.

Hourihane DO'B & Weir DG (1970) Malignant celiac syndrome. *Gastroenterology* **29**: 130–139.

Howell WM, Leung ST, Jones DB et al (1995) HLA-DRB, DQA and DQB polymorphism in celiac disease and enteropathy-associated T-cell lymphoma: commom features and additional risk factors for malignancy. *Human Immunology* (in press).

Isaacson PG (1992) Histopathology of the complications of celiac disease: enteropathy-associated T-cell lymphoma and ulcerative jejunitis. *Frontiers of Gastrointestinal Research* **19**: 194–212.

Isaacson PG & Wright DH (1978a) Intestinal lymphoma associated with malabsorption. *Lancet* **i**: 67–70.

Isaacson PG & Wright DH (1978b) Malignant histiocytosis of the intestine: its relationship to malabsorption and ulcerative jejunitis. *Human Pathology* **9**: 661–677.

Isaacson PG, Spencer J, Connolly CE et al (1985) Malignant histiocytosis of the intestine: a T-cell lymphoma. *Lancet* **ii**: 688–690.

Kagnoff MF (1990) Understanding the molecular basis of coeliac disease. *Gut* **31**: 497–499.

Konig G, Albert E, Dewait M et al (1982) Extrinsic allergic alveolitis combined with celiac disease in childhood. *Respiration* **43**: 444–451.

Levenson SD, Austin RK, Dietler MD et al (1985) Specificity of antigliadin antibody in celiac disease. *Gastroenterology* **89**: 1–5.

Lindberg J, Ahrén C & Iwarson S (1979) Intestinal villous atrophy in chronic active hepatitis. *Scandinavian Journal of Gastroenterology* **14**: 1015–1018.

Loft DE & Marsh MN (1986) Humoral response to wheat protein in patients with coeliac disease and enteropathy-associated T-cell lymphoma. *British Medical Journal* **293**: 1439.

Logan RF, Ferguson A, Finlayson ND & Weir DG (1978) Primary biliary cirrhosis and coeliac disease: an association? *Lancet* **i**: 230–233.

Logan RFA, Rifkind EA, Rutner ID & Ferguson A (1989) Mortality in celiac disease. *Gastroenterology* **97**: 265–271.

McCarthy CF, Fraser ID, Evans KT & Read AE (1966) Lymphoreticular dysfunction in idiopathic steatorrhoea. *Gut* **7**: 140–148.

Maguadda A, Dalla Bernadina B, De Marco P et al (1993) Bilateral occipital calcification, epilepsy and coeliac disease: clinical and neuroimaging features of a new syndrome. *Journal of Neurology, Neurosurgery and Psychiatry* **56**: 885–889.

Matuchansky C, Colin R & Hemet J (1984) Cavitation of mesenteric lymph nodes, splenic atrophy and a flat small intestinal mucosa. *Gastroenterology* **87**: 606–614.

Mead GM, Whitehouse JM, Thompson J et al (1987) Clinical features and management of malignant histiocytosis of the intestine. *Cancer* **60**: 2791–2796.

Mills PR, Brown IL & Wilkinson G (1980) Idiopathic chronic ulcerative enteritis. Report of five cases and review of the literature. *Quarterly Journal of Medicine* **49**: 133–149.

Murray H, Cuevas EC, Jones DB & Wright DH (1995) A study of the immunohistochemistry and T-cell clonality of enteropathy-associated T-cell lymphomas. *American Journal of Pathology* (in press).

Neilsen OH, Jacobsen O, Pedersen ER et al (1985) Non-tropical sprue: malignant disease and mortality rate. *Scandinavian Journal of Gastroenterology* **20**: 13–18.

Nyman E (1949) Ulcerous jejuno-ileitis with symptomatic sprue. *Acta Medica Scandinavica* **134**: 275–285.

O'Driscoll BRC, Stevens FM, O'Gorman TA et al (1982) HLA type of patients with coeliac disease and malignancy in the west of Ireland. *Gut* **23**: 662–665.

O'Farrelly C, Feighery C, O'Briain DS et al (1986) Humoral response to wheat protein in patients with coeliac disease and enteropathy-associated T-cell lymphoma. *British Medical Journal* **293**: 908–910.

O'Grady JG, Stevens FM, Harding B et al (1984) Hyposplenism and gluten-sensitive enteropathy. Natural history, incidence and relationship to diet and small bowel morphology *Gastroenterology* **87**: 1326–1331.

Paulley JW (1954) Observations on the aetiology of idiopathic steatorrhoea. Jejunal and lymph node biopsies. *British Medical Journal* **ii**: 1318–1321.

Pollock DJ (1977) The liver in coeliac disease. *Histopathology* **1**: 421–430.

Salter DM, Krajewski AS & Dewar AE (1986) Immunophenotype analysis of malignant histiocytosis of the intestine. *Journal of Clinical Pathology* **39**: 8–15.

Simmonds JP & Rosenthal FD (1981) Lymphadenopathy in coeliac disease. *Gut* **22**: 555–560.

Spencer J, MacDonald TT, Diss TC et al (1989) Changes in intraepithelial lymphocyte sub-populations in coeliac disease and enteropathy-associated T-cell lymphoma (malignant histiocytosis of the intestine). *Gut* **30**: 339–346.

Sollid LM & Thorsby E (1993) HLA susceptibility genes in celiac disease: genetic mapping and role in pathogenesis. *Gastroenterology* **105**: 910–922.

Stein H, Dienemann D & Sperling M (1988) Identification of a T-cell lymphoma category derived from intestinal mucosa-associated T-cells. *Lancet* **ii**: 1053–1054.

Stevens FM, Connolly CE, Murray JP & McCarthy CF (1990) Lung cavities in patients with coeliac disease. *Digestion* **46**: 72–80.

Swinson CM, Hall PJ, Bedford PA & Booth CC (1983a) HLA antigens in coeliac disease associated with malignancy. *Gut* **24**: 925–928.

Swinson CM, Slavin G, Coles EC & Booth CC (1983b) Coeliac disease and malignancy. *Lancet* **i**: 111–115.

Thompson H (1974) Necropsy studies on adult onset coeliac disease. *Journal of Clinical Pathology* **27**: 710–721.

Trier JS (1991) Celiac sprue. *New England Journal of Medicine* **325**: 1709–1719.

Whitehead R (1968) Primary lymphadenopathy complicating idiopathic steatorrhoea. *Gut* **9**: 569.

Wolber R, Owen D & Freeman H (1990) Colonic lymphocytosis in patients with celiac sprue. *Human Pathology* **21**: 1092–1096.

Wright DH Jones DB, Clark H et al (1991) Is adult onset coeliac disease due to a low-grade lymphoma of intraepithelial T-lymphocytes? *Lancet* **337**: 1373–1374.

Wright PH, Menzies IS, Pound RE et al (1981) Adult idiopathic pulmonary haemosiderosis and coeliac disease. *Quarterly Journal of Medicine* **50**: 95–102.

9

Dermatitis herpetiformis

LIONEL FRY

Dermatitis herpetiformis (DH) was first described as a clinical entity by Louis Duhring, a dermatologist in Philadelphia, in 1884. It was grouped together with pemphigus and pemphigoid and the three disorders were known collectively as the 'bullous diseases' because they all presented with blisters. A clear distinction between pemphigus and the other two disorders was made in 1943 when it was shown that in pemphigus the blister was intraepidermal whereas in DH and pemphigoid it was subepidermal (Civatte, 1943). A distinction between pemphigoid and DH was made on clinical features and response to sulphonamides and dapsone after it was shown that the rash in DH cleared with sulphapyridine (Costello, 1940) and dapsone (Esteves and Brandao, 1950). However, a much more precise distinction between pemphigoid and DH is now possible, based on immuno-fluorescent studies.

CLINICAL FEATURES

Sex incidence

Overall, DH is slightly more common in males (3:2). However, in patients who present early in life, i.e. before the age of 20 years, females predominate (3:2).

Age of onset

DH most commonly presents in late adolescence and early adult life (15–40 years) (Davies and Marks, 1978; Reunala and Lokki, 1978; Gawkrodger et al, 1984; Mobracken et al, 1984; Moi, 1984). However, it may present in childhood, the youngest reported case being 10 months (Ermacora et al, 1986), and at any time in adult life, the oldest reported case being over 90 years (Christensen et al, 1986). In most reported series DH is rare in childhood except for two countries, Italy and Hungary.

Epidemiology

There have been only a few studies on the prevalence of DH in the population. In a study from Edinburgh (Gawkrodger et al, 1984) the prevalence was 11.5 per 100 000 population and a similar prevalence was found in Finland (11.4 per 100 000) (Reunala and Lokki, 1978). Higher prevalences have been reported from Sweden, ranging from 19.6 to 39.2 per 100 000 (Mobracken et al, 1984; Moi, 1984; Christensen et al, 1986). Coeliac disease appears to be more common than DH, the highest prevalence being reported in Ireland (Mylotte et al, 1973; Love, 1981): 1 in 300 in the west of Ireland and 1 in 560 in Northern Ireland. However, strict criteria for diagnosis were not adhered to in the latter study. When these criteria were applied, the prevalence fell to 1 in 1700.

Like coeliac disease, DH is predominantly a European disease, but may be seen in countries to which Europeans have emigrated. Of the 212 patients with DH who attended the DH clinic at St Mary's Hospital, London, none is Afro-Caribbean and only one is half Asian. This particular patient had one Indian and one Portuguese parent. This lack of black patients in our DH clinic is despite large populations attending and living in the hospital's catchment area. I, personally, have not seen a negro with DH.

Morphology of skin lesions

The skin lesions seen in DH are blisters, urticarial plaques and excoriations. The blisters are most commonly present within the urticarial plaques, but may also arise from otherwise normal appearing skin. They are often grouped (hence the term herpetiform) and are usually small, 2–5 mm in diameter. Occasionally larger blisters are seen but they are usually less than 1 cm in diameter. The urticarial plaques may vary in size from one to several centimetres (up to 10 cm). Dermatitis herpetiformis is an intensely irritating eruption and therefore excoriations are a very common feature. Any blisters present are traumatized at an early stage, and thus may not be seen when the patient presents to the physician. It is in fact more common to see scabbed papules than blisters. Thus, the distribution of the eruption may be more suggestive of the diagnosis than the finding of small blisters.

Distribution of the rash

The eruption of DH is usually symmetrical. The commonest site is the extensor surface of the elbows (Figure 1). Approximately 95% of patients will have involvement on the elbows. The eruption also frequently extends to the proximal extensor forearm. The next commonest site is the buttocks, with two thirds of patients having involvement at this site (Figure 2). The third most frequent area is the extensor surface of the knees (Figure 3). The eruption of DH often involves only these sites, and not infrequently only the elbows and buttocks. However, occasionally the eruption is more extensive with involvement of the trunk. Curiously the face and scalp are not usually affected when the eruption first appears, but once the disease is established these are not infrequent sites. The face and scalp are also often involved when there is an exacerbation of the disease.

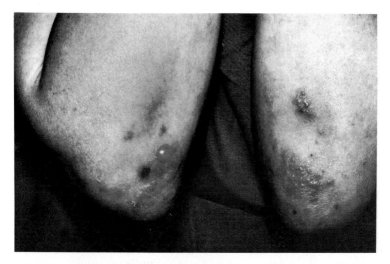

Figure 1. Grouped blisters on the extensor elbows—the commonest site for dermatitis herpetiformis.

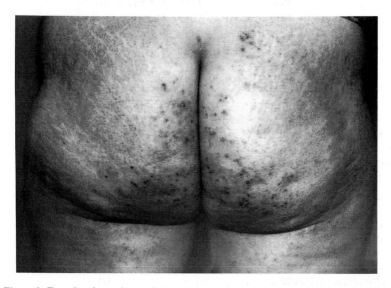

Figure 2. Excoriated papules on the buttocks. No blisters are seen owing to excoriation.

The eruption of DH may also be seen at sites of pressure from clothing, e.g. brassiere straps and tight belts.

Natural history

DH tends to be a persistent and chronic disorder. In patients not treated with a gluten-free diet and followed up for 25 years, the spontaneous

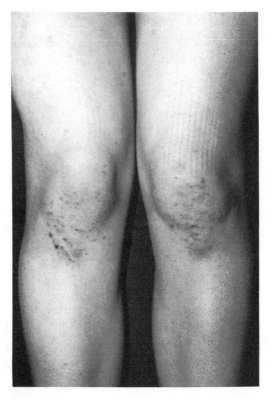

Figure 3. Symmetrical urticarial papules on the knees.

remission rate is 10–15% (Alexander, 1975; Garioch et al, 1994a). In some patients there is a tendency for the rash to become less severe as they become older. There is also a suggestion that in those patients with a late onset the rash is less severe and more likely to remit spontaneously (Christensen et al, 1986).

INVESTIGATIONS

The most important test to establish the diagnosis of DH is a biopsy of uninvolved skin for immunofluorescent studies to detect the presence of immunoglobulin (Ig) A in the upper dermis. If the diagnosis is confirmed by the presence of IgA, the following investigations should also be performed: full blood count and urine analysis, liver function tests, serum creatinine, serum calcium and phosphorus, autoantibody screening including anti-reticulin and anti-endomysial antibodies, and small intestinal biopsy. A biopsy of lesional skin is not necessary for routine purposes.

IgA in the skin in dermatitis herpetiformis

IgA is found in the *uninvolved* skin but not in lesional skin in DH. The presence of IgA at the appropriate site (see below) is the criterion for establishing the diagnosis (Fry and Seah, 1974). If IgA is not found, the diagnosis of DH should not be made. The biopsy may be taken from any site (as IgA is present throughout the skin); however, the upper and outer buttock is recommended as the procedure will leave a small scar. A 4-mm punch biopsy should be taken, imbedded in OCT (Tissue Tek) and snap-frozen in liquid nitrogen or put into an appropriate transport medium for immunofluorescent studies.

IgA is found in two patterns in DH. The most common site is the dermal papillae, where IgA is seen as granular or fibrillar deposits (Figure 4). The other pattern is a linear granular deposition just below the basement membrane (Figure 5). The pattern of deposition may vary in time, i.e. an initial biopsy showing a linear granular pattern of IgA may on a subsequent biopsy show a papillary pattern. The reason for the different patterns of IgA deposition is as yet unknown, but there is no correlation between the pattern and any other features of the disease, such as the severity of the rash or

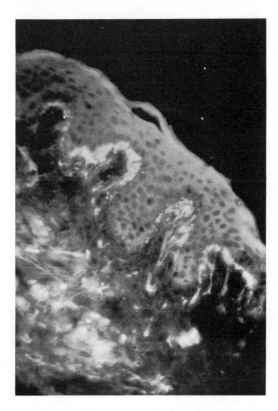

Figure 4. IgA deposits in the dermal papillae.

enteropathy. It is important to distinguish the linear granular pattern of IgA from homogeneous linear IgA deposition (Figure 6). The latter is found in so-called linear IgA disease (LAD). Although there are similar clinical features between LAD and DH, the diseases have a different aetiological basis; the eruption of LAD is not gluten dependent and therefore a gluten-free diet has no role in the management of this disorder. It is therefore of

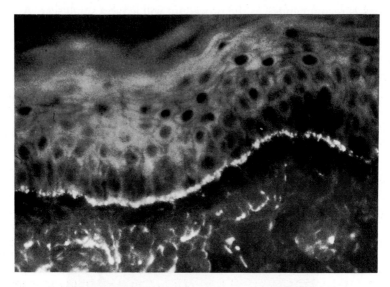

Figure 5. Linear granular deposits of IgA, representing dermatitis herpetiformis.

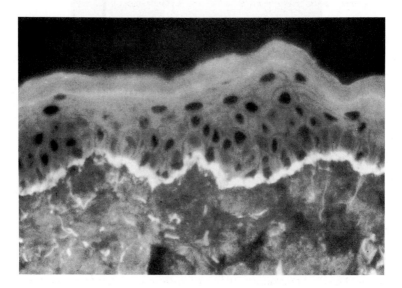

Figure 6. Homogeneous linear deposition of IgA in linear IgA disease.

extreme importance that an experienced immunopathologist familiar with immunofluorescence and the pattern of immunoglobulin deposition in skin disorders reads the slides. Now that transport medium is readily available it is advisable for the biopsies to be sent to a centre with expertise in interpreting the results of immunofluorescent studies on skin biopsies. In the DH clinic at St Mary's Hospital we have had a number of patients referred to us as having DH and not responding to a gluten-free diet. These patients have subsequently been shown on skin biopsy in our laboratory to have LAD.

In experienced hands the chance of finding IgA in a single section of the biopsy is 96% (Seah and Fry, 1975). If no IgA is found and the clinical features are strongly suggestive of the disease, then serial sectioning of the biopsy should be performed, and if still negative a second biopsy should be undertaken. When these two additional procedures were carried out, Seah and Fry (1975) found IgA to be present in the uninvolved skin in all patients with DH. It should be mentioned that IgA is found in the uninvolved skin in patients in spontaneous remission, and in those whose rash is controlled by drug treatment. IgA is also present in those whose rash is controlled by a gluten-free diet, although after many years of this treatment it may disappear in some individuals (Leonard et al, 1983; Garioch et al, 1994a). In the latter study Garioch and colleagues found that 10 (21%) of 48 patients taking a strict diet lost IgA after an average duration of 13 (range 5–24) years. In addition to the IgA, IgM and/or IgG may be found at the same site as the IgA in a small proportion of patients (20% have IgM; 10% have IgG) (Seah and Fry, 1975). The exact significance of this finding is unknown. The C3 component of complement is found in two thirds of patients before treatment with a gluten-free diet. This component of complement tends to disappear from the skin with a gluten-free diet, and is usually not found once control of the rash with the diet alone has been achieved.

Histology

A biopsy of lesional skin of DH is no longer performed for diagnostic purposes. The histological features are not specific for DH, whereas the presence of IgA in uninvolved skin is diagnostic. However, the histological features of a DH skin lesion will be described as they are relevant to the discussion on the pathogenesis of the disease. The initial lesion is a neutrophilic microabscess in the dermal papillae. These abscesses enlarge and coalesce to form a subepidermal blister. Neutrophils are the predominant cell in the blister, and leukocytoclasia and fibrin deposition are commonly seen. Eosinophils are present in approximately 25% of blisters. In the dermis around the blood vessels there is a lymphohistiocytic cell infiltrate.

Small intestinal biopsy

Once the diagnosis of DH has been established by the presence of IgA in uninvolved skin, a small intestinal biopsy should be performed. Approximately two-thirds of patients will show features of coeliac disease, i.e. villous atrophy, crypt hyperplasia, and cellular infiltration of the epithelium and lamina propria (Fry et al, 1974). However, it is likely that all patients with DH have some degree of gluten sensitivity of their small intestine. If multiple biopsies are taken, the incidence of morphological change increases to 95% (Brow et al, 1971) and in those patients with normal villous architecture gluten challenge will induce villous atrophy (Weinstein, 1973). In addition, in patients with normal villous architecture, there is an increase in the number of intraepithelial lymphocytes in 90% and this increase is similar whether villous atrophy is present or not (Fry et al, 1974). Thus, on a single biopsy the majority of patients with DH will have some evidence of a gluten-sensitive enteropathy as judged by villous atrophy and increased intraepithelial lymphocyte count (see also Chapter 5).

Haematological investigations

A full blood count is mandatory. Anaemia may occur as a result of malabsorption of iron or folate, but is most frequently due to haemolysis from treatment with dapsone. Macrocytosis may be present because of haemolysis from dapsone, or as a result of folate deficiency. Because of the high incidence of pernicious anaemia in DH, vitamin B_{12} deficiency may also cause macrocytosis. Thus, appropriate tests for iron, folate and B_{12} deficiency should be performed if indicated. The peripheral blood film may also show the presence of Howell–Jolly bodies, indicating splenic atrophy, which is found in DH as well as coeliac disease.

Liver function tests

Abnormal liver function test results have been reported in 17% of patients with DH (Wojnarowska and Fry, 1981). However, in 8% the raised bilirubin level was attributable to dapsone therapy. Autoimmune liver disease appears to be more common in patients with coeliac disease and, of 212 patients with DH seen in our clinic, one has primary biliary cirrhosis and another has chronic active hepatitis. In addition, abnormal liver function test results do occur in a small proportion of patients with gluten-sensitive enteropathy, which improve following gluten withdrawal.

Autoantibody screening

There is a significant increase in autoimmune disorders in patients with DH, particularly thyroid disease and pernicious anaemia. Thus, screening for thyroid, gastric parietal cell and anti-nuclear antibodies should be performed routinely.

Anti-reticulin antibody (ARA), anti-endomysial antibody (AEMA) and anti-gliadin antibody (AGA) are not of importance in establishing the diagnosis of DH. The incidence of these antibodies in DH is too low (ARA 20% (Seah et al, 1973), AEMA 70% (Sulej and Leonard, 1987) and AGA 50% (Unsworth et al, 1981a)) for them to be used for diagnostic purposes, particularly when the presence of IgA in the uninvolved skin provides a test with a 100% positivity. In addition, the presence of the antibodies is not diagnostic of DH, whereas IgA in the skin at an appropriate site is.

Urine analysis

As there is an increased incidence of diabetes mellitus in DH, it is important that urine is tested routinely.

MANAGEMENT

DH responds rapidly to appropriate drugs and slowly to a gluten-free diet. Thus, initial treatment must be with drugs, because of the severe pruritus associated with the eruption. The three drugs commonly used for controlling the rash are dapsone, sulphapyridine and sulphamethoxypyridazine. Pruritus and the rash often improve within 48 hours, and this rapid response was used in the past to support the clinical diagnosis of DH. However, other eruptions apart from DH also respond to dapsone and the sulphonamides, and the diagnosis should be made only by the finding of IgA in uninvolved skin. With the appropriate dose the eruption should clear within 1 week. However, relapse of the eruption and symptoms is equally rapid when the drug is discontinued. Irritation may return within 24 hours of stopping drug therapy and lesions appear within 2–3 days.

Dapsone

The initial dose of dapsone should be 100 mg daily, and the patient asked to reattend in 2 weeks. If the eruption has cleared, the dose should be reduced to 50 mg daily. If the eruption remains clear, further reduction of dosage should be attempted. This reduction in dosage should be made by increasing the interval of time between each dose, i.e. to alternate days, then every third day, and by further increments of a day until a schedule of once a week is reached. At this dosage it is probable the drug is no longer required. If no control of the rash is achieved with 100 mg daily, the dose should be increased by 100 mg daily every 2 weeks to a maximum of 400 mg daily. If no control is achieved with the maximum dose of dapsone, evidence for the diagnosis should be reviewed, including, if necessary, a second biopsy from uninvolved skin for IgA.

The average dose for control of the rash is 100 mg daily, and the range in our clinic has been from 50 mg twice weekly to 700 mg daily. (The latter is not recommended because of severe side-effects encountered with this dose.) There is no strict correlation between severity of the eruption and dose of dapsone required for control. However, if the eruption is minimal, a low dose of dapsone is often sufficient for control but a severe eruption may also be controlled by a relatively low dose, i.e. 50 mg daily.

Side-effects

Haemolysis is one of the commonest side-effects and occurs to some extent in all patients. In some the haemolysis may be severe, and dapsone must be discontinued. Haemolysis occurs early in the treatment and it is important that a full blood count be carried out 2 weeks after starting dapsone, and then again after a further month. Once patients are established on dapsone without severe haemolysis, a full blood count will be necessary only twice yearly. Although the degree of haemolysis is likely to be dose dependent, some patients are particularly prone to this side-effect, which may occur even with a small dose. The reticulocyte count is a good indicator of the degree of haemolysis and should be performed routinely with a full blood count.

Methaemoglobinaemia is another common side-effect of dapsone, and presents as cyanosis. The degree of methaemoglobinaemia is not directly related to the dose of dapsone. The importance of methaemoglobinaemia is that it will reduce the oxygen-carrying capacity of the blood. It is therefore our policy not to use dapsone (if possible) in patients aged over 50 years as there may be some degree of impaired cardiac or cerebral blood flow, which does not cause symptoms but may with reduced oxygen-carrying capacity of the blood. Agranulocytosis is another haematological side-effect, but fortunately rare.

Headache, lethargy, depression and insomnia are all common symptoms associated with dapsone therapy and, if severe, warrant cessation of therapy.

Peripheral neuropathy, which is usually a mononeuritis of the entrapment type, is a rare but well-recognized complication.

Severe hypoalbuminaemia may also occur rarely.

In our experience 25% of patients will experience side-effects that warrant discontinuation of dapsone.

Sulphapyridine

The initial dose should be 2.0 g daily. Patients should be seen after 2 weeks and the dose adjusted according to the clinical response. The maximum dose should not exceed 4.0 g daily. As with dapsone, there is wide variation in the dosage required to control the eruption ranging from 0.5–4.0 g daily.

Side-effects

There are fewer side-effects with sulphapyridine than with dapsone, but the number of tablets taken per day to control the rash is much higher and patients find this inconvenient.

The side-effects of sulphapyridine are nausea, lethargy and depression. Rarely, agranulocytosis, haemolytic anaemia, renal calculi and CNS abnormalities may occur.

Sulphamethoxypyridazine

This is a relatively little known sulphonamide that has a valuable place in the treatment of DH. The initial dose is 1.0 g daily, and this may be increased to a maximum of 1.5 g daily if necessary. The time interval for change of dosage is the same as that for dapsone. Many patients may have adequate control with 0.5 g daily.

The advantage of sulphamethoxypyridazine is its low incidence of side-effects, and fewer tablets are required for control of the rash compared with sulphapyridine.

Side-effects

These include drug rash, nausea and lethargy. As with all sulphonamides, there is a risk of agranulocytosis.

Combination therapy

If side-effects preclude increasing the dosage, or the maximum dosage has been reached, it is possible to combine any of the three drugs to obtain an increased therapeutic effect. This is frequently done in the DH clinic at St Mary's Hospital.

Gluten-free diet

Gluten withdrawal from the diet was first shown to be of benefit in controlling the rash of DH in 1968 (Fry et al, 1968). It was found that after 6 months of a gluten-free diet there was a decrease in the dose of dapsone required to control the rash. It was subsequently shown (Fry et al, 1969) that on reintroduction of gluten the dapsone requirement increased to its previous levels. Other early reports disputed the beneficial effect of a gluten-free diet on the rash, but these failed to appreciate the length of time the diet was required before improvement became apparent. However, many centres have now confirmed that a gluten-free diet is indeed effective in controlling the eruption. Apart from the length of time taken to control the rash with a gluten-free diet, the strictness of the diet is also important. In our earlier studies (Fry et al, 1973, 1982) we found that, if the diet was very strict, 96% of patients were able to discontinue taking drugs for control of the rash. If patients had occasional gluten intake (less than once a week) then only 45% were able to stop taking drugs, but the majority were able to reduce the dose. Recently we have analysed data on 212 patients seen in the DH clinic over 25 years, of whom 133 have taken the diet (Garioch et al, 1994a). In 44 patients the diet had been completely strict and 41 (93%) of these have been able to discontinue medication. Of the 89 patients taking a gluten-free diet with occasional gluten intake, 37 (42%) were able to discontinue medication. In patients whose diet was completely strict the average time taken to stop medication was 28 (range 4–88) months, whereas in those whose diet was not completely strict the average time was 44 (range 9–106) months. It must be emphasized to the patients starting a gluten-free diet that it will take many months before they will be able to reduce the drug requirement and on average 2 years before they will be able to stop the medication. However, as in patients with coeliac disease, those with DH often have a feeling of 'well-being' after a few weeks of starting the diet.

In our experience, if patients opt to take the diet as part of the treatment, they should do so under the supervision of a dietitian with experience of a gluten-free diet. In our DH clinic the dietitian is part of the team and is present at the consultation. Patients should be encouraged to join the Coeliac Society, and receive the *Coeliac Handbook*.

Advantages of a gluten-free diet

The most obvious advantage is that patients will eventually not require drugs with a relatively high incidence of side-effects to control the rash. In addition, they often experience a feeling of well-being and say they have more energy. The gluten-free diet not only treats the skin rash but also intestinal enteropathy, and this prevents possible malabsorption. Finally, in a combined study of our 212 patients and 275 patients from Finland (under the care of Professor T. Reunala), we have shown that a gluten-free diet does appear to protect patients from developing lymphoma, which is similar to the claim made for the diet in coeliac disease (Holmes et al, 1989).

Reasons for not taking a gluten-free diet

It is our policy to discuss the possibility of treatment with a gluten-free diet with all our patients. However, 40 (19%) of the 212 patients chose not to follow the diet. In addition, a further 39 (18%) did not persist with the diet. The reasons for not taking or continuing with the diet were: (1) it was too difficult and/or unpalatable; (2) it was socially limiting; and (3) it was not practical, e.g. travelling a great deal in their work.

Unlike patients with coeliac disease, those with DH often do not have gastrointestinal symptoms and, providing they can control the rash with drugs without side-effects, they see little point in the inconvenience of a gluten-free diet.

As with coeliac disease, in DH the gluten-free diet must be considered to be life-long. It has been shown that both the skin and small intestine relapse on reintroduction of gluten, even after many years on the diet (Leonard et al, 1983).

ASSOCIATED DISORDERS

There is an increase in so-called autoimmune disorders in DH, and a very high incidence of circulating organ-specific autoantibodies. In a detailed study of thyroid function and antibodies of 115 patients in our department (Weetman et al, 1988), thyroid disease was found in 5% of our patients, and in a further 6% there was a raised level of thyroid-stimulating hormone, implying some degree of failure. Thyroid antibodies were present in 48% of patients. A similar increased incidence of thyroid disease has been reported from two other centres (Reunala and Lokki, 1978; Gawkrodger et al, 1984).

Gastric parietal cell antibodies were found in 62 (29%) of the 212 patients at St Mary's Hospital and pernicious anaemia developed in six (3%). This is a similar figure to that reported in a study from Edinburgh (Gawkrodger et al, 1984). Achlorhydria is a common manifestation of DH and there is a good correlation between the presence of gastric parietal cell antibodies and achlorhydria (Gillberg et al, 1985); more than 90% of patients with achlor-hydria have atrophic gastritis on biopsy.

There is an increased incidence of insulin-dependent diabetes mellitus, being present in five (2%) of our 212 patients, and thus routine testing of urine should be performed at each follow-up visit. Other autoimmune disorders in our group of patients include chronic active hepatitis (one patient), sclerosing cholangitis (one), systemic lupus erythematosus (two) and myasthenia gravis (one). A gluten-free diet does not appear to have any preventive effect on the production of autoantibodies or on the develop-ment of autoimmune disease (McFadden et al, 1991).

Malignancy

As with coeliac disease, there is an increased incidence of lymphoma in DH. In a recent combined study of 212 patients from St Mary's Hospital and 275 from Finland (under the care of Professor T. Reunala), there were four patients with lymphoma in each centre, giving an incidence of 2% and a relative risk of 5.9. This particular study was set up to determine whether a gluten-free diet protected against the development of lymphoma. All patients seen at St Mary's Hospital since 1967, and in Finland from 1978, were followed; a gluten-free diet taken for longer than 5 years was found to be protective against the development of lymphoma. This is similar to the protective effect of a gluten-free diet reported for coeliac disease (Holmes et al, 1989). It should be stressed that this increase in lymphoma is not confined to small intestinal lymphomas: the malignancy may present at sites away from the intestine. The tumours appear to develop from T lymphocytes. In both the Finnish and St Mary's Hospital groups there appeared to be no increase in the incidence of carcinoma, similar to the findings of a recent study by Sigurgeirsson et al (1994), who showed an increase in the incidence in lymphoma but not in carcinoma in 976 patients with DH.

PATHOGENESIS

IgA in the uninvolved skin is the hallmark of DH and is not found in the lesional skin of patients with DH. However, the exact role of the IgA, its origin and persistence despite control of the rash with a gluten-free diet have yet to be explained. It has even been proposed that the IgA may be an epiphenomenon and is not involved in the pathogenesis of the skin lesions as it is present in: (i) uninvolved skin; (ii) patients whose rash is controlled with a gluten-free diet; and (iii) those whose rash undergoes spontaneous resolution. However, it is likely that factors in addition to the IgA are probably necessary for the induction of skin lesions, and these may be affected by a gluten-free diet. It has also been suggested that the quantity of IgA may be important for the skin lesions to be induced. If the concentration of IgA falls below a certain level, skin lesions will not develop. Although IgA is still present in the skin when control of the rash is achieved with a gluten-free diet, it was found to be reduced in amount by this diet (Frodin et al, 1981; Ljunghall and Tjernlund, 1983). It is likely that there is a progressive decrease in the amount of IgA with a strict gluten-free diet, but it takes many years (average 13) for the IgA to disappear (Leonard et al, 1983; Garioch et al, 1994a). This persistence of IgA may be related to the way in which IgA is bound to the skin. Elution studies with the usual substances used to elute immune complexes have not been successful in removing IgA from the skin. It has been proposed that the IgA in DH skin is covalently bound and not deposited as an IgA immune complex. If IgA is covalently bound, this may explain its persistence and very slow disappearance with a gluten-free diet.

It has been assumed that the IgA in the skin comes from the small intestine and that it is deposited as an IgA gluten–antigluten immune complex (Seah et al, 1972). However, gluten has never been found in the skin in DH despite attempts to detect it with anti-gliadin antibodies. This, in itself, may not be conclusive evidence that gluten is not present in the skin; it may be present within the IgA deposits and not be available to react with antibody. Evidence that the IgA is derived from the small intestine was the demonstration of 'J' chain in the IgA deposits in the skin by Unsworth et al (1982). Others, however, have been unable to find J chain (Barghuthy et al, 1988). The IgA in the skin is mainly of subclass IgA_1, and yet secretory IgA from the intestine is composed of equal amounts of IgA_1 and IgA_2, whereas that in serum IgA is mainly IgA_1. However, it has recently been shown that in DH IgA_1 is the predominant subclass in the gastrointestinal secretions of patients with DH (Hall and McKenzie, 1992), so that the observation that the IgA in the skin is IgA_1 subclass does not exclude its origin from the intestine. Originally, it was proposed that the IgA bound to reticulin in the upper dermis (Seah et al, 1972). Subsequent electron microscopic studies (Stingl et al, 1976) reported that the IgA associated with the microfibrillar component of elastic tissue. However, a more recent study using monoclonal antibodies to fibrillin (a component of elastic monofibrillan bundles) could not confirm that IgA was found in association with elastic microfibrils (Lightner et al, 1991). These latter authors considered that the IgA was not associated with any specific structure in the skin, but may bind to a degradation product of the basal lamina. This seems unlikely in view of the fact that the IgA in electron microscopic studies appears to be well below the basal lamina.

In considering the possible binding site of IgA in the skin, the observation that gluten plays a central role in the pathogenesis of the skin lesions should not be overlooked. It has been shown that gluten will bind to reticulin in a non-specific manner to both DH and normal skin (Unsworth et al, 1981b). It was originally proposed that in DH gluten, as found in a gluten–antigluten immune complex, binds to reticulin in the skin (Seah et al, 1972). This damages the reticulin and renders it immunogenic with the subsequent development of anti-reticulin antibody. If this scenario does take place in the skin, it may explain why it takes so long for a gluten-free diet to be effective in DH as new reticulin will have to be formed. A more recent study has again incriminated elastin as the site of deposition (Bodvarsson et al,

1993). Recently, homology has been shown to exist between elastin and glutenin. It is suggested that in DH IgA glutenin antibodies cross-react with elastin in the skin and that this results in the IgA deposition. In support of this hypothesis, Bodvarsson et al found lower levels of IgA antibodies, both to glutenin and elastin, in patients with DH compared with those in normal subjects and patients with coeliac disease. They argued that these lower levels were due to absorption of the antibodies into the skin. Thus, glutenin rather than gliadin may be the cause of the skin lesions in DH. Obviously, studies are now required to prove or disprove this hypothesis.

The characteristic histological features of the skin lesion in DH are neutrophilic microabscesses in the dermal papillae and subepidermal blisters with neutrophil infiltration. It has been assumed since finding IgA and C3 complement in the skin of patients with DH that complement activation is responsible for the chemotactic factors for neutrophil migration into DH skin. Once attracted into the dermal papillae the neutrophils become activated and release enzymes that cause tissue damage and an inflammatory reaction. However, C3 complement, like IgA, is also found in uninvolved skin and therefore complement may not be responsible for the skin lesions.

In a recent study Dahlback et al (1989) investigated the possibility that in DH non-lytic complement complexes are formed, and therefore complement could not be the responsible chemoattractant for neutrophils. These authors investigated the presence of vitronectin in a variety of bullous disorders. Vitronectin is an inhibitor of the membrane attack complex of complement. It binds to nascent C5G-7 complexes, thereby inhibiting C9 polymerization and membrane attack, and results in the formation of non-lytic complexes. These authors found that C9 neo-antigen immunoreactivity co-localizes with C3 immunoreactivity in skin specimens from patients with lupus erythematosus, bullous pemphigoid and DH. In all three disorders, C9 neo-antigens were detected, but in DH and discoid lupus erythematosus vitronectin was found at the same sites. This implies that in DH non-lytic complement complexes are formed and therefore complement does not play a role in neutrophil chemotaxis.

Thus, if complement is not the chemoattractant for neutrophils in DH, another alternative has to be found. Recently, Graeber et al (1993) reported strong expression of interleukin (IL) 8 by the basal keratinocytes in lesional skin compared with uninvolved DH and normal skin. In addition, these workers showed that the dendrites of dermoepidermal dendritic cells expressed granulocyte–macrophage colony-stimulating factor (GM-CSF). These dendrites extend to the dermal papillae where IgA is deposited. IL-8 is a strong chemoattractant for neutrophils and GM-CSF is able to induce Fc–IgA receptors on neutrophils. When neutrophils bind to IgA via their Fc receptors they are activated and produce enzymes causing tissue damage. Thus, in DH, there is now a plausible hypothesis involving cytokines and IgA in the pathogenesis of a DH skin lesion. IL-8 is the chemoattractant and GM-CSF induces the IgA–Fc receptors on the neutrophils, which bind to the IgA and become activated. This explanation involves IgA in the pathological process and accounts for the localization of microabscesses in the dermal papillae. What has still to be explained is the increased expression of IL-8 in basal keratinocytes. It is possible that IL-8 expression is induced by activated T lymphocytes in the skin. It has recently been shown that there is indeed a T-cell infiltrate in the dermis in lesional DH skin (Garioch et al, 1994b). These T cells are predominantly CD4+ and approximately one-third are activated; they are found in close apposition to activated antigen-presenting cells. These activated T cells may also be responsible for inducing the expression of adhesion molecules in the endothelial cells of the capillaries, which act as receptors for neutrophils and account for their migration into the skin. An increased expression of endothelial lymphocyte adhesion molecule (ELAM)-1 has been found in the dermis in lesional DH skin (Graeber et al, 1993). The trigger for the influx and activation of the T cells into the skin in patients with DH has still to be determined. The obvious candidate is gluten, but this has never been found in the skin. It is possible, however, that the T cells respond to another antigen (a self-antigen) that is cross-reactive with gluten (or glutenin). Cross-reactivity on the one hand between gliadins and reticulin and on the other between glutenin and elastin has been suggested. Thus, IgA gliadin–anti-gliadin or IgA glutenin–anti-glutenin complexes could bind to reticulin or elastin, respectively, in the skin, causing damage and release of self-antigens to which T cells respond. This hypothesis implicates gluten, IgA, T cells, neutrophils and cytokines, all of which have been found in the skin.

ASSOCIATION OF DH WITH COELIAC DISEASE

It was suggested in 1967 that the enteropathy in DH (Fry et al, 1967) was likely to be due to gluten as, in addition to the enteropathy, patients had a low serum IgM level, evidence of splenic atrophy, an agglutinating factor to *Lactobacillus casei*, and evidence of folate and iron deficiency, all of which are features of coeliac disease. It was subsequently shown that the enteropathy was indeed due to gluten. Thus, both patients with coeliac disease and DH have a gluten-sensitive enteropathy, but what distinguishes the two groups is that a rash occurs, in association with IgA deposition in the dermis, in DH. The questions to be asked are whether both DH and coeliac disease are basically the same disease; whether all patients have gluten sensitivity, which manifests itself with varying degrees of enteropathy; and whether all have the potential to develop the characteristic rash. Alternatively, are patients with DH and coeliac disease inherently different, with one group (those with coeliac disease) having no potential for the rash. Family, twin and HLA studies suggest that the basic genetic predisposing factor is the same.

Twin studies

Concordance for coeliac disease is well recognized in monozygotic twins and has been reported to approach 100% (Greenberg et al, 1982). DH has also been reported in four pairs of monozygotic twins (Marks et al, 1971; Jepson and Ullman, 1980; Anstey et al, 1991; Reunala and Koskimies, 1991). However, there are four pairs of monozygotic twins in whom one twin has DH and the other coeliac disease (Kosnai et al, 1985; Green et al, 1986; Reunala and Koskimies, 1991). These latter twin studies imply that patients with DH and those with coeliac disease share the same genetic predisposition.

Family studies

There are a number of family studies that also imply a common genetic make-up for DH and coeliac disease. In a study in Finland of 530 patients with DH, 29 (5.5%) had first-degree relatives with coeliac disease, and 24 (4.5%) with DH (Reunala and Koskimies, 1991). This figure for coeliac disease may indeed be higher, because the diagnosis was made only in those with symptoms or signs of the disease (and subsequent small intestinal biopsy). However, it is well known that relatives of patients with DH have a high incidence (40%) of asymptomatic villous atrophy (Marks et al, 1970; Reunala et al, 1976).

In another study in Northern Ireland (Love, 1981), the incidence of DH was 2.4% and coeliac disease 0.6%, in first-degree relatives of 446 patients with DH. The same author studied 435 patients with coeliac disease and found that the incidence of DH was 1% and that of coeliac disease was in the first degree relatives was 5.5%. As in the studies from Finland, the diagnosis of coeliac disease was made only in patients with symptoms and signs and not solely on the basis of intestinal biopsy in all the first-degree relatives.

Further family studies have been carried out in Finland on 'multiple case families' (Reunala and Koskimies, 1991). In all, 53 families were available for study. A single first-degree relative was affected with coeliac disease or DH in 43 families, two relatives in five other families, and three in the remaining families. The disease frequency (DH or coeliac disease) was 19% of parents, 22% of siblings and 24% of children. The overall frequency was 10% for DH and 13% for coeliac disease. Thus, DH and coeliac disease appear to segregate with similar frequency in relatives of patients with DH. Substantiating this finding were 28 sib-pairs, 14 with DH–DH, and 14 with DH–coeliac disease. A further interesting finding in the Finnish study (Reunala and Koskimies, 1991) was of two couples where both parents had DH, and they each had a child with coeliac disease. All these family studies support the twin studies that point to a common genetic factor for DH and coeliac disease.

HLA findings

The original studies showed a significant increase of HLA-B8 in both coeliac disease and DH, and subsequently the class II antigens, HLA-DR3 and HLA-DQW2. The incidence of DQW2 is the highest and has an incidence of approximately 95% in both disorders (Sachs et al, 1986). A more recent report has shown that the same DQB1 and DQA1 alleles that encode the DQW2 molecule in coeliac disease are also overrepresented in DH (Fronek et al, 1991). The same study also reported that both DH and coeliac disease were associated with the HLA-DP region allele DPB1*0301, and negatively associated with a constellation of DPB1 alleles, which include DPB1 *0202, *0901 or *1301. One of the few reported differences between DH and coeliac disease is that in coeliac disease there is an increase in the DPB1*0101 allele which is not present in DH (Kagnoff et al, 1989).

Thus, to date, the HLA associations in both DH and coeliac disease are virtually the same. It is likely that more than one gene is involved with the potential for the enteropathy and skin lesions. If there is a genetic difference between the two diseases, it may be due to an interplay of these gene abnormalities. It has also to be considered that the genes encoding for the HLA antigens are not responsible for gluten sensitivity, but simply represent an association. Alternatively, the HLA genes are just one of several genetic factors predisposing to gluten sensitivity.

The intestine in DH and coeliac disease

It has been said that the difference between coeliac disease and DH is that in DH the enteropathy is less severe. It has been argued that the milder enteropathy may signify a difference in the immunological response to gluten in the two groups of patients. This milder or altered response to gluten may be due to an immune reaction which also leads to deposition of IgA in the skin and subsequent development of skin lesions. However, this proposal may not be correct. It is quite possible that there are varying and similar degrees of enteropathy in both patients destined to develop DH and those who will have coeliac disease alone. In patients with DH there are indeed varying degrees of enteropathy, ranging from a flat (subtotal villous atrophy) to a convoluted (partial villous atrophy) mucosa, to predominantly leafy villi to normal finger-like villi (Fry et al, 1974). This range of variation in architecture is equally distributed, one-third of patients having a flat, one-third a convoluted and one-third an architecturally normal mucosa. However, even in the third with normal villous architecture, the majority of intestinal biopsies show an increase in the number of intraepithelial lymphoid cells, about three times that seen in normals. This degree of infiltration is the same in those with or without change in villous architecture (Fry et al, 1974). In the 5% of patients with DH with normal villous architecture and no increase in the intraepithelial lymphocyte count, sensitivity to gluten can be demonstrated by gluten challenge, where normal villous architecture transforms to a flat mucosa. Thus, all patients with DH have evidence of gluten sensitivity in the small intestine. The varying features of gluten sensitivity seen in the small intestine of patients with DH may also occur in patients with coeliac disease, i.e. those with gluten sensitivity but who are not destined to develop DH. The concept of latent coeliac disease has been known for some time, but because patients are symptomless they do not present to doctors. It has recently been estimated that only 30–40% of patients with gluten-sensitive enteropathy have typical features of coeliac disease, leaving 60–70% with so-called latent enteropathy (Auricchio et al, 1990). In addition 50% of the relatives of patients with coeliac disease (Marsh, 1989) and 40% of the relatives of patients with DH (Marks et al, 1970; Reunala et al, 1976) have asymptomatic flat small intestinal mucosae. If it is accepted that raised intraepithelial lymphocyte counts in patients with normal villous architecture represent mild gluten sensitivity, then the incidence of 'latent' coeliac disease is even higher. It could be argued that in patients with DH the complete range of changes in the intestine due to gluten sensitivity is seen because virtually all patients with DH eventually find their way to a hospital department, because of the rash. However, in patients with gluten sensitivity but no rash (those with coeliac disease), only those with severe enteropathy will attend a hospital. It could also be argued that in those patients destined to develop DH, severe enteropathy may occur. However, because of the severity of the entero- pathy, the patients present to gastroenterology clinics and are treated with a gluten-free diet, so that development of the rash in later life does not occur. There is some evidence to support this suggestion in that a small proportion of patients with DH do give a history of coeliac disease in childhood (Gawkrodger et al, 1993). However, in those who develop DH later, the diet has either not been strict enough or has been given up completely.

Further similarities in the intestine of patients with coeliac disease and DH are an increased incidence of $\gamma\delta$ T cells in the intestinal mucosa (Savilahti et al, 1992) and intestinal humoral immunity (O'Mahony et al, 1990). Thus, there may be no inherent difference in the immune response to gluten in the intestine of patients who develop no skin lesions (coeliac disease) and those who do (DH). The difference may well lie elsewhere. The other candidates usually mentioned are IgA and the skin. It has been suggested that in patients who develop DH there is an abnormality of the IgA compared with that in patients with coeliac disease. This altered IgA has the ability to bind to structures in the skin and subsequently give rise to skin lesions. The other candidate is an abnormality in the skin of patients with DH, which allows the binding of normal IgA. So far, it has not been possible to determine whether either of these possibilities exists.

However, even if there is a similar intestinal response to gluten in both diseases, this does not preclude a difference in the immune response at some stage of the disease. The immune system does change with age and it is possible that these changes influence the response to gluten. This may explain the later onset of DH compared with symptomatic coeliac disease. An analogy can be drawn with another skin disease, namely psoriasis, which is probably triggered by streptococcal infection. The chronic form of the disease, so called 'chronic plaque' disease, develops mainly in the third decade, like DH. Yet, in children, an acute form of the disease is seen (guttate psoriasis) that is different in appearance, but follows streptococcal infection. The development of the immune system may well allow for the different clinical presentations. Thus, although DH and coeliac disease are both due to gluten sensitivity and obviously share a common genetic background, a difference does exist, i.e. the rash. So far, a verifiable explanation for this difference has eluded investigators, but, like most biological secrets, it will eventually be explained.

SUMMARY

Dermatitis herpetiformis (DH) is a relatively rare skin disorder with an estimated incidence of 1 : 10 000 in the UK. It is characterized by urticarial plaques and blisters on the elbows, buttocks, and knees, although other sites may also be involved. The eruption tends to be persistent: only 10–15% of patients have spontaneous remission over a 25-year study period. The disease is characterized by the presence of IgA deposits in the upper dermis of uninvolved skin and the diagnosis should not be made in the absence of these deposits. Two-thirds of patients have a small intestinal enteropathy with villous atrophy as seen in coeliac disease (CD). However, the remaining third also show evidence of a gluten sensitivity in the intestine, as judged by increased lymphocytic infiltration of the epithelium. Villous atrophy also ensues after gluten challenge in those patients with previous normal villous architecture.

The initial treatment of the rash is with one of the following three drugs, dapsone, sulphapyridine or sulphamethoxypyridazine. However, the rash also clears with gluten withdrawal. It must be stressed, however, that the average time to achieve significant reduction in drug requirements is 6 months and it can be over 2 years before drugs are no longer required. On re-introduction of gluten the eruption recurs.

Patients with DH have a high incidence of auto-immune disorders, thyroid disease, pernicious anaemia, and insulin-dependent diabetes, and should be screened for those diseases on a yearly basis. As with coeliac disease there is also an increased incidence of lymphoma and a gluten-free diet appears to protect patients from this complication.

The mechanism by which gluten causes the skin lesions has still to be elucidated, but current investigations implicate lymphocytes and cytokines in the pathogenesis. The original hypothesis of an antigen-antibody reaction in the skin with complement activation causing the skin lesions, may not be correct.

REFERENCES

Alexander JO'D (1975) *Dermatitis Herpetiformis*. London: WB Saunders.
Anstey A, Wilkinson JD & Walshe MM (1991) Dermatitis herpetiformis in monozygotic twins. Concordance for dermatitis herpetiformis and gluten sensitive enteropathy. *Clinical and Experimental Dermatology* **16:** 51–52.
Auricchio S, Greco I & Troncone R (1990) What is the true prevalence of coeliac disease. *Gastroenterology International* **3:** 140–142.
Barghuthy FS, Kumar V, Valeski E et al (1988) Identification of IgA subclasses in skin of dermatitis herpetiformis patients. *International Archives of Allergy and Applied Immunology* **85:** 268–271.
Bodvarsson S, Jonsdottir I, Freysdottir J et al (1993) Dermatitis herpetiformis—an auto-immune disease due to cross-reaction between dietary glutenin and dermal elastin. *Scandinavian Journal of Immunology* **38:** 546–550.
Brow J, Parker F, Weinstein W & Rubin CE (1971) The small intestinal mucosa in dermatitis herpetiformis: severity and distribution of the small intestinal lesion and associated malabsorption. *Gastroenterology* **60:** 355–361.

Christensen OB, Hindsen M & Svensson A (1986) Natural history of dermatitis herpetiformis in southern Sweden. *Dermatologica* **173**: 271–277.

Civatte AC (1943) Diagnostic histopathologique de la dermatite polymorphe douloureuse on Maladie de Duhring–Brocq. *Annals of Dermatology and Syphililogy (Paris)* **3**: 1–30.

Costello M (1940) Dermatitis herpetiformis treated with sulphapyridine. *Archives of Dermatology and Syphilology* **41**: 134.

Dahlback K, Lofberg H & Dahlback B (1989) Vitronection colocalises with Ig deposits and C9 neoantigen in discoid lupus erythematosus and dermatitis herpetiformis, but not in bullous pemphigoid. *British Journal of Dermatology* **120**: 725–733.

Davies MG & Marks R (1978) Dermatitis herpetiformis: a skin manifestation of a generalised disturbance in immunity. *Quarterly Journal of Medicine* **186**: 221–248.

Ermacora E, Prampolini L, Tribbja G et al (1986) Long term follow up of dermatitis herpetiformis in children. *Journal of the American Academy of Dermatology* **15**: 24–30.

Esteves J & Brandao FN (1950) Au sujet de l'action des sulfamides et des sulphones dans la maladie de Duhring. *Trabalhos da Sociedada Portuguesa de Dermatologia e Venerologia* **8**: 209.

Frodin T, Gotthard R, Hed J et al (1981) Gluten free diet for dermatitis herpetiformis: longterm effect on cutaneous, immunological and jejunal manifestations. *Acta Dermato-Venerologica* **61**: 405–411.

Fronek Z, Cheung MM, Hanbury AM & Kagnoff ME (1991) Molecular analysis of HLA-DP and HLA-DQ genes associated with dermatitis herpetiformis. *Journal of Investigative Dermatology* **97**: 799–802.

Fry L & Seah PP (1974) Dermatitis herpetiformis: an evaluation of diagnostic criteria. *British Journal of Dermatology* **90**: 137–146.

Fry L, Keir P, McMinn RMH et al (1967) Small intestinal structure and function, and haematological changes in dermatitis herpetiformis. *Lancet* **ii**: 729–734.

Fry L, McMinn RMH, Cowan JD & Hoffbrand AV (1968) Effect of gluten-free diet on dermatological, intestinal and haematological manifestations of dermatitis herpetiformis. *Lancet* **i**: 557–561.

Fry L, McMinn RMH, Cowan JD & Hoffbrand AV (1969) Gluten-free diet and re-introduction of gluten in dermatitis herpetiformis. *Archives of Dermatology* **100**: 129–135.

Fry L, Seah PP, Riches DJ & Hoffbrand AV (1973) Clearance of skin lesions in dermatitis herpetiformis after gluten withdrawal. *Lancet* **i**: 288–291.

Fry L, Seah PP, Harper PG et al (1974) The small intestine in dermatitis herpetiformis. *Journal of Clinical Pathology* **27**: 817–824.

Fry L, Leonard JN, Swain AF et al (1982) Long term follow up of dermatitis herpetiformis with and without dietary gluten withdrawal. *British Journal of Dermatology* **107**: 631–640.

Garioch JJ, Lewis HM, Sargent SA et al (1994a) 25 years experience of a gluten free diet in the treatment of dermatitis herpetiformis. *British Journal of Dermatology* **131**: 541–545.

Garioch JJ, Baker BS, Leonard JN & Fry L (1994b) T lymphocytes in lesional skin of patients with dermatitis herpetiformis. *British Journal of Dermatology* (in press).

Gawkrodger DJ, Blackwell JN, Gilmore HM et al (1984) Dermatitis herpetiformis: diagnosis, diet and demography. *Gut* **25**: 151–157.

Gawkrodger DJ, Vestey JP, O'Mahoney S & Marks JM (1993) Dermatitis herpetiformis and established coeliac disease. *British Journal of Dermatology* **129**: 694–695.

Gillberg R, Kastrup W, Mobacken H et al (1985) Gastric morphology and function in dermatitis herpetiformis and in coeliac disease. *Scandinavian Journal of Gastroenterology* **20**: 133–140.

Graeber M, Baker BS & Garioch JJ (1993) The role of cytokines in the generation of skin lesions in dermatitis herpetiformis. *British Journal of Dermatology* **129**: 530–532.

Green ST, Natarjan S, Connor JM et al (1986) Monozygotic twins concordant for duodeno-jejunal villous atrophy and dermatitis herpetiformis. *Gut* **29**: 970–971.

Greenberg TA, Hodge SE & Rother JI (1982) Evidence for recessive and against dominant inheritance at the HLA 'linked' locus in coeliac disease. *American Journal of Human Genetics* **34**: 263–277.

Hall RP & McKenzie KD (1992) Comparison of the intestinal and serum antibody response in patients with dermatitis herpetiformis. *Clinical Immunology and Immunopathology* **62**: 33–41.

Holmes GKT, Prior P, Lane MR et al (1989) Malignancy in coeliac disease—effect of a gluten-free diet. *Gut* **30**: 33–38.

Jepson LV & Ullman S (1980) Dermatitis herpetiformis and gluten sensitive enteropathy in monozygotic twins. *Acta Dermato-Venerologica* **60**: 353–355.

Kagnoff ME, Harwood JI, Bugawan T et al (1989) Structural analysis of the HLA-DR, -DQ, and -DP alleles on the associated HLA-DR3 (DRw 17) haplotype. *Proceedings of the National Academy of Sciences of the USA* **86**: 6274–6278.

Kosnai I, Karpati S, Torok E et al (1985) Dermatitis herpetiformis in monozygotic twins: discordance for dermatitis herpetiformis and concordance for gluten sensitive enteropathy. *European Journal of Pediatrics* **144**: 404–405.

Leonard JN, Haffenden GP, Tucker W et al (1983) Gluten challenge in dermatitis herpetiformis. *New England Journal of Medicine* **308**: 816–819.

Lightner VA, Sakai LY & Hall RP (1991) IgA binding structures in dermatitis herpetiformis are independent of elastic microfibrillar bundles. *Journal of Investigative Dermatology* **96**: 88–92.

Ljunghall K & Tjernlund U (1983) Dermatitis herpetiformis: effect of gluten restricted and gluten free diet on dapsone requirements and on IgA and C3 deposits in uninvolved skin. *Acta Dermato-Venereologica* **63**: 129–136.

Love AHG (1981) Epidemiological and genetic aspects of the coeliac syndrome in relation to dermatitis herpetiformis. In McConnell RB (ed.) *The Genetics of Coeliac Disease*, pp 95–99. Lancaster: MTP Press.

McFadden JP, Leonard JN, Powles AV & Fry L (1991) Autoimmunity in dermatitis herpetiformis: effect of a gluten free diet. *Journal of Dermatological Treatment* **2**: 87–90.

Marks J, Birkett D & Shuster S (1970) Small intestinal mucosal abnormalities in relatives of patients with dermatitis herpetiformis. *Gut* **11**: 493–497.

Marks J, May SB & Roberts DF (1971) Dermatitis herpetiformis occurring in monozygotic twins. *British Journal of Dermatology* **84**: 417–419.

Marsh MN (1989) Lymphocyte-mediated intestinal damage—human studies. In Peters TJ (ed.) *The Cell Biology of Inflammation in the Gastrointestinal Tract*, pp 203–229. Hull: Corners Publications.

Mobracken H, Kastrup W & Nilsson LA (1984) Incidence and prevalence of dermatitis herpetiformis in western Sweden. *Acta Dermato-Venereologica* **64**: 400–404.

Moi H (1984) Incidence and prevalence of dermatitis herpetiformis in a county in central Sweden, with comments on the course of the disease and IgA deposits as diagnostic criterion. *Acta Dermato-Venereologica* **64**: 144–150.

Mylotte M, Egan-Mitchell B, McCarthy CF & McNicholl B (1973) Incidence of coeliac disease in the west of Ireland. *British Medical Journal* **1**: 703–705.

O'Mahony S, Vestey VP & Ferguson A (1990) Similarities in intestinal humoral immunity in dermatitis herpetiformis without enteropathy and in coeliac disease. *Lancet* **335**: 1487–1490.

Reunala T & Koskimies S (1991) Familial dermatitis herpetiformis. *Clinics in Dermatology* **9**: 335–340.

Reunala T & Lokki J (1978) Dermatitis herpetiformis in Finland. *Acta Dermato-Venereologica* **58**: 505–510.

Reunala T, Salo OP, Tiilikainen et al (1976) Family studies in dermatitis herpetiformis. *Annals of Clinical Research* **8**: 254–261.

Sachs JA, Awad J, McCloskey D et al (1986) Different HLA associated gene combinations contribute to susceptibility for coeliac disease and dermatitis herpetiformis. *Gut* **27**: 515–520.

Savilahti E, Reunala T & Maki M (1992) Increase of lymphocytes bearing the γδ T cell receptor in the jejunum of patients with dermatitis herpetiformis. *Gut* **33**: 206–211.

Seah PP & Fry L (1975) Immunoglobulins in the skin in dermatitis herpetiformis and their relevance in diagnosis. *British Journal of Dermatology* **92**: 157–166.

Seah PP, Fry L, Stewart JS et al (1972) Immunoglobulins in the skin in dermatitis herpetiformis and coeliac disease. *Lancet* **i**: 611–614.

Seah PP, Fry L, Holborow EJ et al (1973) Antireticulin antibody: incidence and diagnostic significance. *Gut* **14**: 311–315.

Sigurgiersson B, Agnarsson B & Lindelof B (1994) Risk of lymphoma in patients with dermatitis herpetiformis. *British Medical Journal* **308**: 13–15.

Stingl G, Honigsman H, Holubar K & Wolff K (1976) Ultrastructural localisation of immuno-globulins in skin of patients with dermatitis herpetiformis. *Journal of Investigations in Dermatology* **67**: 507–512.

Sulej J & Leonard JN (1987) Anti-endomysial antibodies in dermatitis herpetiformis and coeliac disease. In Chorzelski TP & Kumar VJ (eds) *Immunopathology of the Skin*, pp 477–482. New York: Wiley.

Unsworth DJ, Leonard JN, McMinn RMH et al (1981a) Anti-gliadin antibodies and small intestinal mucosal damage in dermatitis herpetiformis. *British Journal of Dermatology* **105**: 653–658.

Unsworth DJ, Johnson GD, Haffenden GP et al (1981b) Binding of wheat gliadin in vitro to reticulin in normal and dermatitis herpetiformis skin. *Journal of Investigative Dermatology* **76**: 88–93.

Unsworth DJ, Payne AW, Leonard JN et al (1982) IgA in dermatitis herpetiformis skin is dimeric. *Lancet* **i**: 478–480.

Weetman AP, Burrin JM, Mackay D et al (1988) The prevalence of thyroid auto-antibodies in dermatitis herpetiformis. *British Journal of Dermatology* **118**: 377–383.

Weinstein WM (1973) Latent coeliac sprue. *Gastroenterology* **64**: 489–493.

Wojnarowska F & Fry L (1981) Hepatic injury in dermatitis herpetiformis. *Acta Dermato-Venereologica* **61**: 165–168.

10

Coeliac disease research and clinical practice: maintaining momentum into the twenty-first century

ANNE FERGUSON

The First International Conference on Coeliac Disease, organized by Chris Booth, was held a quarter of a century ago. Many of the participants were young clinicians and clinical scientists, beginning careers in a range of relatively new subject areas—epidemiology, genetics, cellular immunology, cereal chemistry. Their subsequent work has profoundly altered our concepts of the aetiology, pathogenesis and complications (but not yet treatment) of gluten sensitivity. Even the definition of coeliac disease is being challenged, in the light of new knowledge of small bowel physiology and of mechanisms of diarrhoea, and as two dimensional histopathology gives way to analyses based on an awareness of the complex cell and tissue kinetics in the separate compartments of the gut mucosa. As we approach the twenty-first century, yet new questions and areas of controversy are arising. Fortunately, both the people and the new techniques will be in place to resolve some of these important outstanding issues in the next few years.

EVOLUTION OF A WORKING CLINICAL DEFINITION OF COELIAC DISEASE

Until the 1950s, the diagnosis of coeliac was made when a child or adult had malabsorption in the absence of infection. During the 1950s it was recognized that treatment with a gluten-free diet produced not only clinical remission but also a reduction in faecal fat excretion. When techniques for peroral small bowel biopsy were introduced during the 1960s, patients with chronic malabsorption syndrome were found to have either an entirely normal or a grossly abnormal jejunal biopsy.

Descriptive terms such as 'flat mucosa', or 'subtotal villous atrophy' became the pathologist's shorthand for a cluster of features (villous and crypt size, epithelial cell damage, intraepithelial and lamina propria lymphoid cell infiltrates), which together characterize the enteropathy of coeliac disease.

At the First International Conference on Coeliac Disease in 1969, Booth

Baillière's Clinical Gastroenterology
Vol. 9, No. 2, June 1995
ISBN 0–7020–1953–4

and Dowling brought together the consensus view of participants (Booth and Dowling, 1970) in a definition of coeliac disease that encompassed *malabsorption with an abnormal small bowel biopsy; both symptoms and biopsy pathology respond to a gluten-free diet.*

At about the same time, European paediatricians were recognizing that abnormal small bowel morphology with villous atrophy occurred fairly frequently in infants with many different infectious, allergic, and other transient or chronic diarrhoeal diseases. Thus, the European Society of Paediatric Gastroenterology proposed strict criteria for coeliac disease (Meuwisse, 1970), namely *malabsorption syndrome with a flat jejunal biopsy which recovers to normal on a gluten-free diet and relapsed on subsequent gluten reintroduction (gluten challenge).* Many thousands of children were submitted to this stringent diagnostic protocol, which could require dietary manipulation over several years and three or more jejunal biopsies. It is now becoming clear that when the original biopsy of such children shows severe enteropathy, gluten challenge produces positive results in 95–99% of them. Accordingly, the criteria have been revised (Walker-Smith et al, 1990) and gluten challenge is no longer considered mandatory.

'Malabsorption' is mentioned in these definitions, in addition to the requirement for abnormal biopsy pathology. However, since there are no specific clinical features identified, and in view of the enormous clinical heterogeneity observed in untreated patients, it has become generally accepted that the criteria for definition and diagnosis should be based on small bowel pathology. In other words, as of 1994, coeliac disease is defined as *a permanent gluten-sensitive enteropathy*, and this has proved useful, practical and acceptable to paediatricians, physicians, pathologists and epidemiologists.

There still is no accurate, non-invasive alternative to small bowel biopsy, although by using a combination of two different candidate screening tests (such as gut permeability and serum immunoglobulin (IgA) anti-gliadin antibody (AGA), or serum AGA and anti-endomysial antibody), it may be possible to identify patients with a very low probability of having significant enteropathy. The best studied immunological tests are serum IgG and IgA class antibodies to gliadin (AGA) (Troncone and Ferguson, 1991a). IgG AGA is usually positive in coeliac disease but often in other gastrointestinal diseases and even in a proportion of normal individuals; the presence of serum IgA AGA is more likely to indicate coeliac disease. This test is positive in the majority of untreated coeliac children but in only 70% of untreated coeliac adults. It also has to be borne in mind that approximately 1 in 50 coeliac patients is IgA deficient. The presence of anti-reticulin antibody in coeliac disease has been recognized for many years; the technical variant of this, based on the use of monkey oesophageal tissue as substrate in an immunofluorescence test, has revealed that IgA endomysial antibody is present in a much higher proportion of untreated coeliac patients than is IgA AGA (Catassi et al, 1994). Anti-endomysial antibody tests are not widely available and the commercially available materials are extremely expensive.

However, despite these criticisms of its use in the diagnostic process for coeliac disease, measurement of AGA has an important role in population screening studies. Furthermore, tests for serum AGA of the IgA class, and various permeability tests, are excellent non-invasive measures to monitor the clinical response of a patient to a gluten-free diet.

When seeking an alternative to small bowel biopsy for the diagnosis of coeliac disease it has to be borne in mind that patients with malabsorption or nutrient abnormalities may have small bowel pathology resulting from diseases other than coeliac disease, including other transient food-sensitive enteropathies, giardiasis, human immunodeficiency virus (HIV) entero- pathy and disaccharidase deficiency. Examination of appropriate biopsy material is essential for diagnosis of these conditions.

Clinical sub-divisions of coeliac disease

The terms silent and active coeliac disease are used by many European physicians and paediatricians but less commonly by British clinicians. *Active coeliac disease* is manifested by unequivocal nutritional deficiencies and/or gastrointestinal symptoms of abdominal distension and diarrhoea; a full- blown malabsorption syndrome is relatively rarely seen nowadays. Clinically *silent coeliac disease* is now being increasingly recognized, for example in asymptomatic people in whom jejunal biopsy has been per- formed as part of a family study or in the screening of blood donors. Strangely, there has been very little research on the factors that differentiate those with symptomatic disease from those with silent disease, who in some way compensate by the function of the distal gut, for the malabsorption and net water secretion proximally. Our careful study of patients with dermatitis herpetiformis showed that heterogeneity of clinical features (and, indeed, severity of enteropathy) could not be explained by the amount of gluten in the diet (Gawkrodger et al, 1991).

Unfortunately, recent research is showing that each word in the definition *permanent gluten-sensitive enteropathy* must now be reviewed, revised or reinterpreted. In this chapter, which concerns future prospects for coeliac disease research, it is useful to structure my suggestions around these four separate topics: enteropathy? permanent? gluten? sensitivity?

ENTEROPATHY?: GLUTEN SENSITIVITY MAY BE EXPRESSED IN A MILD FORM

Careful description and analysis of the architecture of the small bowel mucosa, epithelium of the surface and crypts, and of lymphoid cells in the various microenvironments are much more valuable than a mere verbal summary of the presence or absence of 'enteropathy'. This is becoming increasingly important with changes in clinical practice, biopsy techniques and case mix. Indeed, clinicians who submit endoscopic duodenal biopsies for pathological assessment should use large biopsy forceps, take specimens only from the distal second or, if possible, third part of the duodenum, and emphasize to the pathologist that the site of biopsy is visually un-inflamed. Otherwise, there will be considerable confusion between peptic duodenitis and coeliac disease, particularly when there are a few neutrophils in the lamina propria infiltrate of a coeliac patient.

Mucosal architecture

Original descriptions of the jejunal pathology in coeliac disease concentrated on 'villous atrophy', which could be assessed quickly and inexpensively with a hand lens or dissecting microscope. In the 1970s there were several lines of investigation that directed attention to crypt hyperplasia (not merely an increase in crypt size but also increased proliferative activity). Painstaking and tedious cell-counting methods allowed Wright and colleagues (1973) to construct models of crypts and crypt epithelial cell proliferation kinetics. In the flat mucosa of coeliac disease the crypt mitotic index was double that for crypts of normal mucosa, and the crypt cell production rate was sixfold higher in the coeliac lesion.

We pursued a different approach, based on microdissection of individual crypts and villi (Ferguson et al, 1977), and showed hyperplasia of the crypts with increased numbers of mitotic figures in flat biopsies from coeliac patients.

During the same period, work with animals was showing that a whole range of abnormalities of small intestinal villous and crypt architecture can occur, with virtually any combination of long or short villi, hyperplastic, normal, long, short or hypoplastic crypts, and changes in the number of crypts supplying cells to each villus (Ferguson, 1987). Of particular interest was our demonstration in several model systems that there was a gradient of evolution of T cell-mediated damage to the small bowel mucosa. Crypt hyperplasia, with villi of normal length, preceded the appearance of an enteropathy similar to that of coeliac disease (crypt hyperplasia and villous atrophy); in extreme damage there was a hypoplastic mucosa with short villi and crypts, before final tissue ulceration and destruction (MacDonald and Ferguson, 1976).

Crypt hypoplastic lesions with short or absent villi are also found when crypt cells have been damaged by irradiation, drugs or enteropathic viruses, and in profound malnutrition. The enteropathy of HIV infection is also relatively hypoplastic (Editorial, 1989). The mechanisms of the crypt hypoplastic villous atrophy, occasionally seen in very severe coeliac disease, have not been established and may be via nutrient deficiency or cytotoxic cytokines.

Lymphoid cells

Within the normal small intestinal mucosa there are a number of different compartments, presenting a variety of microenvironments for lymphoid cell migration and interaction with other cells of the lymphoid series, enterocytes and other cell species.

In the flat coeliac lesion, there is little or no villous lamina propria, and the cell densities and cell types within the greatly expanded volume of the lamina propria differ considerably from those of normal mucosa. Immunologists generally agree that the immune signals that are central to the pathogenesis of the T cell-mediated lesion in coeliac disease are likely to arise from T cells within the lamina propria, and studies using immunohistochemical techniques confirm this.

Direct evidence of immune activation of T cells is provided by two key findings. There is expression of CD25 antigen (which identifies the α-chain of the interleukin (IL) 2 receptor) by lamina propria CD4⁺ T cells in coeliac mucosa, and this is linked to gluten exposure (Halstensen and Brandtzaeg, 1993). Human crypt epithelium does not normally express HLA-DR antigens, and the crypt cell HLA-DR expression in coeliac disease, which is gluten dependent (Fais et al,1992), is further evidence that there is activation of T effector cells in the mucosa.

The cells within the microenvironment of the surface or villous epithelium, intraepithelial lymphocytes (IELs), have been studied extensively. Simple counting methods and computer-aided morphometry confirm the subjective observation that in untreated coeliac disease there is a considerably increased density of IEL infiltration within the microenvironment of the surface epithelium. IEL counts drop after treatment with a gluten-free diet; on reintroduction of gluten, as acute challenge or as dietary changes monitored days or weeks later, a rise in IEL count in the surface epithelium is the first and most sensitive index of the effects of gluten on the mucosa.

Spectrum of effects of gluten on the coeliac mucosa

When quantitative histology and computerized image analysis are applied in gluten challenge and gluten withdrawal protocols, and in certain groups of gluten-sensitive individuals, such as those with dermatitis herpetiformis, it becomes clear that features such as villous or crypt architectural changes, lamina propria cell counts and IEL counts form a continuum, with the classical flat lesion at one end of the spectrum and a mucosa with normal villous and crypt architecture at the other end, with the only measurable abnormality being a high density or count of villous IELs (Marsh, 1992). The latter might well be reported as normal by general clinical pathologists, unless formal IEL counts are routinely performed. Other sophisticated studies of intestinal function and immunity show that other features may correlate with a high IEL count, for example increased permeability to large inert probe sugars (Strobel et al, 1984).

In studies of intestinal antibody production, we found that there was overexpression of IgM and IgM antibody responses in patients with mild enteropathy (including the isolated abnormality of a high IEL count), not only in treated coeliac patients but in some with other diagnoses (Arranz and Ferguson, 1993). Overexpression of IgM also occurs in patients with morphometrically absolutely normal biopsies, for example in dermatitis herpetiformis (O'Mahony et al, 1990b), but it must be emphasized that we do not yet know how often this is an even more subtle expression of the mild end of the continuum of pathological expression of gluten sensitivity than is a high IEL count. Since overexpression of IgM also occurs in Crohn's disease (O'Mahoney et al, 1990a), it is certainly not in any way diagnostic of gluten sensitivity. However, mucosal IgM antibodies may be used, with other subtle immune indices, to identify patients who merit careful investigation and perhaps a trial of therapy with a gluten-free diet if their symptoms are severe, as discussed below.

Coeliac disease enteropathy cannot be attributed entirely to T-cell activation. What is the other factor? Perhaps complement?

Most, but not all, of the features of the coeliac lesion can be reproduced in model systems of T-cell activation, such as graft-versus-host reaction in the mouse: crypt hyperplasia, shortening of villi, high density of IEL infiltrate in the villous epithelium, IEL mitosis, HLA class II expression by crypt cells. Different cell activation and cytokine signals may underly these components: interferon γ and IL-2 may influence crypt cells, tumour necrosis factor TNF may be associated with villous flattening, and cytotoxic cells or other cytokines may be involved in the rare, severe, hypoplastic lesion.

However, the striking damage to surface enterocytes that occurs in coeliac disease is not a feature in models of delayed-type hypersensitivity, and cannot merely be attributed to direct gluten toxicity. The cells at the surface of a 'flat' biopsy taken after an overnight fast will have moved out of the crypts on to the surface during the preceding 8–12 hours and therefore have not been exposed to gluten. I am convinced by the evidence for a role of complement in the coeliac lesion (Halstensen et al, 1992) and suggest that IgM–IgG immune complex or complement-mediated damage probably coexists with delayed-type hypersensitivity in untreated patients, and is the major factor responsible for the changes in basal lamina, reduced enterocyte height and derangement of the enterocyte brush border.

Significance of the isolated finding of a high count of IELs

In animal work on delayed-type hypersensitivity in rodent intestine, a rise in the count of villous IELs was a sensitive and early feature of the expression of mucosal T-cell activation (Mowat and Ferguson, 1982) and has been shown to be induced by signals from activated lamina propria CD4+ T cells. By analogy, in clinical practice a high count of IELs in an architecturally small bowel biopsy might also imply a state of T-cell activation, either antigen driven (e.g. by gluten, giardia, histocompatibility antigens) or as a result of aberrant mucosal immunoregulation (as in some theories of the pathogenesis of inflammatory bowel disease). We have recent evidence to support this general point. In a series of non-coeliac biopsies, a high IEL count was found to be associated with crypt cell HLA-DR expression and, in a few cases, also with CD25 expression by lamina propria T cells (Arranz, 1994).

There is plenty of evidence from animal work that IELs are a heterogeneous population, and since it is only a subset (those IELs that utilize the αβ T-cell receptor (TCR)) that rises and falls in number in association with gluten exposure, it still is possible that there are several different signals and stimuli that can produce a high total IEL count, involving different contributing subsets and a variety of mechanisms. Further work on the characteristics of these intriguing cells should lead to new ways of interpreting the isolated finding of a high IEL count in clinical practice.

Gluten-sensitive enteropathy may be manifested only by IEL count

There is now a substantial body of evidence that there are patients who have a high count of IELs in an otherwise normal jejunal biopsy while taking a normal diet, and that their IEL count falls with gluten exclusion and rises on its re-introduction. Some have no gastrointestinal symptoms, for example patients with dermatitis herpetiformis. But there are others who have gluten-sensitive diarrhoea as well as gluten-related IEL counts (Arranz and Ferguson, 1993). It is difficult to escape the conclusion that in these individuals the expression of gluten sensitivity as an enteropathy is minimal, and detected only if a count of IEL is performed. We have suggested that an accepted name for this type of pathology is needed (Ferguson et al, 1993). A candidate term is 'high density IEL enteropathy', and it would be helpful if clinical pathologists could either agree with this or devise a similar, suitable, word or phrase.

In patients with this type of biopsy pathology, it is useful to obtain details of the dietary gluten intake. If this is fairly low, for example because there is another coeliac in the family already on a gluten-free diet, then it may be worth carrying out formal gluten loading with 20 g extra gluten daily for a few weeks, and repeating investigations at the end of this period. There are very few reports of such patients in the literature, and the collecting together of data on individual cases might be the basis of a national or even international collaborative venture, analogous to the highly successful UK collaborative study of malignancy in coeliac disease.

PERMANENT?: BUT THERE ARE NOW WELL-DOCUMENTED CASES OF ACQUIRED DISEASE, AND PERHAPS ALSO PARTIAL RECOVERY OF GLUTEN TOLERANCE

The original simplistic view of gluten sensitivity was that, because of some biochemical defect, the surface of the small bowel, perhaps even the luminal surface of the brush border membrane, was directly damaged by contact with gluten. The main point of controversy was whether the problem in patients with coeliac disease was innate susceptibility of the enterocytes to damage by a particular type of protein, or whether they could not fully digest certain peptide sequences, so that they produced 'toxic' fragments in high concentration. Characterization of the toxic moieties of gliadins has been a holy grail for coeliac researchers for 30 years.

The theories of direct toxicity have been untenable for some time. One key piece of evidence is the delay between gluten re-introduction in a gluten challenge and the development of changes in the gut mucosa; these occur within 3–6 months in most cases, but the change from absolutely normal to flat may occur at any time up to several years. This is the case even when the challenge involves a full dietary load of gluten, 10–20 g daily. Evidence that a degree of clinical and also pathological tolerance to gluten may be acquired in the teenage years has accrued from long-term follow-up of French coeliac children, treated for several years with a gluten-free diet, but later allowed to eat normal food as long as they remained clinically well (Schmitz, 1992). Finally, some studies have shown that gluten and its derivatives do not damage organ cultured biopsies of coeliac patients if they have been taken from a healed mucosa, after gluten-free diet treatment, although other researchers would claim otherwise (Howdle et al, 1981).

Nevertheless, I suspect that, until recently, most of us envisaged that the small bowel mucosa became damaged very shortly after gluten was introduced into a susceptible infants diet, even though clinically evident malabsorption might not develop for months, years or decades. Even when it became evident that the host response to gluten (in the form of tissue-damaging immune reactions) was probably the key to pathogenesis, it still seemed likely that the state of abnormal immunity and associated enteropathy was generated in infancy.

Definition and criteria of latent coeliac disease

The suggestion that there might be a 'pre-coeliac' state was first made by Weinstein (1974), who described two patients with dermatitis herpetiformis and normal jejunal biopsies in whom typical coeliac-like enteropathy developed some weeks after 20 g gluten was added to their already gluten-containing diet. Studies from the UK have confirmed this observation, and the concept is supported by case reports of coeliac patients in whom, by chance, a jejunal biopsy had previously been taken and reported as normal. The term *latent coeliac disease* has been used for 20 years to describe the state of these patients. It is regrettable that the word 'latent' is also used by some for those patients who have unequivocal coeliac disease by the present definition (i.e. a severe enteropathy that is gluten sensitive) but who are not symptomatic. I strongly recommend that this term should be applied only to patients who fulfil the following conditions: (1) have a normal jejunal biopsy while taking a normal diet; and (2) at some other time, before or since, have had a flat jejunal biopsy (or unequivocally severe partial villous atrophy with crypt hyperplasia), which recovers on a gluten-free diet.

Clearly, the patient has latent coeliac disease only at the time that the biopsy is normal, when on a normal diet. There will be relatively few patients who fall into this category because it will usually be only by chance that biopsy (1) has been taken, for example in a research study or if the patient has a disease known to be associated with coeliac disease. Note that this definition is based on the subjective description of the biopsy, and relies on assessment of villous and crypt architecture and lamina propria cellularity. Data on IEL counts are available for only a few of the recorded cases, although some inferences can be made from published photomicrographs of biopsies. It is clear that, in some patients, there is already a high IEL count in biopsy (1), and so they would fit within the evolving concept that there is a spectrum of expression of gluten-sensitive enteropathy. Careful study of these patients might give clues as to what causes a lesion to progress from mild to severe.

Triggering factors for expression of severe enteropathy in a predisposed individual

Work in animals has shown that there may be absolutely no expression of mucosal T-cell immunity in highly sensitized animals. Also, as discussed in detail above, expression of T cell-mediated immunity within the intestinal mucosa occurs across a spectrum of histological and functional abnormalities from minimal to the flat mucosa with crypt hyperplasia. Whether or not these differences can be explained by migration patterns of T cells or by mucosal distribution of different T-cell subsets is still unknown.

Our studies in mice showed that active immunization with gliadin does not trigger the development of a T cell-mediated lesion of the intestine when the diet contains gluten. Additional factors, such as those occurring during intestinal anaphylaxis or a graft-versus-host reaction, were necessary. We suggested that enhanced antigen presentation, recruitment of specific T cells in the mucosa, upregulation of the expression of class II antigens and failure of suppression are all candidate mechanisms for the effects observed (Troncone and Ferguson, 1991b).

By analogy, although mucosal immunological sensitization is an invariable feature of coeliac disease, it is not the precipitating factor for the expression of the full intestinal lesion; there must be another stimulus or co-factor that induces expression of immunity or drives the enteropathy from minimal to overt. Candidate co-factors include an episode of hyperpermeability, nutrient deficiency, increased dietary gluten, impaired intraluminal digestion of ingested gluten, adjuvant effects of intestinal infection and influences of a non-HLA-associated gene.

Despite much research effort, no one has yet found a way to measure antigen-specific T-cell sensitization in the gut mucosa, although cytokine production by antigen-challenged biopsies in organ cultures holds potential. Thus, clinical tests in vivo in patients have to remain the gold standard for testing this theory.

Clinical terminology to be applied to patients with coeliac disease of suspected latent or low-grade pathology

With the exception of dermatitis herpetiformis, it is usually only by chance (e.g. jejunal biopsy performed in a research study) that patients with latent coeliac disease are detected. Now that its existence is accepted, some term is needed to describe patients with a 'normal' biopsy but other features leading to a suspicion of gluten sensitivity. They will need further clinical investigation by a combination of acute gluten challenge (jejunal or rectal), dietary gluten loading and gluten-free diet treatment, all of these monitored closely and objectively.

In the course of our recent research on patients at the mild end of the pathological spectrum of coeliac disease, we found that we were carelessly using the term 'latent coeliacs' in our day-to-day discussion of their clinical progress and research results. In fact, we should have classified them as 'might be latent coeliac disease; we will know in 3–6 months' time after a period of gluten-free diet and/or gluten challenge or gluten loading has been monitored by biopsy'. In other words, they were potentially latent coeliacs, which is a clumsy phrase for an apparently valid concept. We have therefore suggested the term *potential coeliac disease* for patients who need to undergo appropriate dietary manipulation and serial biopsy (Ferguson et al, 1992). A few months later they can confidently be classified as either gluten sensitive or not. If they are not, other avenues of investigation and treatment must be pursued.

Subtle pathological and immunological abnormalities: candidate markers for coeliac disease of latent or low-grade pathology

Coeliac patients whose intestinal lesions have resolved on a gluten-free diet and whose jejunal biopsies are classified as 'normal' for diagnostic purposes may still express subtle pathological or immunological abnormalities similar to those of untreated coeliacs. These abnormalities include a high count of villous IELs, increased $\gamma\delta$ TCR expression by IELs, abnormal jejunal permeability, and high levels of IgM AGA, other IgM class antibodies and IgA AGA (the 'coeliac-like intestinal antibody' (CIA) pattern) (Arranz and Ferguson, 1993) in specimens of jejunal fluid and whole-gut lavage fluid.

Recent studies have revealed that some of the same phenomena may identify cases of latent coeliac disease. High counts of TCR $\gamma\delta$ IELs have been shown in dermatitis herpetiformis (Savilahti et al, 1992) and in latent coeliac disease (Holm et al, 1992); the CIA pattern occurs in patients with dermatitis herpetiformis and normal biopsy on histological examination (O'Mahony et al, 1990b), the total count of IELs may be high as a subtle manifestation of enteropathy (Ferguson and Murray, 1971); anti-reticulin and anti-endomysium antibodies are present in some healthy relatives of coeliac patients (Mäki et al, 1990); and these individuals may also show immunohistochemical evidence of T-cell activation (Holm et al, 1994).

We recently reported that 19% of 217 non-coeliac patients referred for jejunal biopsy had a positive CIA pattern, and that a proportion of these (six of the nine patients who had a trial of a gluten-free diet) were clinically gluten sensitive, particularly when the total IEL count was high (Arranz and Ferguson, 1993). We then proceeded with a comprehensive evaluation of 77 patients referred for jejunal biopsy, in whom biopsy histology was normal (Arranz et al, 1994), to establish the association (or lack of association) between the CIA pattern and high $\gamma\delta$ IEL counts, high total IEL counts, serum IgA AGA and intestinal permeability to the probe sugars lactulose and rhamnose. Twelve patients had high serum AGA level and nine increased permeability. The count of $\gamma\delta$ IELs was high (>5.5 per mm villous epithelium) in nine patients, intestinal antibody pattern was positive in 21, and total IEL count high (>40 per 100 enterocytes) in 13. Overall, there were 31 patients with positive indices, but in 19 only a single test was abnormal. High $\gamma\delta$ IEL counts were found in 6 of the 21 intestinal antibody-positive patients, but only in 2 of 56 who were intestinal antibody negative ($P<0.001$); there were no other significant associations.

Thus, we find that in 40% of patients referred for jejunal biopsy, one or more of the immunological indices of potential coeliac disease is present. If clinical tests establish that even a proportion of these are actually gluten sensitive, there are major implications for gastroenterologists, and the use of tests of subtle immune aberrations will need to be much more widespread than at present.

Such tests present logistic problems. TCR studies by immunohisto-chemistry must be performed on frozen sections. Collection of jejunal fluid and antibody tests on secretions require specialist expertise. We have examined the possible role of anti-endomysial antibody for identification of these patients, in collaboration with Dr Mäki, but the results are disappoint-ing. Anti-endomysial antibody was present in the serum of less than 5% of patients positive for other markers (Arranz, 1994).

THE PROVOKING AGENT, GLUTEN?: HOW CLOSE IS THE IDENTIFICATION OF THE PRECISE TOXIC SEQUENCE? AND HOW WILL THIS LINK IN WITH THE NEW GENETICS?

Proteins and peptides for study

The fact that certain cereal proteins are toxic to coeliac patients has been recognized for 40 years. For most of that time, laboratory and clinical investigators have had to face major logistic problems with the preparation and handling of these large complex molecules, which are insoluble in biological fluids. There is an enormous literature on competing methods for purification, separation, digestion and, of course, on describing the various derivatives of wheat gluten and gliadin. When these preparations have been used for immunological research, the results have often been difficult to interpret, since the measured properties of a harmless, non-immunogenic substance will have been profoundly affected by even trace contamination by immunogenic material.

Today, the methods of structural biochemistry and molecular medicine can be used to describe the precise structure of individual gliadin molecules; to prepare, by synthesis rather than by degradation, gliadin peptides for immunogenicity testing; and by applying the approaches used for other proteins, it will be possible to examine the precise interactions, at an atomic level, between gliadin antigens and antibodies or TCRs.

Antibodies and T cells see and respond to antigen in different ways

There is still a great deal of research to be done on the immunogenicity of gliadins, and particularly whether this is influenced by the individual's genetic make-up. Central to this line of work is the fact that T and B cells recognize different regions of antigens.

Antigens are three dimensional structures and there are usually many polypeptides of the native molecule to which antibodies can bind. Some-times these are concentrated in a particular 'immunodominant' region on the outside of the molecule. Digestion of a food protein in the gut may also reveal new antigenic determinants that have been hidden deep within the native molecule. The key point to note is that antibody and B cells recognize antigens, in solution or on cell surfaces, in their native conformation.

On the other hand, it has been known for many years that T cells recognize both native and denatured antigen, indicating that it is the primary sequences of peptides that are important for the induction of cellular immunity. It is now known that T cells do not see free antigen. The TCR sees only a small fragment of the original antigen, after the latter has been internalized by an antigen-presenting cell, partially degraded by proteolytic enzymes, then carried back to be presented at the cell surface in physical association with a MHC (major histocompatibility complex) molecule. The optimum size of peptides for antigen presentation is 8–24 amino acids, a size that fits well into the grooves of MHC molecules (see Chapters 1 and 2).

By implication, although different MHC molecules can interact with the same antigen, they will present it to T cells in slightly different ways. An individual's genetic make-up may also determine which polypeptide sequences from a single protein the T cells can recognize. Thus, the nature and magnitude of the cellular immune responses to a protein antigen will vary between people of different MHC haplotype.

All cells express class I (HLA-A, HLA-B) MHC molecules, but it is the expression of class II (HLA-D) MHC molecules that controls the development of an immune response in T cells. So-called 'professional' antigen-presenting cells express class II molecules at all times, but there are many cell types that can be induced to express class II if suitably stimulated, and they are then capable of presenting antigen in a way that is recognized by T cells. The fact that class II antigen is expressed on crypt cells in coeliac disease means that, potentially, a whole new range of immune responses can be recruited as part of the evolving lesion. What is critical, however, is to what extent epithelial cell antigen presentation may relate to the initial event, induction of sensitization to gluten rather than tolerance, and this is not yet known.

Linking T-cell recognition and genotype

Many investigators have tried and failed to produce clones of gluten-reactive T cells, but success in this endeavour has now been reported from Norway (Lundin et al, 1993). Interestingly, the clones produced were HLA-DQ restricted, rather than reacting to DR associated with gluten, which might be the way antigen would be presented by the gut epithelium (the crypt cells over-express DR but not DQ in coeliac patients).

Since there may well be contributions both by T cells and antibodies in the fully expressed enteropathy, it will be important that, in these new and exciting lines of research, workers continue to pursue the regulation of B-cell as well as T-cell function.

Other potential uses and applications of new gliadin preparations and peptides

There are many in-house and several commercially available assays for

AGA tests, useful as ancillary diagnostic aids and invaluable for monitoring the effects of diet. As a matter of urgency, we should be introducing some means of monitoring the specificity of reagents, maintaining quality control, and facilitating interlaboratory collaborations and comparisons. Clearly, the availability of precise, chemically defined, antigens will greatly assist these measures. Reference preparations of positive and negative sera would also be invaluable.

Clinicians, investigators and patients must continue to exert pressure on governments and regulatory authorities to ensure accurate labelling of foods in relation to their gluten content. I am uncertain as to the real feasibility of using immunoassay methods to check that foods are gluten free. This is particularly so when we have not yet established the precise disease-provoking antigenic determinants.

SENSITIVITY? OR HYPERSENSITIVITY? BETTER TO CONSIDER MODULATION AND REGULATION OF IMMUNITY TO GLIADIN

We still lack fundamental information on human immune responses to dietary antigens, in normal individuals as well as in coeliac patients. Since the weight of evidence supports T cell-mediated hypersensitivity as central to coeliac disease pathogenesis, techniques for the clinical investigation of the magnitude and modulation of this facet of immunity are urgently required. In planning the experiments that need to be performed, *induction* and *expression* must be considered separately.

Induction of immunity or tolerance to fed antigen

In mammals the form and evolution of specific immunity (i.e. altered reactivity) to an antigen are critically dependent on the circumstances at the first encounter. Important factors include the dose of antigen, its physico-chemical properties, other signals received by reacting cells and the route of administration (Mowat, 1987). Much work has been performed in rodents, showing that feeding of protein antigens, including gliadin, induces the specific immune response of *oral tolerance*. This is a powerful, prolonged suppression and downregulation of the capacity of the animal to mount active antibody- and T cell-mediated immune responses to the antigen concerned. Oral tolerance for T cell-mediated reactions is more profound and of considerably longer duration, and can be induced by much smaller doses of fed antigen, than is oral tolerance for antibody. This is likely to be an important protective mechanism against the development of hyper-sensitivity to dietary antigens.

It is impossible to reproduce the experimental situations used in animals for studies of immunity and tolerance to gliadin in humans. Human infants are born with circulating maternally derived IgG AGA in variable titre and, if breast-fed, will also receive maternal IgA AGA. These will certainly have the capacity to influence subsequent immunity. Small amounts of foods eaten by the mother—milk, eggs and presumably also gluten—are present in human breast milk. Furthermore, there may also be passive transmission of IgG and IgA anti-idiotype antibodies by these routes, i.e. antibodies to the antigen-combining (Fab) site of specific antibodies, which may have the same conformation as the original antigen and can, themselves, act as immunogens.

Thus, although further work is required on weaning diets and the age, amount and patterns of introduction of gluten into infants' diets, research on of the other immunomodulatory influences, such as passively transferred antibody, is also needed.

Are non-coeliacs tolerant?

It is accepted that coeliac patients have an abnormal state of sensitization to gluten. For proper analysis of the pathogenesis of this, we need to know the precise immune status of normal individuals in this respect. Are they actively tolerant or merely not sensitized? There are no such data for humans, but in mice our comparative studies of immune responsiveness of genetically identical animals from gluten-free and gluten-containing diet colonies have clearly shown that mice eating a normal diet are tolerant (Troncone and Ferguson, 1988).

There are scattered anecdotal reports in the literature, recent new data on tolerance to myelin basic protein (Weiner et al, 1993), and to keyhole limpet haemocyanin (Husby et al, 1994), which all provide evidence that oral tolerance can occur in humans.

Expression of cell-mediated immunity in the gut mucosa

When an individual is actively immune to a substance (i.e. has antibodies and/or sensitized T cells), further antigen encounter by feeding leads to immune reactions in the vicinity of the gut mucosa. The effects on intestinal structure and function are critically dependent on the cells and immuno-globulin types involved, the site of reaction (lumen, epithelium, lamina propria, submucosa), and availability and recruitment of non-antigen-specific cells and molecules. Local immune reactions may be entirely harmless, may confer protection (e.g. toxin neutralization) or may have adverse effects—hypersensitivity.

Genetic factors: influence on induction or expression of delayed-type hypersensitivity

Our studies with mice showed that immunological sensitization to gliadin does not trigger the development of a T cell-mediated lesion of the intestine when the diet contains gluten (Troncone and Ferguson, 1991b). Additional co-factors were required, which could act via enhanced antigen present-ation, recruitment of specific T cells in the mucosa, upregulation of the expression of class II antigens, or failure of suppression.

A gene that modulates the expression of mucosal delayed-type hyper-sensitivity, HLA- or non-HLA-associated, is another possible second factor. In other words, the genetic factor in coeliac disease could act not only via induction of abnormal immunity, but also by influencing the severity of pathological effects of expression of cell-mediated immunity in the intestine.

Hypothesis: steps in the pathogenesis of coeliac disease

Integration of knowledge of oral tolerance with recent changes in our perspectives of gluten sensitivity produces the following hypothetical sequence as the pathogenesis of gluten-sensitive enteropathy:

1. Failure of the development of oral tolerance for T cell-mediated immunity, either globally (many antigens) or confined to gluten.
2. The genetically predisposed individual is thus vulnerable to being actively immunized to the food antigen (gluten) if a particular combination of diet, gut permeability, mucosal and systemic immunomodulatory signals coincide. The frequency with which this occurs in non-tolerant individuals, and at what age, will depend on many intrinsic and environmental factors.
3. When active T-cell sensitization has occurred, and there is gluten in the diet, relatively subtle effects on the gut mucosa (low-grade pathology, e.g. high IEL count with normal villi) occur, but only in a proportion of those at risk.
4A. It is then only a matter of time until a critical combination of antigen dose and activated mucosal T-effector cells occurs, and this then precipitates the evolution of severe enteropathy and malabsorption.
4B. Simultaneously with 4A, a wide range of immune effector cells are recruited, other dietary antigens, and possibly autoantigens, become involved, thus perpetuating and worsening the enteropathy and explaining why tissue damage persists for weeks or months after strict dietary exclusion of gluten.

This scheme can accommodate the important advances in coeliac disease research of recent years. There are several steps at which the genetic predisposition may act: via immune response genes, immune recognition of gluten peptides or in the regulation of expression of T cell-mediated enteropathy (Sollid and Thorsby, 1993). The important phenomenon of latent coeliac disease spans stages 2 and 3, depending on whether or not there are subtle immune abnormalities (high IEL count, high $\gamma\delta$ IEL counts, overexpression of mucosal IgM). Our work, and Marsh's, on the evolution of enteropathy from high IEL count to the flat lesion, links stages 3 and 4.

Differences in the proportion of those 'at risk' who progress to the next step, $1\rightarrow2$, $2\rightarrow3$, $3\rightarrow4$, will explain striking differences in disease frequency in groups that share the same genetic make-up, e.g. Swedes and Danes, British infants in the late 1960s and today, healthy and affected relatives of patients with coeliac disease.

I suggest that knowledge of the factors that progress the genetically predisposed individual along this sequence of stages will mean that new approaches for stopping or even reversing the process, and thus curing coeliac disease, can be devised.

PREDICTIONS

There are many new and challenging ideas in the arena of coeliac disease, and several fruitful lines of research are being pursued vigorously. Hopefully, by the turn of the century, the exact nature of coeliac disease will emerge and the pathogenesis of gluten-sensitive enteropathy will be established. I predict the following.

Definition will include descriptions of what the disease-associated gene(s) encodes, the precise molecular conformation of the provoking substance and the trigger for sensitization.

Diagnosis will be based on the demonstration that sensitization has occurred.

Pathogenesis will have been shown to involve failure of oral tolerance, resulting in intestinal sensitization to gluten. Both T cells and immune complexes will be implicated in the severe lesion.

Heterogeneity will have been shown to be genetic as well as clinical, with major (classical) and minor subsets related to genotypic and thus mechanistic differences.

SUMMARY

Recent research shows that each word in the definition of coeliac disease, permanent gluten sensitive enteropathy, must now be reviewed, revised or reinterpreted.

Permanent—but there are now well-documented cases of acquired disease, and perhaps also partial recovery of gut gluten tolerance.

Enteropathy—gluten sensitivity is expressed in a spectrum, with a mild form seen as normal architecture with high count of intraepithelial lymphocytes.

Gluten—the provoking agent—Investigators are intensively working to identify the precise toxic sequence, and to establish how this will link in with new genetic information.

Mechanism of sensitivity? or hypersensitivity?—Critical to this is new knowledge on the modulation and regulation of immunity to intestinal antigens, including gliadin.

A hypothesis is presented, as to the pathogenesis of gluten-sensitive enteropathy, which combines concepts of oral tolerance and of the regulation of expression of delayed type hypersensitivity reactions in the gut mucosa.

REFERENCES

Arranz E & Ferguson A (1993) Intestinal antibody pattern of coeliac disease: occurrence in patients with normal jejunal biopsy histology. *Gastroenterology* **104:** 1263–1272.
Arranz E (1994) Intestinal antibodies and intraepithelial lymphocytes in potential coeliac disease. PhD thesis, University of Edinburgh.

Arranz E, Bode J, Kingstone K & Ferguson A (1994) Intestinal antibody pattern of coeliac disease: association with γδ T cell receptor expression by intraepithelial lymphocytes, and other indices of potential coeliac disease. *Gut* **35:** 476–482.

Booth CC & Dowling RH (1970) Concluding discussion. In Booth CC & Dowling RH (eds) *Coeliac Disease*, pp 244–245. London: Churchill Livingstone.

Catassi C, Ratsch IM, Fabiani E et al (1994) Coeliac disease in the year 2000: exploring the iceberg. *Lancet* **343:** 200–203.

Editorial (1989) HIV-associated enteropathy. *Lancet* **ii:** 777–778.

Fais S, Mauri L, Pallone F et al (1992) Gliadin induced changes in the expression of MHC-class II antigens by human small intestinal epithelium. Organ culture studies with coeliac disease mucosa. *Gut* **33:** 472–475.

Ferguson A (1987) Models of immunologically-driven small intestinal damage. In Marsh MN (ed.) *Immunopathology of the Small Intestine*, pp 225–252. Chichester: John Wiley.

Ferguson A & Murray D (1971) Quantitation of intraepithelial lymphocytes in human jejunum. *Gut* **12:** 988–994.

Ferguson A, Sutherland A, MacDonald TT & Allan F (1977) Technique for microdissection and measurement in biopsies of human small intestine. *Journal of Clinical Pathology* **30:** 1068–1073.

Ferguson A, Arranz E & O'Mahony S (1992) Definitions and diagnostic criteria of latent and potential coeliac disease. In Auricchio S & Visakorpi JK (eds) *Common Food Intolerances 1: Epidemiology of Coeliac Disease*, pp 119–127. Basel: Karger.

Ferguson A, Arranz E & O'Mahony S (1993) Clinical and pathological spectrum of coeliac disease—active, silent, latent, potential. *Gut* **34:** 150–151.

Gawkrodger DJ, McDonald C, O'Mahony S & Ferguson A (1991) Small intestinal function and dietary status in dermatitis herpetiformis. *Gut* **32:** 377–382.

Halstensen TS & Brandtzaeg P (1993) Activated T lymphocytes in the celiac lesion: non-proliferative activation (CD25) of CD4$^+$ α/β cells in the lamina propria but proliferation (Ki-67) of α/β and γ/δ cells in the epithelium. *European Journal of Immunology* **23:** 505–510.

Halstensen TS, Hvatum M, Scott H et al (1992) Association of subepithelial deposition of activated complement and immunoglobulin G and M response to gluten in celiac disease. *Gastroenterology* **102:** 751–759.

Holm K, Maki M, Savilahti E et al (1992) Intraepithelial γ/δ T-cell receptor lymphocytes and genetic susceptibility to coeliac disease. *Lancet* **339:** 1500–1503.

Holm K, Savilahti E, Koskimies S et al (1994) Immuno-histochemical changes in the jejunum in first-degree relatives of coeliac patients and the coeliac disease marker DQ genes. HLA class II antigen expression, interleukin-2-receptor-positive cells and dividing crypt cells. *Gut* **35:** 55–60.

Howdle PD, Carazza GR, Bullen AW & Losowsky MS (1981) Gluten sensitivity of small intestinal mucosa in vitro: quantitative assessment of histologic change. *Gastroenterology* **80:** 442–450.

Husby J, Elson CO, Moldoveanu Z & Mestecky J (1995) Oral tolerance in humans. T cell but not B cell tolerance to a soluble protein antigen. In McGhee JR, Mestecky J, Tlaskalova H & Sterzl J (eds) *Proceedings of 7th International Congress of Mucosal Immunology— Recent Advances in Experimental Medicine and Biology*, New York: Plenum Press (in press).

Lundin KEA, Scott H, Hansen T et al (1993) Gliadin-specific, HLA (α1*0501, β1*0201) restricted T cells isolated from the small intestinal mucosa of celiac disease patients. *Journal of Experimental Medicine* **178:** 187–196.

MacDonald TT & Ferguson A (1976) Hypersensitivity reactions in the small intestine. 2. Effects of allograft rejection on mucosal architecture and lymphoid cell infiltrate. *Gut* **17:** 81–91.

Mäki M, Holm K, Koskinies S et al (1990) Normal small bowel biopsy followed by coeliac disease. *Archives of Disease in Childhood* **65:** 1137–1141.

Marsh MN (1992) Gluten, major histocompatibility complex and the small intestine. *Gastroenterology* **102:** 330–354.

Meuwisse GW (1970) Diagnostic criteria in coeliac disease. *Acta Paediatrica Scandinavica* **59:** 461.

Mowat A (1987) The regulation of immune responses to dietary protein antigens. *Immunology Today* **8:** 193–198.

Mowat AMcI & Ferguson A (1982) Intraepithelial lymphocyte count and crypt hyperplasia measure the mucosal component of the graft-versus-host reaction in mouse small intestine. *Gastroenterology* **83:** 417–423.

O'Mahony S, Barton JR, Crichton S & Ferguson A (1990a) Appraisal of gut lavage in the study of intestinal humoral immunity. *Gut* **31:** 1341–1344.

O'Mahony S, Vestey JP & Ferguson A (1990b) Similarities in intestinal humoral immunity in dermatitis herpetiformis without enteropathy and in coeliac disease. *Lancet* **335:** 1487–1490.

Savilahti E, Reunala T & Maki M (1992) Increase of lymphocytes bearing the γ/δ T cell receptor in the jejunum of patients with dermatitis herpetiformis. *Gut* **33:** 206–211.

Schmitz J (1992) Coeliac disease in childhood. In Marsh MN (ed.) *Coeliac Disease*, pp 17–48. London: Blackwell Scientific Publications.

Sollid LV & Thorsby E (1993) HLA susceptibility genes in celiac disease: genetic mapping and role in pathogenesis. *Gastroenterology* **105:** 910–922.

Strobel S, Brydon WG & Ferguson A (1984) Cellobiose/mannitol sugar permeability test complements biopsy histopathology in clinical investigation of the jejunum. *Gut* **25:** 1241–1246.

Troncone R & Ferguson A (1988) Gliadin presented via the gut induces oral tolerance in mice. *Clinical and Experimental Immunology* **72:** 284–287.

Troncone R & Ferguson A (1991a) Anti-gliadin antibodies. *Journal of Pediatric Gastroenterology and Nutrition* **12:** 150–158.

Troncone R & Ferguson A (1991b) Animal model of gluten induced enteropathy in mice. *Gut* **32:** 871–875.

Walker-Smith JA, Guandalini S, Schmitz J et al (1990) Revised criteria for diagnosis of coeliac disease. *Archives of Disease in Childhood* **65:** 909–911.

Weiner HL, Mackin GA, Matsui M et al (1993) Double blind pilot trial of oral tolerisation with myelin antigens in MS. *Science* **259:** 1321–1324.

Weinstein WM (1974) Latent celiac sprue. *Gastroenterology* **66:** 489–493.

Wright NA, Watson AJ, Morley AR et al (1973) Cell kinetics in the flat (avillous) mucosa of the human small intestine. *Gut* **20:** 701–706.

Index

Note: Page numbers of article titles are in **bold** type.